D0874023

2013
YEAR BOOK OF
**PATHOLOGY
AND LABORATORY
MEDICINE**®

The 2013 Year Book Series

Year Book of Anesthesiology and Pain Management™: Drs Chestnut, Abram, Black, Gravlee, Lien, Mathru, and Roizen

Year Book of Cardiology®: Drs Gersh, Cheitlin, Elliott, Gold, Graham, and Thourani

Year Book of Critical Care Medicine®: Drs Dries, Zanotti-Cavazzoni, Latenser, Martinez, Rincon, and Zwank

Year Book of Dermatology and Dermatologic Surgery™: Dr Del Rosso

Year Book of Diagnostic Radiology®: Drs Elster, Abbara, Oestreich, Offiah, Rosado de Christenson, Stephens, and Strickland

Year Book of Emergency Medicine®: Drs Hamilton, Bruno, Handly, Minczak, Mullin, Quintana, and Ramoska

Year Book of Endocrinology®: Drs Schott, Apovian, Clarke, Eugster, Meikle, Oetgen, Ovalle, Schteingart, and Toth

Year Book of Hand and Upper Limb Surgery®: Drs Yao, Adams, Isaacs, Lee, and Rizzo

Year Book of Medicine®: Drs Barker, Garrick, Gersh, Khardori, LeRoith, Panush, Talley, and Thigpen

Year Book of Neonatal and Perinatal Medicine®: Drs Fanaroff, Benitz, Donn, Neu, Papile, and Van Marter

Year Book of Neurology and Neurosurgery®: Drs Klimo, Minagar, Gandhi, House, Kevill, Liu, Mazia, Panagariya, Ragel, Riesenburger, Robottom, Schwendimann, Shafazand, Uhm, and Yang

Year Book of Obstetrics, Gynecology, and Women's Health®: Drs Dungan and Shulman

Year Book of Oncology®: Drs Arceci, Bauer, Chiorean, Gordon, Lawton, Murphy, Thigpen, and Tsao

Year Book of Ophthalmology®: Drs Rapuano, Cohen, Flanders, Hammersmith, Milman, Myers, Nagra, Nelson, Penne, Pyfer, Sergott, Shields, Talekar, and Vander

Year Book of Orthopedics®: Drs Morrey, Huddleston, Rose, Swiontkowski, and Trigg

Year Book of Otolaryngology-Head and Neck Surgery®: Drs Sindwani, Balough, Franco, Gapany, and Mitchell

Year Book of Pathology and Laboratory Medicine®: Drs Raab and Bissell

Year Book of Pediatrics®: Dr Stockman

Year Book of Plastic and Aesthetic Surgery™: Drs Miller, Boehmler, Gosman, Gutowski, Ruberg, Salisbury, and Smith

Year Book of Psychiatry and Applied Mental Health®: Drs Talbott, Ballenger, Buckley, Frances, Krupnick, and Mack

Year Book of Pulmonary Disease®: Drs Barker, Jones, Maurer, Spradley, Tanoue, and Willsie

Year Book of Sports Medicine®: Drs Shephard, Cantu, Feldman, Galea, Jankowski, Janssen, Lebrun, and Nieman

Year Book of Surgery®: Drs Copeland, Behrns, Daly, Eberlein, Fahey, Huber, Klodell, Mozingo, and Pruett

Year Book of Urology®: Drs Andriole and Coplen

Year Book of Vascular Surgery®: Drs Moneta, Gillespie, Starnes, and Watkins

2013

The Year Book of PATHOLOGY AND LABORATORY MEDICINE®

Editor-in-Chief

Stephen S. Raab, MD

Professor of Pathology, University of Washington, Seattle, Washington, and Memorial University of Newfoundland/Eastern Health Authority, St John's, Newfoundland, Canada

Editor Laboratory Medicine

Michael G. Bissell, MD, PhD, MPH

Professor of Pathology, Ohio State University Medical Center, Columbus, Ohio

Editor

Maxwell L. Smith, MD

Assistant Professor, Director of Liver and Transplant Pathology, Department of Pathology, University of Colorado School of Medicine, Aurora, Colorado

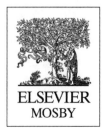

ELSEVIER
MOSBY

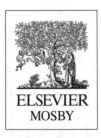

ELSEVIER
MOSBY

Vice President, Continuity: Kimberly Murphy
Editor: Katie Saunders
Supervisor, Electronic Year Books: Donna M. Skelton
Electronic Article Manager: Mike Sheets
Illustrations and Permissions Coordinator: Dawn Vohsen

2013 EDITION
Copyright 2013 Mosby, Inc. All rights reserved.

No part of this publication may be reproduced, stored in a retrieval system, or transmitted, in any form or by any means, electronic, mechanical, photocopying, recording, or otherwise, without prior written permission from the publisher.

Permission to photocopy or reproduce solely for internal or personal use is granted for libraries or other users registered with the Copyright Clearance Center, provided that the base fee of $35.00 per chapter is paid directly to the Copyright Clearance Center, 21 Congress Street, Salem, MA 01970. This consent does not extend to other kinds of copying, such as copying for general distribution, for advertising or promotional purposes, for creating new collected works, or for resale.

Printed in the United States of America
Composition by TNQ Books and Journals Pvt Ltd, India
Printing/binding by Sheridan Books, Inc.

Editorial Office:
Elsevier
Suite 1800
1600 John F. Kennedy Blvd.
Philadelphia, PA 19103-2899

International Standard Serial Number: 1077-9108
International Standard Book Number: 978-1-4557-7285-8

Contributing Editors

Beverley A. Carter, MD, FRCPC
Provincial Director of Pathology and Laboratory Medicine, Government of Newfoundland and Labrador, St John's, Newfoundland, Canada

S. A. Chandrakanth, MD, FRCPC
Staff Pathologist, Clinical Assistant Professor, Eastern Health, Memorial University, Newfoundland and Labrador, St John's, Newfoundland, Canada

Giovanni De Petris, MD
Associate Professor of Laboratory Medicine and Pathology, Mayo Clinic, Scottsdale, Arizona

Dana M. Gryzbicki, MD, PhD
Associate Professor, Pathology, Rocky Vista University, Parker, Colorado

Dora Lam-Himlin, MD
Senior Associate Consultant, Department of Laboratory Medicine and Pathology, Assistant Professor of Pathology, College of Medicine, Mayo Clinic, Scottsdale, Arizona

Ann E. McCullough, MD
Assistant Professor of Laboratory Medicine and Pathology, Mayo Clinic, Scottsdale, Arizona

Miriam D. Post, MD
Assistant Professor, Department of Pathology, University of Colorado School of Medicine, Aurora, Colorado

M. Sherif Said, MD, PhD, FCAP
Associate Professor of Pathology, University of Colorado Denver; Associate Director of Pathology, Denver Health, Denver, Colorado

Heather Signorelli, DO
Pathology Resident at University of Colorado Health Sciences Center, Denver, Colorado

Table of Contents

Journals Represented

Journals represented in this YEAR BOOK are listed below.

Acta Neuropathologica
Acta Oto-Laryngologica
American Journal of Clinical Pathology
American Journal of Gastroenterology
American Journal of Kidney Diseases
American Journal of Medicine
American Journal of Pathology
American Journal of Respiratory and Critical Care Medicine
American Journal of Surgical Pathology
American Journal of Transplantation
Anesthesia & Analgesia
Annals of Diagnostic Pathology
Annals of Emergency Medicine
Annals of Surgical Oncology
Archives of Dermatology
Archives of Internal Medicine
Archives of Pathology & Laboratory Medicine
Arthritis & Rheumatism
Blood
Breast Cancer Research and Treatment
Breast Journal
Cancer
Cancer Epidemiology, Biomarkers & Prevention
Cardiovascular Pathology
Clinical Chemistry
Clinical Infectious Diseases
Clinical & Translational Oncology
Clinics
Clinics in Sports Medicine
Digestive and Liver Disease
Endocrine Pathology
European Journal of Cancer
Gut
Head & Neck
Heart
Hepatology
Histopathology
Human Pathology
Human Reproduction
International Journal of Gynecology & Pathology
International Journal of Otolaryngology
Journal of Clinical Microbiology
Journal of Clinical Oncology
Journal of Clinical Pathology
Journal of Emergency Medicine
Journal of Hypertension
Journal of Immunology

Journal of Lower Genital Tract Disease
Journal of Molecular Diagnostics
Journal of Pediatric Gastroenterology and Nutrition
Journal of Rheumatology
Journal of the American Academy of Dermatology
Journal of the American Medical Association
Journal of the National Cancer Institute
Journal of Thoracic and Cardiovascular Surgery
Journal of Thoracic Oncology
Journal of Urology
Kidney International
Lancet
Lancet Neurology
Liver Transplantation
Mayo Clinic Proceedings
Modern Pathology
Nature
Nature Genetics
Nephrology Dialysis Transplantation
New England Journal of Medicine
Orthopedics
Pediatric and Developmental Pathology
Pediatrics
Proceedings of the National Academy of Sciences of the United States of America
Proteome Science
Public Library of Science One
Radiology
Science Translational Medicine
Southern Medical Journal
Thorax
Thrombosis Research
Transfusion
Virchows Archiv

STANDARD ABBREVIATIONS

The following terms are abbreviated in this edition: acquired immunodeficiency syndrome (AIDS), cardiopulmonary resuscitation (CPR), central nervous system (CNS), cerebrospinal fluid (CSF), computed tomography (CT), deoxyribonucleic acid (DNA), electrocardiography (ECG), health maintenance organization (HMO), human immunodeficiency virus (HIV), intensive care unit (ICU), intramuscular (IM), intravenous (IV), magnetic resonance (MR) imaging (MRI), ribonucleic acid (RNA), ultrasound (US), and ultraviolet (UV).

NOTE

The YEAR BOOK OF PATHOLOGY AND LABORATORY MEDICINE is a literature survey service providing abstracts of articles published in the professional literature. Every effort is made to assure the accuracy of the information presented in these pages. Neither the editors nor the publisher of the YEAR BOOK OF PATHOLOGY AND LABORATORY MEDICINE can be responsible for errors in the original materials. The editors' comments are their own opinions. Mention of specific products within this publication does not constitute endorsement.

To facilitate the use of the YEAR BOOK OF PATHOLOGY AND LABORATORY MEDICINE as a reference tool, all illustrations and tables included in this publication are now identified as they appear in the original article. This change is meant to help the reader recognize that any illustration or table appearing in the YEAR BOOK OF PATHOLOGY AND LABORATORY MEDICINE may be only one of many in the original article. For this reason, figure and table numbers will often appear to be out of sequence within the YEAR BOOK OF PATHOLOGY AND LABORATORY MEDICINE.

PART I

ANATOMIC PATHOLOGY

1 Outcomes Analysis

Two Hundred Years of Hospital Costs and Mortality — MGH and Four Eras of Value in Medicine
Meyer GS, Demehin AA, Liu X, et al (Dartmouth-Hitchcock Med Ctr, Lebanon, NH; Natl Quality Forum, Washington, DC; Massachusetts General Hosp, Boston; et al)
N Engl J Med 366:2147-2149, 2012

Background.—One parameter for assessing health care delivery is value. The Massachusetts General Hospital (MGH) has maintained mortality and cost data since its opening. A review of these data shows national trends in health care that can speak to the value obtained.

Method.—The data on quality of care were collected from 1821 through the present day and included a report on the condition of patients leaving the hospital and the inpatient cost per patient discharged alive. Analysis yielded a run chart on value. Caution was exercised in assessing mortality, since it can be altered by patient demographics, case mix, severity, chance, historical trends, assess to care, secular events such as epidemics and wars, declining length of stay, and the available services provided.

Results.—The data indicate four distinct eras of hospital care value. The first was 1821 through 1910 and was characterized by random variation in inpatient mortality around a standard mean and stable costs for care. The second era was from 1911 through 1960 and was marked by modest declines in mortality and modest increases in costs. The third era, 1961 through 2000, demonstrated a steeper decline in mortality and a steeper rise in costs. Since 2001, mortality has been level but the cost per patient has escalated dramatically, constituting the fourth era of health care value.

Conclusions.—The eras of value seen through the analysis of data from a single academic medical center demonstrate changes in US medicine. The beginning era had relatively high inpatient mortality with low costs that increased generally in response to events such as wars and epidemics rather than as a result of care quality. The second era saw a modest increase in value with increased use of high-impact therapies and medical breakthroughs that allowed physicians to treat a wider spectrum of patients. The third era reflected the growing research-industrial complex's introduction of diagnostics and therapeutics that could be used for many more diseases. Each of these first three eras reflected the overcoming of challenges in ways that produced greater value. The post-2000 era has produced diminishing returns, however. The growth in costs has far outstripped reductions in inpatient mortality. Some of the increased cost reflects

3

treatment of severely ill patients with complex conditions, but for the first time, improved mortality appears to be achieved at unsustainable costs.

▶ In 2012, the *New England Journal of Medicine* published a series of articles under the topic of 200 Years of Hospital Costs and Mortality. Although a number of these articles are fascinating, I find this one by Meyer and colleagues shocking in terms of costs and mortality rates (Fig 1 in the original article). Since the 1960s, the adjusted cost per patient alive at discharge has skyrocketed. Meyer et al question whether these costs are unsustainable. Because many medical decisions are based on laboratory test results, the potential for pathologists to play a role beyond just reporting these test results is huge. Clearly, much of the costs are related to treatment and often for treating complex conditions. However, laboratory results often are critical for monitoring treatment and leading to the treatment conditions in the first place. Thus, laboratory testing is the gateway for current treating paradigms. I can imagine a future in which pathologists and clinicians work as a team to determine the optimal management strategies, with cost as an element in decision making. Pathologists could be key players for health care reform. For additional reading, please see reference list.[1,2]

S. S. Raab, MD

References

1. Shahian DM, Wolf RE, Iezzoni LI, Kirle L, Normand SL. Variability in the measurement of hospital-wide mortality rates. *N Engl J Med.* 2010;363: 2530-2539. [*Erratum, N Engl J Med 2011;364:1382*].
2. Shactman D, Altman SH, Eilat E, Thorpe KE, Doonan M. The outlook for hospital spending. *Health Aff (Millwood).* 2003;22:12-26.

Quality Assurance Measures for Critical Diagnoses in Anatomic Pathology
Renshaw A, Gould EW (Baptist Hosp, Miami, FL)
Am J Clin Pathol 137:466-469, 2012

We sought to characterize how well computerized "case flags" performed in evaluating critical diagnoses in anatomic pathology. All cases identified by a pathologist at sign-out and flagged as a critical diagnosis in anatomic pathology in 2 hospital laboratories during a 3-year period were reviewed. A subset of all critical diagnoses consisting of only treatable, immediately life-threatening (TILT) diagnoses was selected, and a text search for key words was used to evaluate performance during a 6-month period. During a 3-year period, there were 635 cases (0.5% of all cases) that were flagged as critical diagnoses. A key word search identified 269 TILT cases, which represented 1.8% of all cases during this time; 30 (11.2%) were critical diagnoses, of which 24 (80%) had documentation of a call to the clinician and only 2 (7%) were flagged as a critical diagnosis. Critical diagnoses in anatomic pathology remain poorly defined. Computerized case flags underestimate the number of critical diagnosis cases in a laboratory and cannot identify missed critical diagnoses. A more limited and clearly defined approach to quality assurance of critical diagnoses emphasizing

TILT diagnoses and selected key word searches can be performed and requires reviewing only 1.8% of all cases.

▶ The term *critical value* originated in clinical pathology and was developed to alert clinicians of laboratory test results that could affect "life or limb." A clinical laboratory critical value does not require the laboratory to know patient history or the clinician understanding that a diagnosis is expected or unexpected. Some have the view that critical anatomic pathology diagnoses depend on history and clinician expectations, indicating that a critical anatomic pathology diagnosis depends on preanalytic information and in this view is not just the diagnosis itself. Renshaw and Gould are correct in asserting that critical diagnoses are poorly defined in anatomic pathology. From a workflow perspective, failed communication is a large source of medical error and "critical" anatomic diagnoses are only a subset of diagnoses that need to be communicated in a better fashion to clinicians. I think pathologists need to perform a deeper root cause analysis of why specific anatomic diagnoses (eg, all malignancies) are not communicated immediately to clinicians. The pathology profession also needs to understand what clinicians want and need to know. For additional reading, please see reference list.[1]

S. S. Raab, MD

Reference

1. College of American Pathologists. Inspection checklist in anatomic pathology. http://www.cap.org/apps/capportal2010:ANP.12175. Accessed August 1, 2011.

Enhanced biomedical scientist cut-up role in colonic cancer reporting
Sanders SA, Smith A, Carr RA, et al (Cellular Pathology Laboratory, Warwick, UK)
J Clin Pathol 65:517-521, 2012

Aims.—To extend the biomedical scientist (BMS) cut-up role to include gastrointestinal category D colorectal cancer resection specimens, and to address issues of quality and safety by presenting performance data from the first 50 BMS cut-up specimens in comparison with national guidelines and pathologist performance over the same timeframe.

Methods.—Close mentoring and consultant supervision was carried out for every case with adherence to standard operating procedures and following colorectal cancer dataset guidelines as published by the Royal College of Pathologists. Performance targets were audited including anticipated spread of Dukes' stage, targets for mean lymph node harvest, percentage extramural vascular invasion and serosal involvement, and mean tumour blocks sampled. Histological pre-reporting of 20 cases was encouraged, and time spent by BMS and consultant at all stages of specimen reporting was noted.

Results.—Performance targets were all exceeded by the BMS and compared favourably with pathologist performance. A measure of consultant cut-up and histology reporting time saved was identified.

Conclusions.—Benefits of extending the BMS role to category D specimens may include BMS professional advancement, efficient use of consultant time and the development of a team approach to cancer reporting. The achievement of colorectal cancer performance targets and favourable comparison with pathologist performance implies there was no perceived detrimental effect on quality or safety and thus patient management.

▶ Although pathologists still debate the laboratory role of pathologist extenders (ie, pathologists' assistants [PA] or biomedical scientists [BMS]), I think this article primarily underlines the challenges in the education of all pathologist trainees. Sanders and colleagues provide a UK perspective of the on-the-job education in the BMS profession, which has less responsibility compared with the North American PA profession. The mean amount of time for a BMS (in training) to perform the gross tissue examination, sampling, and reporting is longer than the mean time for a pathologist to perform these tasks and a pathologist needs to supervise the BMS while on the job. Of course, this is not surprising. I believe that our profession needs to reorganize our training paradigms, in which training is less about using real specimens for practice and more simulation-based. Sanders et al report that the BMS microscopic prereporting of cases had errors (similar to the errors reported for beginning residents in the United States), and a training program based on simulated specimens could be taken offline and used to improve this practice or the practice of North American residents. The effort to build this program is not insurmountable. For additional reading, please see reference list.[1-3]

S. S. Raab, MD

References

1. Galvis CO, Raab SS, D'Amico F, Grzybicki DM. Pathologist's assistants practice: a measurement of performance. *Am J Clin Pathol.* 2001;116:816-822.
2. Horton L. Implementation of the extended role of biomedical scientists in specimen description, dissection and sampling—final report. *R Coll Pathol.* 2004. http://www.rcpath.org.
3. Hughes R, Treacy A, Gulmann C. The search for lymph nodes; does a second search influence the staging and/or management in mesorectal cancer excisions? *Histopathology.* 2009;54:768-770.

Addenda in Pathology Reports: Trends and Their Implications
Finkelstein A, Levy GH, Cohen P, et al (Yale Univ School of Medicine, New Haven, CT)
Am J Clin Pathol 137:606-611, 2012

Addenda are typically used to report results of additional studies that are delayed relative to histopathologic studies. However, the frequency and pattern of use of addenda have not been previously reported. We studied the dynamics of addenda creation within the same month at 5-year intervals during a 15-year period at our institution. The number of addenda and type and impact of information communicated in addenda were assessed in the month of July in 1993, 1998, 2003, and 2008, and the possible role of addenda in quality improvement was evaluated. Cases with addenda increased from 0.9% in 1993 to 8.6% in 2008. In 5.6% of addenda, there was information that might have been better reported in an amendment, suggesting that criteria for amendments need to be universally implemented. Charting trends and types of addenda offered opportunities for quality improvement by identifying weaknesses in the workflow organization of the laboratory.

▶ The data presented by Finkelstein and coauthors show the rising rate of addendum reports over a 15-year timeframe at 1 institution (Table 1 in the original article). The authors suggest that the increase in addenda is caused by 2 main factors: the growth of ancillary tests and the clinical necessity for information in a quicker fashion. I have yet to read an evaluation of clinician opinion of addenda and if a portion of the growth in numbers is secondary to pathologist or pathology group focus on turnaround time (apart from the clinical need). The authors also report that a number of addenda should have been issued as amended reports because the diagnostic information (eg, diagnosis, stage of disease) was changed. Finkelstein et al discuss the meaning and challenges in differentiating amended and addendum reports. This discussion reveals issues related to our pathology culture, which often has an undercurrent of blame and fear. Some pathologists will record an error as an addendum report, rather than an amended report, because they are fearful of the consequences of error reporting. This culture is also the reason why pathologists are reluctant to issue an amended report if "it doesn't affect the patient." As the culture moves from a focus on reporting to a focus on preventing, the method of reporting will become less of an issue. For additional reading, please see reference list.[1,2]

S. S. Raab, MD

References

1. Meier FA, Zarbo RJ, Varney RC, et al. Amended reports: development and validation of a taxonomy of defects. *Am J Clin Pathol.* 2008;130:238-246.
2. Association of the Directors of Anatomic and Surgical Pathology, Nakhleh R, Coffin C, Cooper K. Recommendations for quality assurance and improvement in surgical and autopsy pathology. *Hum Pathol.* 2006;37:985-988.

Clinical Implication of an Insufficient Number of Examined Lymph Nodes After Curative Resection for Gastric Cancer
Son T, Hyung WJ, Lee JH, et al (Yonsei Univ College of Medicine, Seoul, Korea)
Cancer 118:4687-4693, 2012

Background.—The seventh edition of the tumor, lymph node (LN), metastasis (TNM) staging system increased the required number of examined LNs in gastric cancer from 15 to 16. However, the same staging system defines lymph node-negative gastric cancer regardless of the number of examined LNs. In this study, the authors evaluated whether gastric cancer can be staged properly with fewer than 15 examined LNs.

Methods.—The survival rates of 10,010 patients who underwent curative gastrectomy from 1987 to 2007 were analyzed. The patients were divided into 2 groups according to the number of examined LNs, termed the "insufficient" group (≤ 15 examined LNs) and the "sufficient" group (≥ 16 examined LNs). The survival curves of patients from both groups were compared according to the seventh edition of the TNM classification.

Results.—Three hundred sixteen patients (3.2%) had ≤ 15 examined LNs for staging after they underwent standard, curative lymphadenectomy. Patients who had T1 tumor classification, N0 lymph node status, and stage I disease with an insufficient number of examined LNs after curative gastrectomy had a significantly worse prognosis than patients who had ≥ 16 examined LNs. Moreover, having an insufficient number of examined LNs was an independent prognostic factor for patients who had T1, N0, and stage I disease.

Conclusions.—LN-negative cancers in which ≥ 15 LNs were examined, classified as N0 in the new TNM staging system, could not adequately predict patient survival after curative gastrectomy, especially in patients with early stage gastric cancer.

▶ For at least 1 group of patients with gastric cancer, Son et al show that the number of lymph nodes sampled affects the ability to predict survival after gastrectomy. The issue of appropriate lymph node sampling reflects the team approach that surgeons and pathologists must use to improve patient care quality. Although we know certain factors that correlate with the number of lymph nodes sampled, I do not know of a well-performed root cause analysis that evaluates the wide range of system factors that lead to low numbers of sampled lymph nodes. These factors would include experience of pathologist (or pathologist extender), experience of surgeon, and patient-related factors (eg, some patients may have fewer lymph nodes based on probability), and the countermeasures that pathologists would take if low numbers of lymph nodes are sampled. For example, reexamination of the gross tissue, additional sampling, and use of agents to highlight missed lymph nodes all could lead to greater lymph node harvesting. Yet, laboratories do not have best practices of gross tissue examination that are mandatorily practiced. Manuscripts such as the one by Son et al highlight the continued importance of gross tissue examination techniques. For further reading, see reference list.[1,2]

S. S. Raab, MD

References

1. Seto Y, Nagawa H, Muto T. Impact of lymph node metastasis on survival with early gastric cancer. *World J Surg.* 1997;21:186-189.
2. Wu CW, Hsieh MC, Lo SS, Tsay SH, Lui WY, P'eng FK. Relation of number of positive lymph nodes to the prognosis of patients with primary gastric adenocarcinoma. *Gut.* 1996;38:525-527.

Observer Variation in the Application of the Pheochromocytoma of the Adrenal Gland Scaled Score

Wu D, Tischler AS, Lloyd RV, et al (Brigham and Women's Hosp, Boston, MA; Tufts Med Ctr, Boston, MA; Mayo Clinic, Rochester, MN; et al)
Am J Surg Pathol 33:599-608, 2009

Morphologic determination of the malignant potential of adrenal pheochromocytoma is a challenging problem in surgical pathology. A multiparameter Pheochromocytoma of the Adrenal Gland Scaled Score (PASS) was recently developed based on a comprehensive study of a single institutional cohort of 100 cases. Assignment of a PASS was proposed to be useful for identifying pheochromocytomas with potential to metastasize, which defines malignancy according to the current World Health Organization terminology. A PASS is derived by evaluating multiple morphologic parameters to obtain a scaled score based on the summed weighted importance of each. Despite the proposal of this system several years ago, few studies have since examined its robustness and, in particular, the potential for observer variation inherent in the interpretation and assessment of these morphologic criteria. We further examined the utility of PASS by reviewing an independent single institutional cohort of adrenal pheochromocytomas as evaluated by 5 multi-institutional pathologists with at least 10 years experience in endocrine pathology. We found significant interobserver and intraobserver variation in assignment of PASS with variable interpretation of the underlying components. We consequently suggest that PASS requires further refinement and validation. We cannot currently recommend its use for clinical prognostication.

▶ The findings of Wu et al show the importance of performing validation studies on schemes that are designed to link pathology criteria to clinical outcomes. Some tumors, such as adrenal pheochromocytomas, are difficult (if not impossible) to separate into benign and malignant subtypes based on histologic features. Thompson proposed using the PASS scheme and Wu and colleagues tested this scheme in "practice." Wu et al did not convene a consensus conference to provide education or discussion of the criteria, which I think is a major weakness in this study. Pathology is rife with experts who purport to use specific criteria for diagnosis, and different experts use different criteria. Without consensus, the field is left with nonstandardized diagnostic systems and unacceptable levels of diagnostic variability, or failures in precision. Consequently, Wu and colleagues can use these study data to report that the PASS system lacks validity. However, the more important study would be an attempt to reach consensus on the PASS criteria (or at least education using examples of the PASS criteria) and then test for validity. Maybe the PASS system lacks validity, and pheochromocytomas cannot be subclassified. However, until experts reach consensus through education and testing, I do not think we will really know. For additional reading, please see reference list.[1,2]

S. S. Raab, MD

References

1. Thompson LD. Pheochromocytoma of the Adrenal gland Scaled Score (PASS) to separate benign from malignant neoplasms: a clinicopathologic and immunophenotypic study of 100 cases. *Am J Surg Pathol.* 2002;26:551-566.
2. Gao B, Meng F, Bian W, et al. Development and validation of pheochromocytoma of the adrenal gland scaled score for predicting malignant pheochromocytomas. *Urology.* 2006;68:282-286.

Preoperative Diagnosis of Benign Thyroid Nodules with Indeterminate Cytology

Alexander EK, Kennedy GC, Baloch ZW, et al (Harvard Med School, Boston, MA; Veracyte, South San Francisco, CA; Univ of Pennsylvania, Philadelphia; et al)
N Engl J Med 367:705-715, 2012

Background.—Approximately 15 to 30% of thyroid nodules evaluated by means of fine-needle aspiration are not clearly benign or malignant. Patients with cytologically indeterminate nodules are often referred for diagnostic surgery, though most of these nodules prove to be benign. A novel diagnostic test that measures the expression of 167 genes has shown promise in improving preoperative risk assessment.

Methods.—We performed a 19-month, prospective, multicenter validation study involving 49 clinical sites, 3789 patients, and 4812 fine-needle aspirates from thyroid nodules 1 cm or larger that required evaluation. We obtained 577 cytologically indeterminate aspirates, 413 of which had corresponding histopathological specimens from excised lesions. Results of a central, blinded histopathological review served as the reference standard. After inclusion criteria were met, a gene-expression classifier was used to test 265 indeterminate nodules in this analysis, and its performance was assessed.

Results.—Of the 265 indeterminate nodules, 85 were malignant. The gene-expression classifier correctly identified 78 of the 85 nodules as suspicious (92% sensitivity; 95% confidence interval [CI], 84 to 97), with a specificity of 52% (95% CI, 44 to 59). The negative predictive values for "atypia (or follicular lesion) of undetermined clinical significance," "follicular neoplasm or lesion suspicious for follicular neoplasm," or "suspicious cytologic findings" were 95%, 94%, and 85%, respectively. Analysis of 7 aspirates with false negative results revealed that 6 had a paucity of thyroid follicular cells, suggesting insufficient sampling of the nodule.

Conclusions.—These data suggest consideration of a more conservative approach for most patients with thyroid nodules that are cytologically indeterminate on fine-needle aspiration and benign according to gene-expression classifier results. (Funded by Veracyte.)

▶ Here we have a report of use of microarray data as an adjunct to standard diagnosis in the evaluation of cytologically indeterminate thyroid nodules. Tested fine-needle aspirate (FNA) samples were prospectively submitted from multiple institutions to be analyzed by the proprietary Veracyte gene-expression classifier (Affirma Thyroid FNA analysis) in a study funded by Veracyte. The authors include Veracyte employees and array developers with oversight by a steering committee of non-Veracyte expert thyroid pathologists and clinicians. An extensive supplementary appendix, marked "privileged and confidential," describes the technical details and company methods.

The goal here is to attempt to distinguish molecularly suspicious from nonsuspicious samples in a group of cytologically atypical or suspicious specimens. If successful, the promise is that those genetically nonsuspicious might avoid thyroid surgery typically prompted by an indeterminate thyroid FNA. Your thyroid nodule screened as atypical/suspicious cytologically; is the RNA from that same nodule as suspicious?

What is interesting about this approach is what it does not tell us. The test does not purport to make a diagnosis, establish malignancy or benignancy, or even to completely exclude a diagnosis. Rather, the authors are careful to keep the publication focused on a specific purpose, stratifying by the degree of genetic abnormality in a challenging management group. Reports suggestive of a high risk for malignancy in an atypical or suspicious thyroid FNA are reported as "suspicious."

This approach seems to have some promise and it will be interesting to see if wider use in daily practice allows such differentiation or muddies the water. A nice aspect of the assay is the stability of the sample for RNA recovery, described in the supplementary material to the article, allowing FNA sampling and brief storage in RNA preservative. Such an approach gives time for the cytology to be examined, discussed, and reexamined, allowing a post-reporting decision about the use of the assay to be made by pathologist and clinician together. The potential strength in the assay lies in the high negative predictive value (NPV) for thyroid malignancy (85% to 95% depending on the indeterminate thyroid Bethesda classification of the tested specimen). A more robust assay would have an NPV closer to 100%. But even with comprehensive molecular testing, each test will have its own performance characteristic shortcomings. Potential drawbacks in the assay are similar to those with the thyroid FNA cytological method in general: lack of concordance in the diagnosis of cytologically indeterminate nodules (agreement on some cytologically atypical specimens was not always concordant among very knowledgeable pathologist authors), obtaining an adequate sample (early inadequacies in specimens prompted a change in collection requiring an additional FNA pass), and the small possibility of falsely negative samples (several specimens were thyroid carcinomas, not suggested by the gene expression array results).

An important point about such technology, especially with preliminary reports, is to know the limitations of such an approach and the components of the marketed package. This assay is pitched to find those thyroid nodules that are more likely to be benign among indeterminate specimens. Will everyone remember and know that? Use of the Veracyte method may show promise within the limits defined by this concept but it remains to be seen whether wider use of this technology will develop only in that context. Included in the approximately $3500.00 cost for the test is an expert cytological consultation to verify the indeterminate classification of the thyroid FNA, presumably a built-in control against use in misinterpreted benign or malignant samples. The obligatory consultation included in the Veracyte test may well change thyroid FNA practice patterns from submitting hospitals and lead to increased discordant cytological opinions. Practitioners using this test should be well aware of the narrowly defined performance parameters described herein.

A. McCullough, MD

The Effect of a Lean Quality Improvement Implementation Program on Surgical Pathology Specimen Accessioning and Gross Preparation Error Frequency
Smith ML, Wilkerson T, Grzybicki DM, et al (Univ of Colorado, Aurora; Univ of Washington, Seattle)
Am J Clin Pathol 138:367-373, 2012

Few reports have documented the effectiveness of Lean quality improvement in changing anatomic pathology patient safety. We used Lean methods of education; hoshin kanri goal setting and culture change; kaizen events; observation of work activities, hand-offs, and pathways; A3-problem solving, metric development, and measurement; and frontline work redesign in the accessioning and gross examination areas of an anatomic pathology laboratory. We compared the pre- and post-Lean implementation proportion of near-miss events and changes made in specific work processes. In the implementation phase, we documented 29 individual A3-root cause analyses. The pre- and postimplementation proportions of process- and operator-dependent near-miss events were 5.5 and 1.8 ($P < .002$) and 0.6 and 0.6, respectively. We conclude that through culture change and implementation of specific work process changes, Lean implementation may improve pathology patient safety.

▶ This manuscript by Smith and colleagues is a follow-up to previously published data outlining the level of latent problems in the accessioning and gross examination phases of an anatomic pathology laboratory. Smith et al use a variety of Lean tools and principles to drive culture change leading to front-line improvement. The investigators used the method of observation to document the large number of latent factors that contributed to active error and inefficiency and found that the front-line personnel who participated in the redesign of their own work environment were able to eliminate a large number of the latent problems (Table 2 in the original article). The majority of these problems was system-related and affected workflow and connections between personnel. Interestingly, the near-miss events classified as operator-dependent were difficult to reduce, perhaps indicating that different latent factors, such as training and environmental conditions, contribute to these event types. Effective quality improvement requires a number of initiatives targeting a large number of component causes. Some of these initiatives may be undertaken by the front-line personnel who are empowered to drive change, whereas others require support from top levels of management. For additional reading, please see reference list.[1,2]

S. S. Raab, MD

References

1. Smith ML, Raab SS. Assessment of latent factors contributing to error: addressing surgical pathology error wisely. *Arch Pathol Lab Med.* 2011;135:1436-1440.
2. Kotter JP. *Leading Change: Why Transformation Efforts Fail.* Boston, MA: Harvard Business Press; 2006.

Diagnostic errors in the new millennium: a follow-up autopsy study

Schwanda-Burger S, Moch H, Muntwyler J, et al (Med Clinic, Zurich, Switzerland; Univ of Zurich, Switzerland)
Mod Pathol 25:777-783, 2012

A systematic review of the second half of the last century suggested that diagnostic errors have decreased over time. Our previous study covering the years 1972–1992 was then the only time series showing a significant reduction of diagnostic errors from a single institution. We report here the results of a follow-up study a decade later. We analyzed discrepancies between clinical and autoptic diagnoses in 100 randomly selected medical patients who died in the wards and in the medical intensive care unit at a tertiary-care teaching hospital in Switzerland in the year 2002. Autopsy rate declined from around 90% in the years from 1972 to 1992 to 54% in the present study. Major diagnostic errors (class I and II) declined significantly from 30 to 7% ($P < 0.001$) over the last 30 years. Class I errors decreased from 16 to 2% ($P < 0.001$) in the year 2002. Sensitivity for cardiovascular diseases increased from 69 to 92% ($P = 0.006$), for infectious diseases from 25 to 90% ($P = 0.013$) and for neoplastic diseases from 89 to 100% ($P = 0.053$). Specificity for cardiovascular diseases increased from 85 to 98% ($P < 0.001$) but was unchanged at a high level for infectious diseases and neoplastic diseases. The number of diagnostic procedures increased from 144 to 281 ($P < 0.001$) with an increase in the number of computer tomography investigations and of tissue sampling in the last decade. The frequency of major diagnostic errors has been further reduced at the beginning of the new millennium probably due in large part to new diagnostic tools (Fig 1).

▶ It has been said that autopsies are the ultimate quality assurance tool, and in the era of focus on patient safety, the decline of the autopsy is lamentable. Several studies have shown that the frequency of medical error, as detected by the autopsy, has not decreased over time. Schwanda-Burger and colleagues challenge this concept in this single-institutional study from Zurich, Switzerland (Fig 1). This study has several strengths and weaknesses and the foray of the authors into hypothesizing on the causes of detected errors ignores some of the currently accepted thoughts on the system nature of medical error. However, I believe that articles such as this one strongly support the notion that autopsies provide a critical tool for error detection and improvement. Interestingly, the authors suggest that improvement may have been secondary to the use of new diagnostic tools, rather than data provided by the autopsy service itself. In the

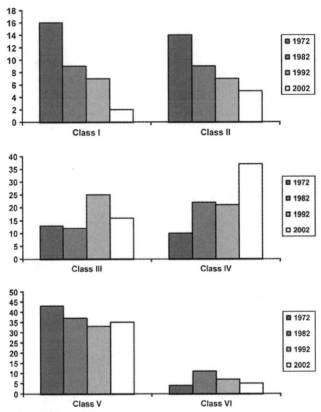

FIGURE 1.—Changes in discrepancy classes I–VI over the study years. Class I decreased from 16 to 2% ($P < 0.001$) and class II decreased from 14 to 5% ($P = 0.026$). Major diagnostic errors (class I and II) decreased from 30 to 7% ($P < 0.001$). Class III increased from 13 to 16% ($P = 0.207$) and class IV from 10 to 37% ($P < 0.001$). Minor diagnostic errors increased from 23 to 53% ($P < 0.001$). Class V decreased from 43 to 35% ($P = 0.212$) and class VI from 4 to 5% ($P = 1.000$). (Reprinted by permission from Macmillan Publishers Ltd: Modern Pathology. Schwanda-Burger S, Moch H, Muntwyler J, et al. Diagnostic errors in the new millennium: a follow-up autopsy study. *Mod Pathol.* 2012;25:777-783, Copyright 2012 by USCAP, Inc)

patient safety world, most errors are secondary to failures in process, which technology may or may not fix. From this point of view, autopsies may be used to monitor system quality improvement progress, rather than detecting a failed process and then designing an improvement initiative. For additional reading, please see reference list.[1-3]

S. S. Raab, MD

References

1. Goldman L, Sayson R, Robbins S, Cohn LH, Bettmann M, Weisberg M. The value of the autopsy in three medical eras. *N Engl J Med.* 1983;308:1000-1005.
2. Shojania KG, Burton EC, McDonald KM, Goldman L. Changes in rates of autopsy-detected diagnostic errors over time: a systematic review. *JAMA.* 2003; 289:2849-2856.

3. Veress B, Alafuzoff I. A retrospective analysis of clinical diagnoses and autopsy findings in 3,042 cases during two different time periods. *Hum Pathol.* 1994;25: 140-145.

Concordance Between Whole-Slide Imaging and Light Microscopy for Routine Surgical Pathology

Campbell WS, Lele SM, West WW, et al (Univ of Nebraska Med Ctr, Omaha)
Hum Pathol 43:1739-1744, 2012

The use of high-resolution digital images of histopathology slides as a routine diagnostic tool for surgical pathology was investigated. The study purpose was to determine the diagnostic concordance between pathologic interpretations using whole-slide imaging and standard light microscopy. Two hundred fifty-one consecutive surgical pathology cases (312 parts, 1085 slides) from a single pathology service were included in the study after cases had been signed out and reports generated. A broad array of diagnostic challenges and tissue sources were represented, including 52 neoplastic cases. All cases were digitized at ×20 and presented to 2 pathologists for diagnosis using whole-slide imaging as the sole diagnostic tool. Diagnoses rendered by the whole-slide imaging pathologists were compared with the original light microscopy diagnoses. Overall concordance between whole-slide imaging and light microscopy as determined by a third pathologist and jury panel was 96.5% (95% confidence interval, 94.8%-98.3%). Concordance between whole-slide imaging pathologists was 97.7% (95% confidence interval, 94.7%-99.2%). Five cases were discordant between the whole-slide imaging diagnosis and the original light microscopy diagnosis, of which 2 were clinically significant. Discordance resulted from interpretive criteria or diagnostic error. The whole-slide imaging modality did not contribute to diagnostic differences. Problems encountered by the whole-slide imaging pathologists primarily involved the inability to clearly visualize nuclear detail or microscopic organisms. Technical difficulties associated with image scanning required at least 1 slide be rescanned in 13% of the cases. Technical and operational issues associated with whole-slide imaging scanning devices used in this study were found to be the most significant obstacle to the use of whole-slide imaging in general surgical pathology (Table 2).

▶ The data presented by Campbell et al confirm that the accuracy of digital diagnosis is comparable to that of light microscopy (Table 2). In my opinion, these data have been known for quite a long time, because diagnostic accuracy and precision are the first issues that needed to be addressed. The main problems in fully moving to a digitally based system revolve around process issues and the lack of understanding the sociotechnical components of work. In regard to process problems, Campbell and colleagues report the relatively high frequency of errors in slide scanning and the length of time to scan large "batches" of slides. Sociotechnically, we have yet to understand how pathologists and technologists will work to adopt these technologies effectively. Consequently, we will use

TABLE 2.—Concordance Rates with Original LM Diagnoses and Between Study Pathologists

	Pathologist A to Original Dx	Pathologist B to Original Dx	Between Study Pathologists
Concordant—equivalent diagnoses	84.7%	81.9%	90.2%
Concordant—minor, clinically insignificant differences	12.1%	14.4%	7.4%
Discordant—clinically significant	1.9%	2.3%	0.9%
Read failures—could not evaluate	1.4%	1.4%	1.4%
% Total concordance	96.7%	96.3%	97.7%

Abbreviation: Dx, diagnosis.

these technologies to render consult (secondary opinions), prior to use as a primary diagnostic tool, which also has regulatory restrictions. As the field progresses, the daily work issues (eg, integration into laboratory information systems, workflow, image storage) will be addressed. For further reading, see reference list.[1,2]

S. S. Raab, MD

References

1. Graham AR, Bhattacharyya AK, Scott KM, et al. Virtual slide telepathology for an academic teaching hospital surgical pathology quality assurance program. *Hum Pathol.* 2009;40:1129-1136.
2. Ho J, Parwani AV, Jukic DM, Yagi Y, Anthony L, Gilbertson JR. Use of whole slide imaging in surgical pathology quality assurance: design and pilot validation studies. *Hum Pathol.* 2006;37:322-331.

Papillary Lesions of the Breast: Impact of Breast Pathology Subspecialization on Core Biopsy and Excision Diagnoses
Jakate K, De Brot M, Goldberg F, et al (Univ of Toronto, Ontario, Canada; Mount Sinai Hosp, Toronto, Ontario, Canada; St Michael's Hosp, Toronto, Ontario, Canada)
Am J Surg Pathol 36:544-551, 2012

Background.—Classifying papillary lesions of the breast on core biopsy (CB) is challenging. Although traditionally all such lesions were surgically excised, at present, conservative management of benign lesions is being advocated; therefore, accurately classifying papillary lesions on CB is all the more imperative. The extent to which subspecialty training in breast pathology might mitigate such difficulties in diagnosis has not yet been reported. We investigated change in diagnoses from CB to surgical excision according to subspecialist training in breast pathology and interobserver agreement between specialized breast pathologists (BPs) and nonbreast pathologists (NBPs) in classifying these lesions.

Design.—CBs of 281 papillary lesions from 266 patients diagnosed between 2000 and 2010 were classified by both a BP and NBP into benign, atypical, ductal carcinoma in situ/encapsulated papillary carcinoma, or invasive carcinoma categories. Rates of change in diagnostic category in the surgical excision specimen were calculated on the basis of (i) the original diagnosis, (ii) diagnosis made by the BP, and (iii) diagnosis made by the NBP. Comparisons were made using the χ^2 test. Kappa values were calculated for interobserver agreement.

Results.—Of 162 lesions with subsequent excision, 90 were originally diagnosed as benign, 38 as atypical, 25 as ductal carcinoma in situ/encapsulated papillary carcinoma, and 9 as invasive on CB. The upgrade rate for benign papillomas to an atypical or malignant lesion on surgical excision was 22.2% according to the original diagnosis. This rate fell to 16.3% when the BP diagnoses were considered, compared with 26.3% for the NBP diagnoses. There was no significant difference between BPs and NBPs in the rate of upgrade from a benign to an atypical/malignant diagnosis, although downgrades from atypical/malignant to benign papillomas were more commonly seen among NBPs ($P = 0.002$). Overall, the BP diagnosis on CB was less likely to differ from the excision diagnosis ($P = 0.0001$). Benign papillomas upgraded on excision were more likely to occur with larger radiologic mass size ($P = 0.033$) compared with those that were not upgraded. Of 8 benign papillomas upgraded to a malignant lesion on excision, 7 were discordant on radiology. Interobserver agreement between BP and NBP diagnoses was in the "fair agreement" range ($\kappa = 0.38$), with perfect agreement in 66.4% of cases.

Conclusions.—Correlation between CB and excision diagnoses for breast papillary lesions is significantly greater for BPs than for NBPs. This is largely because of a tendency to overcall atypia or malignancy on CB by NBPs. However, upgrades from benign to atypical or malignant did not significantly differ according to subspecialization. With accurate pathologic assessment and radiologic-pathologic correlation, the upgrade rate of benign papillomas to malignancy can be minimized significantly.

▶ More focused study of subspecialization in pathology is critical to determine its strengths and weaknesses. Articles such as the one by Jakate et al compare subspecialists with nonsubspecialists, but the characteristics of the pathologists in the 2 groups often are poorly characterized. In addition, such manuscripts do not examine other models of pathology sign-out, such as team sign-out with 2 pathologists, referral of specific case types to internal expertise, or other quality methods that serve to address the potential weaknesses of nonsubspecialists. I think the assumption is that subspecialty allows for the greater study of the range of diseases in certain organ systems and produces experts. However, we do not know what types of cases require an expert, if we could identify these cases in some specific manner prior to sign-out, or if practice patterns could deal with the lack of subspecialty expertise in other ways. For example, Jakate et al point out that radiologic-pathologic correlation is critical in improving patient care. Because many subspecialists have cultivated this relationship and some nonsubspecialists have not, would improving this relationship in nonsub-specialists make the 2 groups more equivalent (rather than becoming a subspe-cialist)? For additional reading, please see reference list.[1,2]

S. S. Raab, MD

References

1. Arora N, Hill C, Hoda SA, Rosenblatt R, Pigalarga R, Tousimis EA. Clinicopath-ologic features of papillary lesions on core needle biopsy of the breast predictive of malignancy. *Am J Surg.* 2007;194:444-449.
2. Tse GM, Tan PH, Lacambra MD, et al. Papillary lesions of the breast—accuracy of core biopsy. *Histopathology.* 2010;56:481-488.

2 Breast

Network meta-analysis of margin threshold for women with ductal carcinoma in situ
Wang SY, Chu H, Shamliyan T, et al (Univ of Minnesota School of Public Health, Minneapolis)
J Natl Cancer Inst 104:507-516, 2012

Background.—Negative margins are associated with reduced risk of ipsilateral breast tumor recurrence (IBTR) for women with ductal carcinoma in situ (DCIS) treated with breast-conserving surgery (BCS). However, there is no consensus about the best minimum margin width.

Methods.—We searched the PubMed database for studies of DCIS published in English between January 1970 and July 2010 and examined the relationship between IBTR and margin status after BCS for DCIS. Women with DCIS were stratified into two groups, BCS with or without radiotherapy. We used frequentist and Bayesian approaches to estimate the odds ratios (OR) of IBTR for groups with negative margins and positive margins. We further examined specific margin thresholds using mixed treatment comparisons and meta-regression techniques. All statistical tests were two-sided.

Results.—We identified 21 studies published in 24 articles. A total of 1066 IBTR events occurred in 7564 patients, including BCS alone (565 IBTR events in 3098 patients) and BCS with radiotherapy (501 IBTR events in 4466 patients). Compared with positive margins, negative margins were associated with reduced risk of IBTR in patients with radiotherapy (OR = 0.46, 95% credible interval [CrI] = 0.35 to 0.59), and in patients without radiotherapy (OR = 0.34, 95% CrI = 0.24 to 0.47). Compared with patients with positive margins, the risk of IBTR for patients with negative margins was smaller (negative margin > 0 mm, OR = 0.45, 95% CrI = 0.38 to 0.53; > 2 mm, OR = 0.38, 95% CrI = 0.28 to 0.51; > 5 mm, OR = 0.55, 95% CrI = 0.15 to 1.30; and > 10 mm, OR = 0.17, 95% CrI = 0.12 to 0.24). Compared with a negative margin greater than 2 mm, a negative margin of at least 10 mm was associated with a lower risk of IBTR (OR = 0.46, 95% CrI = 0.29 to 0.69). We found a probability of .96 that a negative margin threshold greater than 10 mm is the best option compared with other margin thresholds.

Conclusions.—Negative surgical margins should be obtained for DCIS patients after BCS regardless of radiotherapy. Within cosmetic constraint, surgeons should attempt to achieve negative margins as wide as possible in their first attempt. More studies are needed to understand whether margin thresholds greater than 10 mm are warranted.

▶ This article has spurned much discussion on the appropriate width of surgical margins in patients being treated for ductal carcinoma in situ. The authors have concluded that surgeons should attempt to achieve negative margins as wide as possible for these patients. Several editorials were immediately published calling the findings into question. There are large issues with Wang et al's study, such as the lack of random assignment of patients in many of the studies included and uncertainty about the inference of causality. The most significant observation on the work is that in almost all of the studies included surgeons did not achieve "wide" margins. It has been previously shown that patients in large trials (NSABP B17 and B24) in which a negative margin was defined as no tumor at ink have done well with long-term follow-up. I would recommend that pathologists review this article as well as the intelligent editorial by Morrow included in the same issue.

B. A. Carter, MD, FRCPC

Ki-67: Level of Evidence and Methodological Considerations for Its Role in the Clinical Management of Breast Cancer: Analytical and Critical Review
Luporsi E, André F, Spyratos F, et al (CHU Nancy & Nancy-Université, Vandoeuvre-les-Nancy, France; Institut Gustave Roussy, Villejuif, France; Institut Curie—Hôpital René Huguenin, St-Cloud, France; et al)
Breast Cancer Res Treat 132:895-915, 2012

Clinicians can use biomarkers to guide therapeutic decisions in estrogen receptor positive (ER+) breast cancer. One such biomarker is cellular proliferation as evaluated by Ki-67. This biomarker has been extensively studied and is easily assayed by histopathologists but it is not currently accepted as a standard. This review focuses on its prognostic and predictive value, and on methodological considerations for its measurement and the cut-points used for treatment decision. Data describing study design, patients' characteristics, methods used and results were extracted from papers published between January 1990 and July 2010. In addition, the studies were assessed using the REMARK tool. Ki-67 is an independent prognostic factor for disease-free survival (HR 1.05—1.72) in multivariate analyses studies using samples from randomized clinical trials with secondary central analysis of the biomarker. The level of evidence (LOE) was judged to be I-B with the recently revised definition of Simon. However, standardization of the techniques and scoring methods are needed for the integration of this biomarker in everyday practice. Ki-67 was not found to be predictive for long-term follow-up after chemotherapy. Nevertheless, high KI-67 was found to be associated with immediate pathological complete response in the neoadjuvant setting, with an LOE of II-B. The REMARK score improved over time (with a range of 6—13/20 vs. 10—18/20, before and after 2005, respectively). KI-67 could be considered as a prognostic biomarker for

TABLE 5.—Summary of Assessment of Various Markers as Prognostic Factors for DFS in Women with Breast Cancer

Reference[a]	Marker	HR (95% CI)
Stuart-Harris et al. [100]	Ki-67	1.76 (1.56—1.98)
Rakha et al. [94]	SBR grade (3 vs. 1)	1.6 (1.3—2.0)
Look et al. [64]	uPA/PAI-1 (pN0)	2.37 (1.78—3.16)
Rakha et al. [94]	Node status	1.5 (1.4—1.7)
Wirapati et al. [113]	ER (neg. vs. high)	2.2 (1.6—3.0)
Blows et al. [10]	HER2	1.55 (1.23—1.96)

SBR Scarf—Bloom—Richardson histological grading system.
Editor's Note: Please refer to original journal article for full references.
[a]Not all patients received systemic adjuvant treatment.

therapeutic decision. It is assessed with a simple assay that could be standardized. However, international guidelines are needed for routine clinical use (Table 5).

▶ This article contributes to the discussion of the value of Ki-67 assessment in breast cancer and will be of great interest to breast pathologists, general pathologists, and immunohistochemists. While multiple previous articles have shown the value of Ki-67 as a prognosticator, uptake into surgical pathology laboratories has been slow. This report clarifies some of the reasons that is so. Luporsi et al, in a systematic review of 71 randomized clinical trials, cohort studies, and case control studies, looked at the evidence supporting the use of Ki-67 in breast cancer patients. Overall, they found that it does have value as a prognosticator of disease-free survival with a hazard ratio similar to grade and nodal status (Table 5).[1] More important is that they discuss the many problems that practicing pathologists have encountered when attempting to include Ki-67 testing in their breast cancer arsenal. Varying cut points for positivity, varying numbers of cells counted, use of automated imaging technology, and use of molecular methods instead of immunohistochemistry are all discussed. No definitive recommendations are made, but the authors press for international guidelines to standardize the preanalytic phase, the staining techniques, the cut points for positivity, and the counting methods. This standardized approach will be helpful for the practicing pathologist.

B. A. Carter, MD, FRCPC

Reference

1. Rakha EA, El-Sayed ME, Lee AH, et al. Prognostic significance of Nottingham histologic grade in invasive breast carcinoma. *J Clin Oncol.* 2008;26: 3153-3158.

Clinicopathologic Characteristics of Carcinomas That Develop After a Biopsy Containing Columnar Cell Lesions: Evidence Against a Precursor Role

Boulos FI, Dupont WD, Schuyler PA, et al (American Univ of Beirut Med Ctr, Lebanon; Vanderbilt Univ Med Ctr, Nashville, TN)
Cancer 118:2372-2377, 2012

Background.—Columnar cell lesions are frequently associated with atypical ductal hyperplasia, lobular neoplasia, and tubular carcinoma, and have been suggested as a precursor lesion for low-grade carcinomas. However, in long-term follow-up studies, columnar cell lesions are associated with only a slight increase in later breast cancer development. If columnar cell lesions are precursor lesions, one would expect subsequent cancers to develop at the same site as the biopsy and to be preferentially of low grade. The goal of this article is to review the clinical and pathologic features of carcinomas that develop after a diagnosis of columnar cell lesion to try to establish whether these lesions are precursors to low-grade invasive carcinoma.

Methods.—The authors reviewed biopsies containing columnar cell lesions, using the criteria of Schnitt and Vincent-Salomon, from 77 women in the Nashville Breast Cohort who developed subsequent breast carcinoma. Clinicopathologic features including laterality, type, and grade of the subsequent cancer were recorded.

Results.—Breast cancer developed a median of 11 years after initial biopsy. The median age at diagnosis was 60 years. The majority of invasive carcinomas were of no special type and of intermediate grade. Moreover, the carcinomas were as likely to occur in the contralateral breast as in the breast that was originally diagnosed with columnar cell lesion, regardless of columnar cell lesion subtype ($P = .48$).

Conclusions.—Carcinoma subsequent to columnar cell lesions may occur in either breast and tends to show a similar grade and type distribution as sporadic breast cancer. These findings argue against columnar cell lesions being a true precursor for low-grade invasive carcinoma (Table 1).

▶ This study will be helpful for those pathologists who are active members of the pathology–radiology breast correlation teams at their institutions and for any surgical pathologist who provides consultation and advice to patients and

TABLE 1.—Clinicopathologic Characteristics of Cancer Cases Following CCL Subtypes

Type	I/lat	C/lat	Grade 1	Grade 2	Grade 3	Size, cm (Range)	LNM
CCC	9[a]	4[a]	3/14	7/14	4/14	1.8 (0.1-4.0)	4/14
CCH	12	15	10/27	12/27	5/27	1.6 (0.2-4.5)	8/27
CCA	6	7	3/13	4/13	6/13	1.5 (0.7-3.0)	7/13
CCL	27[a]	26[a]	16 [30%]	23 [42%]	15 [28%]	1.56 (0.1-4.5)	19/54

Abbreviations: C/lat, contralateral; CCA, columnar cell atypia; CCC, columnar cell change; CCH, columnar cell hyperplasia; CCL, columnar cell lesion; I/lat, ipsilateral; LNM, lymph node metastasis.
[a]One woman had bilateral cancer and contributed to cancer information but not to laterality with respect to CCC.

practitioners involved in breast needle core biopsy clinics. As more women undergo breast screening internationally and as mammography equipment improves, the rate of nonmalignant diagnoses on tissue core biopsies for mammographic abnormalities has risen. The diagnosis of columnar cell lesions, largely unheard of before the 1990s, is increasingly common. The recent breast literature has likewise followed with hundreds of articles on the subject published in the past 2 decades. Despite the attention that columnar cell atypia has attracted recently, 2 important questions remain: 1) should isolated columnar cell atypia be excised after identification on a core needle biopsy and 2) does columnar cell atypia represent a precursor lesion to low-grade in situ and invasive carcinoma. Using the Nashville Breast Cohort and its long-term follow-up data this study attempts to clarify the second question using entry biopsies between 1965 and 1982. An elegant discussion of Page's argument that proof of a precursor lesion is documentation of progression is included. The authors find no evidence for precursor status (Table 1) and reinforce the idea that columnar cell atypia confers a slight increase in the risk of future development of breast cancer for patients with that diagnosis.

B. A. Carter, MD, FRCPC

Lobular In-Situ Neoplasia on Breast Core Needle Biopsy: Imaging Indication and Pathologic Extent Can Identify Which Patients Require Excisional Biopsy

Rendi MH, Dintzis SM, Lehman CD, et al (Univ of Washington Med Ctr, Seattle)
Ann Surg Oncol 19:914-921, 2012

Background.—The surgical management of lobular in-situ neoplasia (LN) identified by core needle biopsy (CNB) is currently variable. Our institution has routinely excised LN on CNB since 2003, allowing for an unbiased assessment of upgrade rates.

Methods.—Cases of LN on CNB, including atypical lobular hyperplasia (ALH) and lobular carcinoma-in-situ (LCIS), were identified in our pathology database. CNBs with concurrent pleomorphic LCIS, ductal carcinoma-in-situ (DCIS), and invasive carcinoma were excluded. Imaging indication/modality, biopsy indication, and radiologic concordance were determined. Pathology review included scoring total foci of LN in each CNB. Upgrade rates to invasive carcinoma or DCIS at excision were calculated.

Results.—A total of 106 cases of LN (73 ALH and 33 LCIS) on CNB were identified. Thirty patients had concurrent atypical ductal hyperplasia (ADH) and 76 had LN alone; 93 (88%) of the patients had available surgical follow-up (25 LN + ADH and 68 LN alone). The upgrade rate at excision was 16% (4 of 25) for LN + ADH and 4.4% (3 of 68) for LN alone. Patients with LN alone and discordant imaging, imaging for high-risk indications, or extensive LCIS (> 4 foci) accounted for all the upgrades. Normal-risk

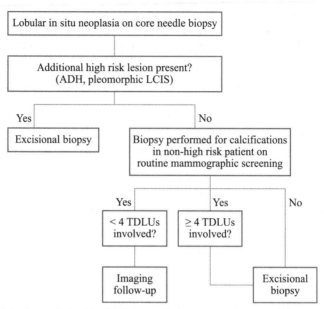

FIGURE 2.—Proposed algorithm for deciding which patients with LN should be recommended to undergo surgical excisional biopsy. A high-risk patient is defined as a patient with any of the following: *1* a strong family history or personal history of breast cancer, *2* imaging performed for extent of disease evaluation, and *3* a patient with a clinical finding at breast examination. (Reprinted from Rendi MH, Dintzis SM, Lehman CD, et al. Lobular in-situ neoplasia on breast core needle biopsy: Imaging indication and pathologic extent can identify which patients require excisional biopsy. *Ann Surg Oncol.* 2012;19:914-921, with kind permission from Springer Science+Business Media.)

TABLE 1.—Imaging/Biopsy Indication and Imaging Modality

Characteristic	n (%)
Imaging indication	
Routine mammographic screening	54 (51%)
High-risk screening	18 (17%)
Clinical finding evaluation	6 (6%)
Follow-up after lumpectomy	5 (5%)
Extent of disease evaluation	23 (21%)
Biopsy indication	
Calcification	73 (69%)
Mass	15 (14%)
MRI enhancement	17 (16%)
Architectural distortion	1 (1%)
Imaging modality	
Mammogram	79 (74%)
MRI	25 (24%)
Ultrasound	2 (2%)

patients who underwent biopsy to assess calcifications found by routine mammographic screening with LN alone did not result in upgrade.

Conclusions.—Women with a CNB diagnosis of LN for calcifications found on routine, normal-risk mammographic screening have a negligible risk of upgrade and may not require excisional biopsy. However, excisional biopsy should be offered to women undergoing imaging for other indications or with > 4 foci of LN on CNB (Fig 2, Table 1).

▶ This article provides insight into the appropriate management of a diagnosis of lobular neoplasia (LN) on needle core biopsies. It will be of interest to breast pathologists, general pathologists, radiologists, and residents. The diagnosis of lobular neoplasia on needle core biopsy is rare, accounting for less than 5% of all diagnoses rendered. The small sample size at most institutions as well as the frequent co-occurrence of LN with other lesions of risk has contributed to the general lack of guidelines on management of this entity. However, as the use of breast magnetic resonance imaging increases, this diagnosis is likely to become more common. In this study at a large institution there were only 106 cases of LN identified over a 6-year period. These cases were usually identified through the screening mammography program and were diagnosed after a biopsy for calcification (Table 1). Based on their findings, the authors propose an algorithm for recommending excisional biopsy in cases of LN (Fig 2). A significant proportion of women with this diagnosis on needle core biopsy can be spared further surgery and be placed in a follow-up program. For additional reading, please see reference list.[1,2]

B. A. Carter, MD, FRCPC

References

1. Elsheikh TM, Silverman JF. Follow-up surgical excision is indicated when breast core needle biopsies show atypical lobular hyperplasia or lobular carcinoma in situ: correlative study of 33 patients with review of the literature. *Am J Surg Pathol.* 2005;29:534-543.
2. Arpino G, Allred DC, Mohsin SK, Weiss HL, Conrow D, Elledge RM. Lobular neoplasia on core-needle biopsy—clinical significance. *Cancer.* 2004;101:242-250.

Impact of Routine Pathology Review on Treatment for Node-Negative Breast Cancer

Kennecke HF, Speers CH, Ennis CA, et al (British Columbia Cancer Agency, Vancouver, Canada)
J Clin Oncol 30:2227-2231, 2012

Purpose.—Routine secondary pathology review influences diagnosis and treatment among patients diagnosed with breast cancer. The impact of review on patients with node-negative breast cancer and the nature of the pathology elements leading to management changes are not well described.

Methods.—Patients with node-negative, invasive, or in situ breast cancer and evaluable nodes referred to the British Columbia Cancer Agency during two time periods between 2004 and 2007 were included. Pathologists with expertise in breast cancer reviewed the original reports and slides. Biomarker testing was not routinely repeated. Medical record review was conducted to determine whether original pathology was changed and whether recommended therapy was affected.

TABLE 2.—Type and Frequency of 102 Changes on Central Pathology Review Among 405 Patients With Node-Negative Invasive or in Situ Breast Cancer

Change on Pathology Review	Direction of Change		Overall Frequency	
	Negative → Positive	Positive → Negative	No.	%
Tumor grade	28 (grade increased)	13 (grade decreased)	41	40
Lymphovascular invasion	17	10	27	26
Nodal status	6 (N0 to N1) 9 (N0 to N0i+)	0	15	15
Margin status	11	1	12	2
PR status	3	0	3	3
ER and/or PR	2	0	2	2
Invasive v in situ	0	2	2	2

Abbreviations: ER, estrogen receptor; PR, progesterone receptor.

TABLE 3.—Frequency of Changes in Systemic and Radiation Therapy Among 81 Patients With at Least One Change on Secondary Pathology Review

Patients	Systemic Therapy		Radiation Therapy		Total
	Added	Modified	Added	Modified	
No.	12	3	4	8	27

Results.—Among 906 eligible patients, 405 (45%) received a pathology review. Univariate comparisons revealed that reviewed patients were younger ($P < .001$) and more likely to have close margins ($P < .001$), whereas other characteristics were similar. A total of 102 pathology changes were documented among 81 patients (20%). The most frequently changed elements were grade (40%) and lymphovascular (26%), nodal (15%), and margin (12%) status. These changes resulted in 27 treatment modifications among 25 patients (6%). Treatment changes were primarily related to nodal and margin status, and only two of 27 were related to measurement of tumor biology in women with estrogen receptor–positive, node-negative breast cancer.

Conclusion.—Reported rates of change are significant and warrant routine secondary pathology review among patients with node-negative breast cancer or ductal carcinoma in situ before final treatment is recommended. Review remains relevant in the era of gene expression signatures to determine margin and nodal status (Tables 2 and 3).

▶ This study reinforces the role of oncologic pathologists in the care of the cancer patient. Although multiple studies[1,2] have documented the impact of secondary pathology review on clinical management of patients with cancer, many institutions have not yet implemented this practice. Lack of availability to timely pathology review is the most common reason for low uptake. This is the case at the British Columbia Cancer Agency. Because of a lack of resources in their pathology department, the blanket review policy was revised to include only selected oncology diagnoses. For breast cancer patients, only those diagnosed with ductal carcinoma in situ or lymph node—negative invasive breast cancer have access to a pathologist's review. This study was designed to investigate whether this limited practice was of benefit to the patients. In this subgroup Kennecke et al show (Table 2) that 81 women had at least 1 change in their pathologic diagnosis on central pathology review. Significant changes in the recommendations for systemic and/or radiation therapy were made in a small number of cases (6% of 405) as a result of this review (Table 3). The authors note that in the setting of limited pathology resources, patients with node-negative breast cancer or ductal carcinoma in situ are a relevant subgroup to undergo routine pathology review. The main strength of this article is that is supports the necessity of pathology review for all cancer patients.

B. A. Carter, MD, FRCPC

References

1. Price JA, Grunfeld E, Barnes PJ, Rheaume DE, Rayson D. Inter-institutional pathology consultations for breast cancer: impact on clinical oncology therapy recommendations. *Curr Oncol.* 2010;17:25-32.
2. Tsung JS. Institutional pathology consultation. *Am J Surg Pathol.* 2004;28: 399-402.

Encapsulated papillary carcinoma of the breast: a study of invasion associated markers
Rakha EA, Tun M, Junainah E, et al (Univ of Nottingham, UK)
J Clin Pathol 65:710-714, 2012

Encapsulated papillary carcinoma (EPC) of the breast is a distinct histological subtype characterised by malignant epithelial proliferation supported by fibrovascular stalks. Although EPC typically lacks myoepithelial cells, it shows indolent clinical course. The classification of EPC as an in situ, or invasive disease, remains a matter of debate.

Methods.—In this study, the authors investigated a panel of invasion-associated markers in a series of EPC and compared their expression with control groups of nonpapillary ductal carcinoma in situ (DCIS) and conventional invasive carcinomas. The expression pattern of four matrix metalloproteinases (MMP-1, MMP-2, MMP-7 and MMP-9), transforming growth factor receptor beta, vascular endothelial growth factor (VEGF) and E-cadherin were assessed in the tumour cell and/or stromal tissue, and the results were analysed.

Results.—EPC showed higher expression levels of both MMP-1 and MMP-9 compared with DCIS, and no significant differences were observed between EPC and invasive carcinoma. Expression of MMP-2 and MMP-7 levels were similar in EPC and DCIS, but both showed lower levels compared

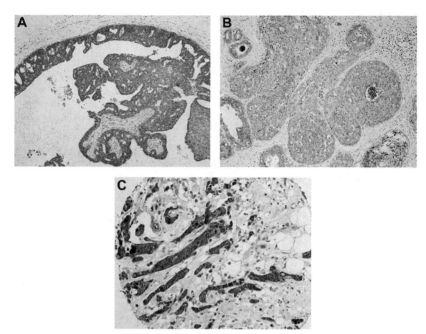

FIGURE 1.—Expression of matrix metalloproteinase 9: (A) A case of encapsulated papillary carcinoma showing moderate cytoplasmic expression. (B) A case of low-grade non-papillary duct carcinoma in situ showing weak cytoplasmic expression. (C) A case of invasive carcinoma showing moderate to strong cytoplasmic expression of matrix metalloproteinase 9. (Reprinted from Rakha EA, Tun M, Junainah E, et al. Encapsulated papillary carcinoma of the breast: a study of invasion associated markers. *J Clin Pathol.* 2012;65:710-714.)

with invasive tumours. EPC showed higher expression of E-cadherin and transforming growth factor receptor ß1 compared with both DCIS and invasive cancer. No difference in the stromal expression of MMPs or tumour expression of VEGF was detected.

Conclusion.—EPC exhibits an expression pattern of invasion-associated markers, which is intermediate in nature between DCIS and invasive cancer, providing further support of the unique biological features of EPC, and which may explain its clinically indolent behaviour (Figs 1 and 2, Table 2).

▶ Encapsulated papillary carcinoma is a recently introduced diagnosis in breast cancers and this entity is often a puzzle for pathologists and oncologists alike. Under its previous name, encysted papillary carcinoma, it was initially perceived as a variant of in situ carcinoma. However, confounding its noninvasive status, as the literature grew, there was always a rare, but significant risk of invasive and/or metastatic behavior. This article provides supportive evidence for the new categorization of this lesion as an invasive carcinoma with expansile growth and indolent behavior. Using a panel of invasion associated immunohistochemical markers (Figs 1 and 2, Table 2) the authors show that encapsulated papillary

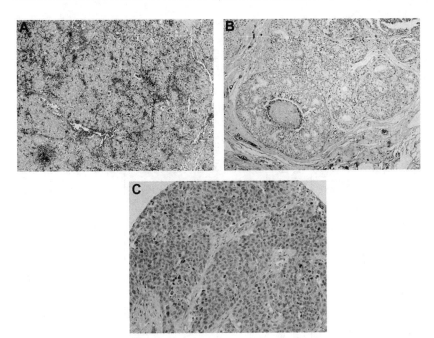

FIGURE 2.—Expression of transforming growth factor receptor β (TGFβ): (A) A case of encapsulated papillary carcinoma showing strong cytoplasmic expression of TGFβ. (B) A case of low-grade non-papillary duct carcinoma in situ showing negative TGFβ expression. (C) A case of invasive carcinoma showing weak to moderate cytoplasmic expression of TGFβ. (Reprinted from Rakha EA, Tun M, Junainah E, et al. Encapsulated papillary carcinoma of the breast: a study of invasion associated markers. *J Clin Pathol.* 2012;65:710-714, with permission from the BMJ Publishing Group Ltd.)

carcinoma has an expression profile midway between ductal carcinoma in situ and invasive carcinoma of the breast. An interesting discussion of the role of transforming growth factor-b1 in the development of the thick fibrous, possibly reactive capsule commonly present in this lesion is included. The study is limited by its small sample size. For additional reading, please see the reference list.[1,2]

B. A. Carter, MD, FRCPC

References

1. Collins LC, Carlo VP, Hwang H, Barry TS, Gown AM, Schnitt SJ. Intracystic papillary carcinomas of the breast: a reevaluation using a panel of myoepithelial cell markers. *Am J Surg Pathol.* 2006;30:1002-1007.
2. Rakha EA, Gandhi N, Climent F, et al. Encapsulated papillary carcinoma of the breast: an invasive tumor with excellent prognosis. *Am J Surg Pathol.* 2011;35: 1093-1103.

TABLE 2.—The Percentages of Tumour Expression (%) of the Seven Biomarkers in Malignant Cells of Encapsulated Papillary Carcinoma (EPC), Non-Papillary Ductal Carcinoma In Situ (DCIS) and Conventional invasive Carcinoma of the Breast

Biomarker	EPC %; Median (Range)	DCIS %; Median (Range)	p Value EPC Versus DCIS	Invasive Carcinoma %; Median (Range)	p Value EPC Versus Invasive	p Value DCIS Versus Invasive
MMP-1	65%; 15 (0–170)	10%; 0 (0–10)	0.009	80%; 60 (0–300)	0.024	<0.001
MMP-2	77%; 30 (0–160)	70%; 13 (0–140)	0.115	86%; 80 (0–300)	0.002	0.001
MMP-7	100%; 140 (20–300)	90%; 105 (0–270)	0.537	86%; 200 (0–300)	<0.001	<0.001
MMP-9	77%; 40 (0–160)	60%; 5 (0–150)	0.046	80%; 80 (0–200)	0.083	0.003
TGF-β1	65%; 30 (0–150)	10%; 0 (0–20)	0.001	13%; 0 (0–160)	<0.001	0.631
VEGF	100%; 160 (20–160)	100%; 160 (30–160)	0.786	83%; 120 (0–300)	0.603	0.483
E-cadherin	100%; 170 (120–300)	100%; 200 (200–300)	0.059	89%; 200 (0–300)	0.502	0.244

% = percentage of positivity of expression as defined by ≥10% expression.
p Value is estimated using H-score as continuous variables; however, the same results were obtained using percentage of expression.
MMP, matrix metalloproteinase; TGF, transforming growth factor receptor; VEGF, vascular endothelial growth factor.

Papillary Lesions of the Breast: Impact of Breast Pathology Subspecialization on Core Biopsy and Excision Diagnoses

Jakate K, De Brot M, Goldberg F, et al (Univ of Toronto, Ontario, Canada; Mount Sinai Hosp, NY; St Michael's Hosp, Toronto, Ontario, Canada)
Am J Surg Pathol 36:544-551, 2012

Background.—Classifying papillary lesions of the breast on core biopsy (CB) is challenging. Although traditionally all such lesions were surgically excised, at present, conservative management of benign lesions is being advocated; therefore, accurately classifying papillary lesions on CB is all the more imperative. The extent to which subspecialty training in breast pathology might mitigate such difficulties in diagnosis has not yet been reported. We investigated change in diagnoses from CB to surgical excision according to subspecialist training in breast pathology and interobserver agreement between specialized breast pathologists (BPs) and nonbreast pathologists (NBPs) in classifying these lesions.

Design.—CBs of 281 papillary lesions from 266 patients diagnosed between 2000 and 2010 were classified by both a BP and NBP into benign, atypical, ductal carcinoma in situ/encapsulated papillary carcinoma, or invasive carcinoma categories. Rates of change in diagnostic category in the surgical excision specimen were calculated on the basis of: (i) the original diagnosis, (ii) diagnosis made by the BP, and (iii) diagnosis made by the NBP. Comparisons were made using the χ^2 test. Kappa values were calculated for interobserver agreement.

Results.—Of 162 lesions with subsequent excision, 90 were originally diagnosed as benign, 38 as atypical, 25 as ductal carcinoma in situ/encapsulated papillary carcinoma, and 9 as invasive on CB. The upgrade rate for benign papillomas to an atypical or malignant lesion on surgical excision was 22.2% according to the original diagnosis. This rate fell to 16.3% when the BP diagnoses were considered, compared with 26.3% for the NBP diagnoses. There was no significant difference between BPs and NBPs in the rate of upgrade from a benign to an atypical/malignant diagnosis, although downgrades from atypical/malignant to benign papillomas were more commonly seen among NBPs ($P = 0.002$). Overall, the BP diagnosis on CB was less likely to differ from the excision diagnosis ($P = 0.0001$). Benign papillomas upgraded on excision were more likely to occur with larger radiologic mass size ($P = 0.033$) compared with those that were not upgraded. Of 8 benign papillomas upgraded to a malignant lesion on excision, 7 were discordant on radiology. Interobserver agreement between BP and NBP diagnoses was in the "fair agreement" range ($\kappa = 0.38$), with perfect agreement in 66.4% of cases.

Conclusions.—Correlation between CB and excision diagnoses for breast papillary lesions is significantly greater for BPs than for NBPs. This is largely because of a tendency to overcall atypia or malignancy on CB by NBPs. However, upgrades from benign to atypical or malignant did not significantly differ according to subspecialization. With accurate pathologic assessment and radiologic-pathologic correlation, the upgrade rate of benign papillomas to malignancy can be minimized significantly (Fig 1, Table 3).

▶ Because of assumed associated risk of malignancy, the diagnosis of papillary lesion on a needle core biopsy of the breast usually mandates a complete excision.

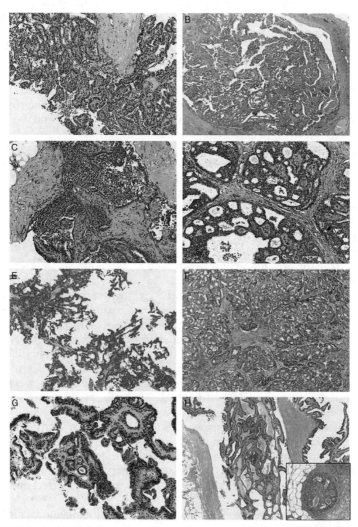

FIGURE 1.—Benign CB diagnoses upgraded to malignant on excision (refer to Table 3) (hematoxylin and eosin): (A) CB of case 1. (B) EPC found on excision of case 1. (C) CB of case 3. (D) DCIS within a papilloma found on excision of case 3. (E) CB of case 6. (F) Invasive ductal carcinoma with papillary features found on excision of case 6. (G) CB of case 7. (H) Benign papilloma found on excision of case 7 with conventional DCIS in the background breast (inset). (Reprinted from Jakate K, De Brot M, Goldberg F, et al. Papillary lesions of the breast: impact of breast pathology subspecialization on core biopsy and excision diagnoses. *Am J Surg Pathol.* 2012;36:544-551, with permission from Lippincott Williams & Wilkins.)

TABLE 3.—Benign Papillomas Upgraded to Malignancy on Surgical Excision

Case Number	Original Diagnosis	NBP Diagnosis	BP Diagnosis	Surgical Excision Diagnosis	BI-RADS Score/Radiologic Impression	Radiologic- Pathologic Correlation
1	NBP	**Benign**	**DCIS/EPC**	EPC	4b	Discordant
2	NBP	**Benign**	Benign	DCIS within a papilloma	4b	Discordant
3	NBP	**Benign**	**Atypical**	DCIS within a papilloma	4a	Concordant
4	NBP	**Benign**	**Atypical**	DCIS within a papilloma	Suspicious calcifications	Discordant (calcifications not seen in CB)
5*	NBP	Benign	—	4mm focus of Invasive ductal carcinoma NST; no papillomas	5	Discordant
6	NBP	**Benign**	**DCIS/EPC**	Invasive ductal carcinoma with papillary features	4c	Discordant
7	BP	Benign	Benign	DCIS (cribriform and micropapillary types) with adjacent benign papilloma	4b	Discordant
8	NBP	Benign	Benign	DCIS (micropapillary, papillary,solid, cribriform, and comedo types) with adjacent benign papillomas	Suspicious calcifications	Discordant (calcifications not seen in CB)

Cases with NBP and BP disagreement are in bold.
NST indicates no special type.
*Slides not available for review by BP.

In the recent literature,[1,2] authors have questioned this practice, with some screening centers advocating for watchful waiting for benign papillary lesions. However, papillary lesions are very challenging to classify into benign or malignant categories on needle core biopsy specimens. The authors of this article, in a retrospective review, sought to explore the value of subspecialty signout for papillary lesions of the breast. In 162 cases with excisional follow-up they found that subspecialty trained breast pathologists had a significantly lower rate of change of diagnosis than generalist pathologists. And generalist pathologists overcalled atypia and malignancy on needle core biopsy, resulting in downgraded diagnoses on excisional specimens. Upgrade rates were not significantly different between the 2 groups. Discordant radiology was found to be a significant factor in lesions called benign on needle core and found to be atypical or malignant on excisional biopsy (Table 3). The authors stress the importance of radiology/pathology correlation.

B. A. Carter, MD, FRCPC

References

1. Ivan D, Selinko V, Sahin AA, Sneige N, Middleton LP. Accuracy of core needle biopsy diagnosis in assessing papillary breast lesions: histologic predictors of malignancy. *Mod Pathol.* 2004;17:165-171.
2. Jung SY, Kang HS, Kwon Y, et al. Risk factors for malignancy in benign papillomas of the breast on core needle biopsy. *World J Surg.* 2010;34:261-265.

Pathology of breast and ovarian cancers among *BRCA1* and *BRCA2* mutation carriers: results from the Consortium of Investigators of Modifiers of *BRCA1/2* (CIMBA)

Mavaddat N, for the Consortium of Investigators of Modifiers of *BRCA1/2* (Univ of Cambridge, UK; et al)

Cancer Epidemiol Biomarkers Prev 21:134-147, 2012

Background.—Previously, small studies have found that *BRCA1* and *BRCA2* breast tumors differ in their pathology. Analysis of larger datasets of mutation carriers should allow further tumor characterization.

Methods.—We used data from 4,325 *BRCA1* and 2,568 *BRCA2* mutation carriers to analyze the pathology of invasive breast, ovarian, and contralateral breast cancers.

Results.—There was strong evidence that the proportion of estrogen receptor (ER)-negative breast tumors decreased with age at diagnosis among *BRCA1* (p-$trend = 1.2 \times 10^{-5}$), but increased with age at diagnosis among *BRCA2*, carriers (p-$trend = 6.8 \times 10^{-6}$). The proportion of triple-negative tumors decreased with age at diagnosis in *BRCA1* carriers but increased with age at diagnosis of *BRCA2* carriers. In both *BRCA1* and *BRCA2* carriers, ER-negative tumors were of higher histologic grade than ER-positive tumors (Grade 3 vs. Grade 1; $p = 1.2 \times 10^{-13}$ for *BRCA1* and $p = 0.001$ for *BRCA2*). ER and progesterone receptor (PR) expression were independently associated with mutation carrier status (ER-positive odds ratio (OR) for *BRCA2* = 9.4, 95% CI: 7.0-12.6 and

PR-positive OR = 1.7, 95% CI: 1.3-2.3, under joint analysis). Lobular tumors were more likely to be *BRCA2*-related (OR for *BRCA2* = 3.3, 95% CI: 2.4-4.4; $p = 4.4 \times 10^{-14}$), and medullary tumors *BRCA1*-related (OR for *BRCA2* = 0.25, 95% CI: 0.18-0.35; $p = 2.3 \times 10^{-15}$). ER-status of the first breast cancer was predictive of ER-status of asynchronous contralateral breast cancer ($p = 0.0004$ for *BRCA1*; $p = 0.002$ for *BRCA2*). There were no significant differences in ovarian cancer morphology between *BRCA1* and *BRCA2* carriers (serous: 67%; mucinous: 1%; endometrioid: 12%; clear-cell: 2%).

Conclusions/Impact.—Pathologic characteristics of *BRCA1* and *BRCA2* tumors may be useful for improving risk prediction algorithms and informing clinical strategies for screening and prophylaxis (Tables 1 and 2).

▶ Pathologists who act as consultants to cancer centers are often asked to identify, via histologic analysis, patients with many types of hereditary cancers. The authors used the large database of the Consortium of Investigators of *BRCA1* and *BRCA2* (CIMBA), an international collaboration of 37 centers in 20 different countries, to define the histopathologic features of breast and ovarian cancers in these women (Tables 1 and 2). There are 4000 *BRCA1* carriers and 2000 *BRCA2* carriers included. Previous studies, especially on *BRCA2*, carriers have been limited by their small size. This study provides a more precise characterization of the pathology of *BRCA1* and *BRCA2* tumors. Although they largely confirmed the findings of previous investigators, now those findings can be confidently widely applied. Using this report's age-specific histopathologic data in risk

TABLE 1.—Pathology of Invasive Breast Cancer in *BRCA1* and *BRCA2* Mutation Carriers and Odds Ratios for Predicting *BRCA2* Mutation Carrier Status

	BRCA1 n (%)*	*BRCA2* n (%)*	OR[†]	95% CI	OR[‡]	95% CI
Morphology						
Invasive Ductal	2,387 (80)	1,515 (83)	1.00	-	-	-
Invasive Lobular	67 (2.2)	153 (8.4)	3.3	(2.4-4.4)	-	-
Medullary [§]	281 (9.4)	40 (2.2)	0.25	(0.18-0.35)	-	-
Other	258 (8.6)	116 (6.4)	0.81	(0.63-1.02)	-	-
ER, PR, HER2, TN						
ER-positive	625 (22)	1,475 (77)	11.4	9.8-13.2	10.0	8.2-12.1
PR-positive	539 (21)	1,084 (64)	6.8	5.8-7.9	5.5	4.5-6.6
HER2-positive	138 (10)	121 (13)	1.5	1.1-2.1	1.3	0.9-1.9
Non-TN (vs. TN)	411 (31)	700 (84)	11.0	8.8-13.8	9.0	6.8-11.8
Grade						
Grade 1	64 (3)	100 (7)	1.0	-	1.0	-
Grade 2	481 (20)	603 (43)	1.01	0.72-1.44	1.1	0.67-1.8
Grade 3	1,822 (77)	711 (50)	0.32	0.23-0.45	0.71	0.44-1.17

OR, odds ratio; CI, confidence interval; estrogen receptor, ER; progesterone receptor, PR; Human epidermal growth factor receptor 2, HER2; TN, triple negative

*Number of tumors (n) of each morphology type or tumor grade, or number of receptor positive tumors, and as percentage (%) of all *BRCA1* or *BRCA2*-related tumors.

[†]Odds ratios for *BRCA2* mutation carrier status, compared with *BRCA1* mutation carrier status, associated with tumor morphology, receptor positive tumors, or Grade 2 vs. Grade 1, and Grade 3 vs. Grade 1 tumors; analyses were adjusted for country and age at diagnosis.

[‡]analyses adjusted for country, age at diagnosis, and tumor grade; OR for analysis of grade, adjusted for country, age at diagnosis and ER status.

[§]includes atypical medullary carcinomas.

TABLE 2.—Distribution of Grade and Morphology of ER-Positive and ER-Negative Tumours in *BRCA1* and *BRCA2* Mutation Carriers

Type	BRCA1 Mutation Carriers			BRCA2 Mutation Carriers		
	ER-Negative n (%)*	ER-Positive n (%)	OR† (95% CI)	ER-Negative n (%)	ER-Positive n (%)	OR (95% CI)
Grade						
Grade 1	18 (1.2)	28 (6.9)	1.00	12 (4.3)	68 (7.4)	1.00
Grade 2	191 (13.1)	170 (41.6)	0.57 (0.31-1.05)	67 (24)	442 (48.2)	1.2 (0.60-2.4)
Grade 3	1246 (85.7)	210 (51.5)	0.12 (0.07-0.21)	200 (71.7)	408 (44.4)	0.33 (0.17-0.6)
Morphology						
Ductal	1,353 (58.8)	385 (86.5)	-	266 (85.8)	889 (84)	-
Lobular	16 (2.7)	21 (4.7)	-	15 (4.8)	110 (10.4)	-
Medullary §	141 (23.5)	17 (3.8)	-	14 (4.6)	13 (1.2)	-
Other	91 (15)	22 (5)	-	15 (4.8)	46 (4.3)	-

ER, estrogen receptor; OR, odds ratio; CI, confidence intervals.
*Number of tumors (n) of each grade or morphology type by ER-status as a percentage (%) of all ER-negative or ER-positive tumors where this information is available.
†OR and 95% CI are for ER-positive vs. ER-negative disease in Grade 2 or Grade 3 tumors are compared with Grade 1 tumors. These analyses were adjusted for age at diagnosis of breast cancer and country of origin.
§includes medullary and atypical medullary tumours.

prediction models will provide more accurate mutation carrier predictions. This can, in turn, influence screening and treatment strategies. Weaknesses of the study are the lack of central review of all pathology materials and the lack of a comparative control group. For further reading, please see Evans et al[1] and Tai et al.[2]

B. A. Carter, MD, FRCPC

References

1. Evans DG, Lalloo F, Cramer A, et al. Addition of pathology and biomarker information significantly improves the performance of the Manchester scoring system for BRCA1 and BRCA2 testing. *J Med Genet.* 2009;46:811-817.
2. Tai YC, Chen S, Parmigiani G, Klein AP. Incorporating tumor immunohistochemical markers in BRCA1 and BRCA2 carrier prediction. *Breast Cancer Res.* 2008; 10:401.

Fine Needle Aspiration Cytology in Symptomatic Breast Lesions: Still an Important Diagnostic Modality?

Smith MJ, Heffron CC, Rothwell JR, et al (Adelaide and Meath Incorporating the Natl Children's Hosp (AMNCH), Tallaght, Dublin, Ireland)
Breast J 18:103-110, 2012

The objective of this study was to make an assessment of the utility of fine needle aspiration cytology (FNAC), in a "one-stop" symptomatic breast triple assessment clinic. Controversy surrounds the optimal tissue biopsy methodology in the diagnosis of symptomatic breast cancer and the identification of benign disease. FNAC in the context of a Rapid Assessment Breast Clinic (RABC) allows the same day diagnosis and early treatment of breast cancer, with the immediate reassurance and discharge of those with benign disease. We analyzed prospective data accrued at a RABC, over a 4-year period from 2004 to 2007. All patients were triple assessed, with FNACs performed on site by two consultant cytopathologists. Investigations were reported immediately, and clinical data were captured via a database using compulsory data field entry. There were 4487 attendances at our RABC, with 1572 FNACs were performed. The positive predictive value of FNAC with a C5 cancer diagnosis was 100%, 95.6% for a C4 report, with a complete sensitivity of 94%. The full specificity of correctly identified benign lesions was 77.4%, with a false negative rate of 3.85%. This enabled 66% of patients attending the RABC to receive a same day diagnosis of benign disease and discharge. FNAC is highly accurate in the diagnosis of symptomatic breast cancer in an RABC. FNAC allows accurate diagnosis of benign disease and immediate discharge of the majority of patients. In this era, when a large majority of patients have benign disease, we believe that FNAC provides an equivalent, if not better, method of evaluation of patients in a triple assessment RABC (Table 2).

▶ This is an important article for those pathologists who practice cytopathology or perform fine-needle aspiration (FNA) biopsy. Most pathology practitioners

TABLE 2.—Histology of FNAC Samples

	C5	C4	C3	C2	C1	Total
			FNAC Classification			
Histology						
Malignant	190	23	8	9	7	232
Invasive	189	19	8	9	7	229
Noninvasive	1	4	0	0	0	2
Total benign	0	1	32	128	100	261
No histology	2	0	3	904	165	1079
Total FNAC results	192 (12.2%)	24 (1.5%)	43 (2.7%)	1041 (66.2%)	272 (17.3%)	1572

FNAC, fine needle aspiration cytology.

agree that the role of FNA in the assessment of breast cancer patients is controversial. Over the past few decades, there has also been a drop in the number of pathologists with expertise in this modality. Many centers have switched solely to tissue core biopsy. In a prospectively acquired cohort of 4487 symptomatic breast patients attending a triple assessment clinic, the authors sought to identify groups of patients that could benefit from this easy to carry out diagnostic tool. Its value was best in patients with benign disease. For those with malignant disease long-standing issues such as tumor grade, histologic subtype (invasive vs noninvasive) and biomarker status were not resolved. Although the FNA biopsy was satisfactorily accurate (Table 2), these patients still required tissue diagnosis and this is the major weakness of the study. The strengths of the study are the large cohort size and its prospective design.

B. A. Carter, MD, FRCPC

Semi-quantitative immunohistochemical assay *versus* onco*type* DX® qRT-PCR assay for estrogen and progesterone receptors: an independent quality assurance study
Kraus JA, Dabbs DJ, Beriwal S, et al (Dept of Pathology, Pittsburgh, PA; Magee-Womens Hosp of UPMC, Pittsburgh, PA)
Mod Pathol 25:869-876, 2012

Estrogen receptor (ER) status is a strong predictor of response to hormonal therapy in breast cancer patients. Presence of ER and level of expression have been shown to correlate with time to recurrence in patients undergoing therapy with tamoxifen or aromatase inhibitors. Risk reduction is also known to occur in ER-negative, progesterone receptor (PR)-positive patients treated with hormonal therapy. Since the 1990s, immunohistochemistry has been the primary method for assessing hormone receptor status. Recently, as a component of its onco*type* DX® assay, Genomic Health began reporting quantitative estrogen and PR results determined by quantitative reverse transcription polymerase chain reaction (qRT-PCR). As part of an ongoing quality assurance program at our institution, we reviewed 464 breast cancer cases evaluated by both immunohistochemistry and onco*type*

DX® assay for estrogen and PR. We found good correlation for ER status between both assays (98.9% concordance), with immunohistochemistry being slightly more sensitive. Concordance for PR was 94.2% between immunohistochemistry and qRT-PCR with immunohistochemistry again more sensitive than RT-PCR. The results also showed linear correlation between immunohistochemistry H-scores and qRT-PCR expression values for ER (correlation coefficient of 0.579), and PR (correlation coefficient of 0.685). Due to the higher sensitivity of hormone receptor immunohisto-chemistry and additional advantages (ie preservation of morphology, less expensive, faster, more convenient), we conclude immunohistochemistry is preferable to qRT-PCR for determination of estrogen and PR expression.

▶ Almost universally, patients with breast cancer have immunohistochemical (IHC) determination of estrogen receptor (ER) and progesterone receptor (PR) to determine response to therapeutic options. The past few years have seen the introduction and unprecedented rapid clinical adaptation of multigene profile assays for breast cancer prognostication.[1,2] These assays usually test for ER and PR expression as part of the profile. In an era of laboratory efficiencies, some laboratories are being asked to consider stopping IHC staining for ER and PR. Although the concordance rate in this study is acceptably high for ER stain-ing, it drops for PR staining and, as in many previously published reports, IHC stains were found more sensitive that reverse transcription-polymerase chain reaction. Kraus wisely discusses the contamination disadvantage of quantitative reverse transcription-polymerase chain reaction which requires tissue microdis-section and grinding. In the 1990s, pathologists moved from biochemical assess-ment of hormone receptors for this very reason. Once again normal ductal breast tissue, fibroadipose tissue, inflammatory cells, biopsy cavities, and in situ carci-noma may in fact be tested and not the invasive carcinoma. Hormone receptor testing for breast cancer patients is best determined by immunohistochemistry.

B. A. Carter, MD, FRCPC

References

1. O'Connor SM, Beriwal S, Dabbs DJ, Bhargava R. Concordance between semi-quantitative immunohistochemical assay and oncotype DX RT-PCR assay for estrogen and progesterone receptors. *Appl Immunohistochem Mol Morphol.* 2010;18:268-272.
2. Flanagan MB, Dabbs DJ, Brufsky AM, Beriwal S, Bhargava R. Histopathologic variables predict Oncotype DX recurrence score. *Mod Pathol.* 2008;21: 1255-1261.

3 Gastrointestinal System

Objective Quantification of the Ki67 Proliferative Index in Neuroendocrine Tumors of the Gastroenteropancreatic System: A Comparison of Digital Image Analysis With Manual Methods

Tang LH, Gonen M, Hedvat C, et al (Memorial Sloan-Kettering Cancer Ctr, NY; et al)

Am J Surg Pathol 2012 [Epub ahead of print]

Pathologic grading for prognostic stratification of neuroendocrine tumors (NETs) is critical but presents a challenging interpretive dilemma. Tumor cell proliferative rate is an important factor in the determination of prognosis, and immunohistochemical analysis with Ki67 is becoming more widely used to quantify the proliferative rate. However, Ki67 assessment has limitations due to lack of uniformity and consistency in quantification. These limitations are accentuated in well-differentiated NETs, as differences in the range of 1% to 5% can alter tumor grade, with potential implications for treatment. We therefore performed a concordance study to assess different Ki67 quantification techniques including: (a) digital image analysis (DIA); (b) manual counting (MC) of > 2000 cells; and (c) "eyeballed" estimate (EE) of labeling percentage by pathologists (n = 18), including individuals experienced in evaluating Ki67 labeling as well as others who had little prior experience assessing Ki67 percentages. Forty-five Ki67 images were selected and analyzed using the 3 methods. On the basis of the recommendations of the World health Organization (WHO) for grading NETs, MC of 2000 cells was used as the "gold standard" reference against which the other techniques were compared. Three images were presented twice, the second being inverted, to assess intraobserver consistency. Statistical analyses were performed to evaluate: (a) the concordance between methods; (b) intraobserver and interobserver consistency; and (c) correlation of NET grades on the basis of Ki67 scores by EE versus the gold standard. Agreement between scores was assessed by intraclass correlation (ICC). DIA and MC were highly concordant (ICC = 0.98). The ICC between DIA and the mean EE of all observers was 0.88. However, there was discordance among individual observers on all cases quantified by EE (ICC = 0.13). The ICC for intraobserver consistency was 0.39 = 0.26. With Ki67 in the ranges of < 1%, 2% to 3%, and > 20%, the mean of Ki67 by EE was, respectively, 93% = 2%, 55% = 7%, and 55% = 15% correct against the gold standard. The κ statistics for EE exhibited low agreement (κ = 0.24; 95% confidence interval, 0.23-0.25) for all WHO NET grades. Incorrect assessment by EE resulted in upgrading of all WHO G1 group tumors (n = 14); in the WHO G2 group, downgrading of 41% cases occurred (n = 11) when Ki67 was < 5% (by DIA or MC), and upgrading of 59% cases occurred (n = 16) when Ki67 was > 5%. We conclude that DIA and MC are the acceptable standards for Ki67 assessment. Given the inherent discordance in determining the grade, the use of an approximate EE of the Ki67-labeling index requires critical reevaluation, especially for NETs with a labeling index straddling the cut-points between grades. Consequently, determination of therapeutic strategies should be guided by an amalgamation of clinicopathologic characteristics, including but not limited to the Ki67 index.

▶ Following the European Neuroendocrine Tumor Society (ENETS) recommendation for histologic grading of gastroenteropancreatic neuroendocrine tumors (GEP-NETs) the World Health Organization (WHO) issued the classification of GEP-NETs in 2010.

The classification is based primarily on mitotic activity or the Ki67 proliferative index expressed as the percentage of tumor cells showing nuclear immunoreactivity.

The well-differentiated GEP-NETs are divided in 2 grades: G1 or low grade (mitoses < 2/10 HPF or $2/mm^2$, or Ki67 < 3%) and G2 or intermediate grade (mitoses of 2 to 20/10/HPF, or Ki67 labeling index of 3% to 20%).

It is apparent that standardization and reproducibility can be a problem in separating (eg, 2.99% from 3% Ki67 labeling) and distinguish grade 1 from grade 2 GEP-NETs.

The ENETS/WHO 2 groups suggest counting a minimum of 500 to 2000 tumor cells manually. In reality, an eyeball estimate is much more common in practice.

The study is relevant because it compares the various methods available to the pathologists and indicates which are concordant and reproducible against the gold standard (the manual count of 2000 cells).

Eyeball estimate proves to be poorly reproducible especially in the cutoff values that allow distinction between grade 1 and grade 2 (see Fig 5 in the original article).

Although Ki67 use as an indication of proliferative rate is important, we do not know if it overrides prognostic parameters such as mitotic rates or vascular invasion. To use KI67 properly in studies and understand its value, the study indicates that eyeball estimates in GEP-NETs should likely not be relied on, especially in the very subtle differences in labeling rate between G1 and G2 grades.

G. De Petris, MD

Gastric Adenocarcinoma and Proximal Polyposis of the Stomach (GAPPS): A New Autosomal Dominant Syndrome
Worthley DL, Phillips KD, Wayte N, et al (Columbia Univ, NY; SA Clinical Genetics Service, South Australia, Australia; Univ of Queensland, Australia; et al)
Gut 61:774-779, 2012

Objective.—The purpose of this study was the clinical and pathological characterisation of a new autosomal dominant gastric polyposis syndrome, gastric adenocarcinoma and proximal polyposis of the stomach (GAPPS).

Methods.—Case series were examined, documenting GAPPS in three families from Australia, the USA and Canada. The affected families were identified through referral to centralised clinical genetics centres.

Results.—The report identifies the clinical and pathological features of this syndrome, including the predominant dysplastic fundic gland polyp histology, the exclusive involvement of the gastric body and fundus, the apparent inverse association with current *Helicobacter pylori* infection and the autosomal dominant mode of inheritance.

Conclusions.—GAPPS is a unique gastric polyposis syndrome with a significant risk of gastric adenocarcinoma. It is characterised by the autosomal dominant transmission of fundic gland polyposis, including areas of dysplasia or intestinal-type gastric adenocarcinoma, restricted to the proximal stomach, and with no evidence of colorectal or duodenal polyposis or other heritable gastrointestinal cancer syndromes.

▶ The presence of multiple fundic polyps elicits the differential diagnosis of multiple carcinoids, fundic gland polyps (FGPs) associated with proton pump inhibitors, FGPs associated with familial adenomatous polyposis (FAP), and that of other hereditary and nonhereditary polyposis syndromes. Sporadic FGPs have a very low rate of dysplasia. Syndromic ones are capable of progression to adenoma and adenocarcinoma, an event that remains, however, distinctly unusual.

The novel observation of a hereditary gastric polyposis from 3 families (in the United States, Australia, and Canada) with a distinct risk of adenocarcinoma arising from dysplastic fundic gland polyps will complicate the approach to the patients with multiple FGPs. No distinctive histopathological features were found beside the presence of dysplasia or malignancy in the affected patients or in family members. For the time being, we will have to rely on the clinical criteria introduced by the authors, be aware of this new entity, and collect additional families to find its genetic basis.

G. De Petris, MD

Management of precancerous conditions and lesions in the stomach (MAPS): guideline from the European Society of Gastrointestinal Endoscopy (ESGE), European Helicobacter Study Group (EHSG), European Society of Pathology (ESP), and the Sociedade Portuguesa de Endoscopia Digestiva (SPED)
Dinis-Ribeiro M, on behalf of MAPS Participants (Portuguese Oncology Inst of Porto, Portugal; et al)
Virchows Arch 460:19-46, 2012

Atrophic gastritis, intestinal metaplasia, and epithelial dysplasia of the stomach are common and are associated with an increased risk for gastric cancer. In the absence of guidelines, there is wide disparity in the management of patients with these premalignant conditions. The European Society of Gastrointestinal Endoscopy, the European Helicobacter Study Group, the European Society of Pathology, and the Sociedade Portuguesa de Endoscopia Digestiva have therefore combined efforts to develop evidence-based guidelines on the management of patients with precancerous conditions and lesions of the stomach. A multidisciplinary group of 63 experts from 24 countries developed these recommendations by means of repeat online voting and a meeting in June 2011 in Porto, Portugal. The recommendations emphasize the increased cancer risk in patients with gastric atrophy and metaplasia and the need for adequate staging in the case of high-grade dysplasia, and they focus on treatment and surveillance indications and methods.

▶ There is a lack of surveillance and management guidelines for precancerous conditions and lesions in the stomach, such as atrophy, intestinal metaplasia, and dysplasia. However, a strong body of evidence has shown that these conditions predispose patients to carcinoma. This multidisciplinary group of experts has created a consensus guideline for surveillance based on review of the literature and a voting scheme.

This guideline is welcome and should be required reading for all pathologists signing out gastric biopsies—not just those who consider themselves as gastrointestinal pathologists or subspecialists. Although we in the United States do not typically stage atrophy or routinely use the OLGA (operative link for gastritis assessment) or OLGIM (operative link for gastric intestinal metaplasia) systems in daily practice, the most basic concepts of gastritis are summarized nicely in this article and should be recognized by the general pathologist.

Gastritis has been known by variable nomenclature, but standard terms are used within this article and, for those who are just familiarizing themselves with gastritis, this article is a gold mine and a great place to get started with standardization of terminology. Recommendations are also made regarding standard biopsy protocols, which are in line with previous recommendations (ie, Updated Sydney System), which can be useful to clinicians. This article represents a wonderful summary and can be used as a tool to educate pathology colleagues and clinicians and get them on board with shared terminology and an understanding of gastritis beyond simply chronic gastritis or chronic inflammation.

D. Lam-Himlin, MD

Ampullary Region Carcinomas: Definition and Site Specific Classification With Delineation of Four Clinicopathologically and Prognostically Distinct Subsets in an Analysis of 249 Cases
Adsay V, Ohike N, Tajiri T, et al (Emory Univ School of Medicine, Atlanta, GA; Showa Univ School of Medicine, Tokyo, Japan; et al)
Am J Surg Pathol 36:1592-1608, 2012

Ampullary (AMP) carcinomas comprise a heterogenous group of cancers lacking adequate subcategorization. In the present study, 249 strictly defined primary AMP carcinomas (ACs) identified in 1469 malignant pancreatoduodenectomy specimens were analyzed for defining features. Gross and microscopic findings were used to determine tumor epicenter and extent of preinvasive component. ACs were classified into 4 distinct subtypes based on location: (1) *Intra-AMP* (25%): Invasive carcinomas arising in intra-ampullary papillary-tubular neoplasms with zero to minimal, duodenal surface involvement (< 25% of the tumor). These tumors were more commonly found in men, they had a relatively large overall size (mean, 2.9 cm) but had smaller invasive component (mean, 1.5 cm), and were predominantly of a lower TNM stage (85%, T1/2; and 72% N0). They carried the best prognosis among the 4 groups (3-y survival, 73%). (2) *AMP-ductal* (15%): These were tumors forming constrictive, sclerotic, plaque-like thickening of the walls of the common bile duct and/or pancreatic duct resulting in mucosa-covered, button-like elevations of the papilla into the duodenal lumen. There was no significant exophytic (preinvasive) growth. These were the smallest tumors (mean overall size, 1.9 cm; mean invasion size 1.7 cm), but carried the worst prognosis (3-y survival, 41%), presumably due to the pancreatobiliary histology/origin (in 86%); however, even this group had significantly better prognosis when compared with 113 ordinary pancreatic ductal adenocarcinomas (3 y, 11%; $P < 0.0001$). (3) *Peri-AMP-duodenal* (5%): Massive exophytic, ulcerofungating tumors growing into the duodenal lumen and eccentrically encasing the ampullary orifice with only minimal intra-ampullary luminal involvement. These were mostly of intestinal phenotype (75%) and some had mucinous features. Although these tumors were the largest (mean overall size 4.7 cm; and mean invasion size 3.4 cm), and had the highest incidence of lymph node metastasis (50%), they carried an intermediate prognosis (3-y survival, 69%) to that seen among a group of 55 nonampullary duodenal carcinoma controls. (4) *AC—not otherwise specified* (*"papilla of Vater"*; 55%): Ulcero-nodular tumors located at the papilla of Vater, which do not show the specific characteristics identified among the other 3 subtypes. In conclusion, ACs comprise 4 clinicopathologic subtypes that are prognostically distinct (Fig 7).

▶ Adsay and colleagues have conducted perhaps one of the most necessary and important studies in gastrointestinal pathology this year. Ampullary cancers have been poorly defined in the past, and even definitive resources, such as the College of American Pathologists (CAP) synoptic reporting protocol, have had internal variations on the exact definition. Carcinomas arising in this area have been confusing for pathologists to properly categorize, and recognition of differing prognoses for this broad category of cancers has not been addressed adequately. For example, although the CAP recognizes 3 categories of ampulla of Vater cancers, the AJCC (American Joint Cancer Committee/Union Internationale Contre le Cancer) staging manual regards only the intra-ampullary category as an ampullary cancer.

This study not only clearly defines the 4 categories of ampullary cancer, but it does so in a manner that is easily and intuitively understood. The authors categorize the lesions based on their anatomic location and gross appearance. Their simple illustrations (Fig 7) make categorization surprisingly straightforward, while their histologic examples of each tumor category also emphasize the morphologic differences. As one might expect, given the differing location, gross morphology, and microscopic appearance of these cancers, each category demonstrates a separate clinicopathologic subtype with distinct prognostic implications.

INTRA-AMP : 25%

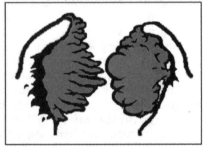

AMP-DUCTAL : 15%

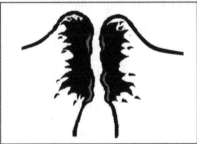

PERIAMP-DUODENAL : 5%

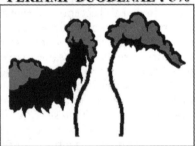

AMP-NOS : 55%

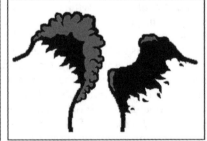

FIGURE 7.—Ampullary region carcinomas comprise 4 distinct types discernible by correlation of gross and microscopic findings and by determining the distribution of the preinvasive (gray colored) and invasive components (black colored) of the lesion whether they show significant preinvasive component within the ampullary channel (INTRA-AMP); or forming infiltrative tumors on the walls of the distal ends of the CBD or pancreatic duct (AMP-DUCTAL); or growing predominantly on the duodenal surfaces with significant "adenoma" component (PERIAMP-DUODENAL); or located at the edge of the papilla of Vater (AMPNOS). (Reprinted from Adsay V, Ohike N, Tajiri T, et al. Ampullary region carcinomas: definition and site specific classification with delineation of four clinicopathologically and prognostically distinct subsets in an analysis of 249 cases. *Am J Surg Pathol.* 2012;36:1592-1608, with permission from Lippincott Williams & Wilkins.)

Other authors have addressed some of these issues in previous studies, but this large series is worth keeping at arm's length and referencing while working at both the gross station and the microscope. For those pathologists who have pathologists' assistants gross in their specimens, it is worthwhile to review the anatomy and categories presented in this article together. More studies showing additional clinicopathologic features of each category are needed and are sure to follow. In time, with additional strong studies such as this, the AJCC staging manual and the CAP synoptic reporting protocol will become concordant on their definitions, staging, and prognoses.

D. Lam-Himlin, MD

Endoscopic Surveillance of Patients With Hereditary Diffuse Gastric Cancer: Biopsy Recommendations After Topographic Distribution of Cancer Foci in a Series of 10 CDH1-mutated Gastrectomies

Fujita H, Lennerz JKM, Chung DC, et al (Massachusetts General Hosp and Harvard Med School, Boston)
Am J Surg Pathol 36:1709-1717, 2012

The management of hereditary diffuse-type gastric cancer revolves around surveillance biopsies and the timing of prophylactic gastrectomy. In the absence of a validated surveillance biopsy protocol, we modeled bioptic diagnostic yield on the basis of the topographic distribution of cancer foci in a series of 10 gastrectomies in *CDH1*-mutation carriers. Complete histologic examination was performed in all cases, and 1817 slides were evaluated for the presence of in situ, intramucosal, or submucosal diffuse-type carcinoma. Detailed maps determined the density of cancer foci. On the basis of the number of sampled glands per biopsy in routine surveillance preoperative endoscopy, we estimated the theoretical number of biopsies necessary for a 90% rate of detection of neoplastic foci, and we evaluated this number, taking into account the regional distribution of these foci. A total of 96 m of gastric mucosa with $\sim 1\,193\,453$ gastric glands yielded 302 cancer foci [in situ ($n = 89$), intramucosal ($n = 209$), and submucosal ($n = 4$)] spanning the width of a total of 1820 glands (8 to 1205 per case; average 182 ± 115). On the basis of the number of glands per stomach and the average number of glands sampled during surveillance biopsy (28.7 ± 1.7; range, 0 to 79; $n = 112$), the theoretical number of biopsies necessary to capture at least 1 cancer focus was estimated to be 1768 (range, 50 to 5832) to assure a 90% detection rate. Mapping of cancer foci showed the highest density in the anterior proximal fundus (37%) and cardia/proximal fundus (27%). Our results argue for the incorporation of cancer focus distribution into any biopsy protocol, although detection is likely to remain extremely low, and they call into question the validity of endoscopic surveillance.

▶ The autosomal dominant *CDH1* gene germline mutation resulting in hereditary diffuse gastric cancer (HDGC) results in early and diffuse-type gastric cancer. Although endoscopic surveillance has been the mainstay of early detection, no studies confirm their utility. This study shows that to assure a 90% detection rate of at least 1 cancer focus, a minimum of 1768 biopsies are necessary. Clearly, this number is impractical for endoscopists and pathologists alike, and it brings into question the usefulness of endoscopic surveillance biopsies.

This study does not close the door on surveillance biopsies, particularly in very young patients, but it does bring into question the utility of the practice in patients who are considering long-term surveillance over gastrectomy. In addition, as optical contrast techniques improve, the role of endoscopic surveillance will likely be bolstered, but further study is required in this area.

The authors also found that the early foci of diffuse gastric cancer have a predilection for the proximal stomach, particularly the oxyntic mucosa. This finding is important for 3 reasons: (1) This information can be used to guide clinicians who perform surveillance biopsies, as additional sampling of the cardia and proximal fundus would be of interest and will likely have a higher yield; (2) this finding confirms the observation that HDGC may have a precursor lesion arising from cells of the oxyntic mucosa—another clue to the biology of these deadly tumors; and (3) the data suggest that pathology sampling of propylactic gastrectomy specimens should concentrate on extensive samples of the gastric cardio-oxyntic mucosa, as 74% of tumor foci are found in these areas.

D. Lam-Himlin, MD

Serrated Lesions of the Colorectum: Review and Recommendations From an Expert Panel
Rex DK, Ahnen DJ, Baron JA, et al (Indiana Univ, Indianapolis; Univ of Colorado School of Medicine, Denver; Univ of North Carolina at Chapel Hill; et al)
Am J Gastroenterol 107:1315-1329, 2012

Serrated lesions of the colorectum are the precursors of perhaps one-third of colorectal cancers (CRCs). Cancers arising in serrated lesions are usually in the proximal colon, and account for a disproportionate fraction of cancer identified after colonoscopy. We sought to provide guidance for the clinical management of serrated colorectal lesions based on current evidence and expert opinion regarding definitions, classification, and significance of serrated lesions. A consensus conference was held over 2 days reviewing the topic of serrated lesions from the perspectives of histology, molecular biology, epidemiology, clinical aspects, and serrated polyposis. Serrated lesions should be classified pathologically according to the World Health Organization criteria as hyperplastic polyp, sessile serrated adenoma/polyp (SSA/P) with or without cytological dysplasia, or traditional serrated adenoma (TSA). SSA/P and TSA are premalignant lesions, but SSA/P is the principal serrated precursor of CRCs. Serrated lesions have a distinct endoscopic appearance, and several lines of evidence suggest that on average they are more difficult to detect than conventional adenomatous polyps. Effective colonoscopy requires an endoscopist trained in the endoscopic appearance of serrated lesions. We recommend that all serrated lesions proximal to the sigmoid colon and all serrated lesions in the rectosigmoid > 5 mm in size, be completely removed. Recommendations are made for post-polypectomy surveillance of serrated lesions and for surveillance of serrated polyposis patients and their relatives (Table 2).

▶ This article should be considered required reading by both pathologists and clinicians alike. In addition to providing a brief history and summary of the dilemmas surrounding these neoplasms, this group of experts in the field offer guidelines for the diagnosis and surveillance of serrated lesions (Table 2). Although the World Health Organization set the standard for terminology in 2010,[1] this article provides

TABLE 2.—Key Conclusions and Recommendations of the Consensus Group[a]

Pathology

1   Serrated lesions of the colorectum should be classified histologically as hyperplastic polyp (HP), sessile serrated adenoma/polyp (SSA/P) with or without cytologic dysplasia, or traditional serrated adenoma (TSA). Exceptions and subcategories are discussed in the text. Clinicians and pathologists within institutions should work collaboratively to achieve a common usage and understanding of terminology of serrated lesions.

2   SSA/P and TSA are pre-cancerous lesions. SSA/P is the principal precursor of hypermethylated colorectal cancers (cancers with the CpG island methylator phenotype). This pathway occurs primarily in the proximal colon.

3   SSA/P is distinguished from HP pathologically by findings of crypt distortion, particularly in the crypt base, in SSA/P. We recommend that a single unequivocal architecturally distorted, dilated, and/or horizontally branched crypt, particularly if it is associated with inverted maturation, is sufficient for a diagnosis of SSA/P. Most large serrated lesions in the proximal colon are SSA/Ps.

4   SSA/P with cytological dysplasia is a more advanced lesion in the progression to cancer compared with SSA/P without cytological dysplasia.

Endoscopy

5   SSA/P and hyperplastic polyps in the proximal colon have a distinct endoscopic appearance, which includes a "mucus cap", color usually similar to normal mucosa, and indistinct edges. All colonoscopists should be able to recognize serrated lesions.

6   Detection of proximal colon serrated lesions by individual endoscopists is highly correlated with adenoma detection. Pending development of specific detection targets for proximal colon serrated lesions, endoscopists should measure their adenoma detection rates as a check on adequate detection of serrated lesions.

7   All serrated lesions proximal to the sigmoid colon should be fully resected during colonoscopy. All serrated lesions in the rectosigmoid colon >5 mm in size should be fully resected.

Surveillance

8   Serrated polyposis is defined by the World Health Organization (see text for details). Patients with serrated polyposis require close endoscopic follow up with control of polyp burden by endoscopy or by surgical resection if the number, size, or location of serrated polyps precludes endoscopic resection or if a cancer is diagnosed.

9   First degree relatives of patients with SPS should undergo colonoscopy at age 40 or 10 years before the age at diagnosis of SPS. Colonoscopy should be at 5-year intervals or more often if polyps are found.

10   There are few longitudinal observational studies after removal of serrated lesions on which recommendations for postpolypectomy surveillance can be based. Recommendations are mostly based on features of serrated lesions for which there is evidence of an association with increased risk of cancer or advanced neoplasms, including proximal colon location, large size, increasing number, and histological features, including SSA/P histology (see text and Table 5, Figure 7 for details).

SPS, Serrated polyposis syndrome.
[a]Clinical recommendations made here are considered strong by the panel, but are supported by low quality or very low quality evidence, and are likely to change when higher quality evidence becomes available.

practical sign-out guidance for pathologists, including a most useful recommendation of a new "serrated polyp, unclassified" category.

The interval surveillance recommendations for clinicians represent consensus opinion by a group of experts in the field. However, this is based on low-quality or very low-quality evidence and personal experience. As higher quality evidence becomes available through longitudinal studies, these guidelines are likely to evolve. In addition, readers should be apprised that the US Multi-Society Task Force updated its guidelines for surveillance and screening intervals in individuals with baseline average risk in September 2012,[2] only a few months after the release of the above expert consensus recommendation. There are variations in recommendations between the two documents, but both offer improved guidance for surveillance of patients with completely excised serrated polyps and recommendations to follow the shortest appropriate surveillance interval for patients with multiple polyps.

This article is an outstanding resource for pathologists in understanding the current terminology and molecular underpinnings of serrated neoplasms as well as the current concepts surrounding surveillance strategies. Despite the lack of high-quality evidence, this article can be used as an effective tool to aid pathologists within a department to improve uniformity in sign-outs; although, admittedly, there remains significant interobserver variability in these lesions, even among experts. Clinicians, too, can be engaged via this article such that all physicians who are involved in a patient's care are on the same page, and up to date, on this rapidly evolving topic.

D. Lam-Himlin, MD

References

1. Snover D, Ahnen DJ, Burt RW, et al. Serrated polyps of the colon and rectum and serrated ("hyperplastic") polyposis. In: Bozman FT, Carneiro F, Hruban RH, et al, eds. *WHO Classification of Tumours Pathology and genetics Tumours of the digestive system.* 4th edition. Berlin: Springer-Verlag; 2010.
2. Leiberman DA, Rex DK, Winawer SJ, Glardiello FM, Johnson DA, Levin TR; United States Multi-society Task Force on Colorectal Cancer. Guidelines for Colonoscopy surveillance after screening and polypectomy: a consensus updated by the US Multi-Society Task Force on Colorectal Cancer. *Gasteroenterology.* 2012 Sep; 3(143):844-57. http://dx.doi.org/10.1053/j.gastro.2012.06.001. Epub 2012 Jul 13. Review. PubMed PMID: 22763141.

MicroRNA Expression Patterns in Indeterminate Inflammatory Bowel Disease

Lin J, Cao Q, Zhang J, et al (Indiana Univ School of Medicine, Indianapolis; Univ of Michigan, Ann Arbor; et al)
Mod Pathol 1-7, 2012

A diagnosis of idiopathic inflammatory bowel disease requires synthesis of clinical, radiographic, endoscopic, surgical, and histologic data. While most cases of inflammatory bowel disease can be specifically classified as either ulcerative colitis or Crohn's disease, 5—10% of patients have equivocal features placing them into the indeterminate colitis category. This study examines whether microRNA biomarkers assist in the classification of classically diagnosed indeterminate inflammatory bowel disease. Fresh frozen colonic mucosa from the distal-most part of the colectomy from 53 patients was used (16 indeterminate colitis, 14 Crohn's disease, 12 ulcerative colitis, and 11 diverticular disease controls). Total RNA extraction and quantitative reverse-transcription-PCR was performed using five pairs of microRNA primers (miR-19b, miR-23b, miR-106a, miR-191, and miR-629). Analysis of variance was performed assessing differences among the groups. A significant difference in expressions of miR-19b, miR-106a, and miR-629 was detected between ulcerative colitis and Crohn's disease groups ($P < 0.05$). The average expression level of all five microRNAs was statistically different between indeterminate colitis and Crohn's disease groups ($P < 0.05$); no significant difference was present between indeterminate and ulcerative colitis groups. Among the 16 indeterminate colitis patients, 15 showed ulcerative colitis-like and one Crohn's disease-like microRNA pattern. MicroRNA expression patterns in indeterminate colitis are far more similar to those of ulcerative colitis than Crohn's disease. MicroRNA expression patterns of indeterminate colitis provide molecular evidence indicating that most cases are probably ulcerative colitis—similar to the data from long-term clinical follow-up studies. Validation of microRNA results by additional long-term outcome data is needed, but the data presented show promise for improved classification of indeterminate inflammatory bowel disease.

▶ The frequency of indeterminate colitis (IC) in patients clearly affected by inflammatory bowel disease has remained around 10% in the past few decades, unchanged by the introduction of newer diagnostic techniques. We do not know if IC is an independent disease or a not yet fully manifested ulcerative colitis (UC) or Crohn disease (CD) because of the lack of a positive identifier of IC. The importance of IC is clear when the gold standard therapy of UC (procto-colectomy with ileal pouch-anal anastomosis [IPAA]) is considered. Patients with IC (complication rate after IPAA: 20%) do not do as well as patients with UC (complication rate: 10%); they do better, however, than patients with CD (complication rate: 30% to 45%)[1] in which IPAA is generally contraindicated. The results regarding the natural history and outcomes of IC patients undergoing IPAA, however, are greatly variable due to the variety of the defining criteria of IC. Several studies have suggested a closer similitude of IC to UC.[1] When the diagnosis of IC was changed to CD and these patients were removed from analysis, it appeared that the remainders showed behaviors identical to UC. Other studies[2] supported the notion that most patients with IC likely have UC. The current study is interesting because it employs the colonic mucosa biopsies (easily obtainable and capable of providing information before resection) for a novel test with an attempt to compare microRNA of IC in well-defined IC patients and controls consisting of UC, CD, and diverticulosis.

It is interesting to see how previous clinical follow-up studies find confirmation in this novel methodology: Most of the IC patients display expression patterns of UC rather than CD. If confirmed with follow-up studies, the possibility of determining the IC characteristics before resection would prove quite helpful as a prognostic marker.

G. De Petris, MD

References

1. Yu CS, Pemberton JH, Larson D. Ileal pouch-anal anastomosis in patients with indeterminate colitis: long-term results. *Dis Colon Rectum.* 2000;43:1487-1496.
2. Gramlich T, Delaney CP, Lynch AC, Remzi FH, Fazio VW. Pathological subgroups may predict complications but not late failure after ileal pouch-anal anastomosis for indeterminate colitis. *Colorectal Dis.* 2003;5:315-319.

Unusual DNA Mismatch Repair–Deficient Tumors in Lynch Syndrome: a Report of New Cases and Review of the Literature
Karamurzin Y, Zeng Z, Stadler ZK, et al (Memorial Sloan-Kettering Cancer Ctr, NY; et al)
Hum Pathol 43:1677-1687, 2012

Immunohistochemical detection of DNA mismatch repair proteins and polymerase chain reaction detection of microsatellite instability have enhanced the recognition of mismatch repair–deficient neoplasms in patients with Lynch syndrome and, consequently, led to the identification of tumors that have not been included in the currently known Lynch syndrome tumor spectrum. Here, we report 4 such unusual tumors. Three of the 4, a peritoneal mesothelioma, a pancreatic acinar cell carcinoma, and a pancreatic well-differentiated neuroendocrine tumor, represented tumor types that, to the best of our knowledge, have not been previously reported in Lynch syndrome. The fourth tumor was an adrenocortical carcinoma, which has rarely been reported previously in Lynch syndrome. Three of our 4 patients carried a pathogenic germ-line mutation in a mismatch repair gene. The unusual tumor in each of the 3 patients showed loss of the mismatch repair protein corresponding to the mutation. The fourth patient did not have mutation information but had a history of colonic and endometrial carcinomas; both lacked MSH2 and MSH6 proteins. Interestingly, none of the 4 unusual tumors revealed microsatellite instability on polymerase chain reaction testing, whereas an appendiceal carcinoma from 1 of the study patients who was tested simultaneously did. The recognition of such tumors expands the repertoire of usable test samples for the workup of high-risk families. As yet, however, there are no data to support the inclusion of these tumors into general screening guidelines for detecting Lynch syndrome, nor are there data to warrant surveillance for these tumors in patients with Lynch syndrome (Fig 1, Table 1).

▶ Lynch syndrome (LS) patients are at risk of colon, uterus, ovary, stomach, small intestine, hepatobiliary, sebaceous, and urothelial tumors. These tumors

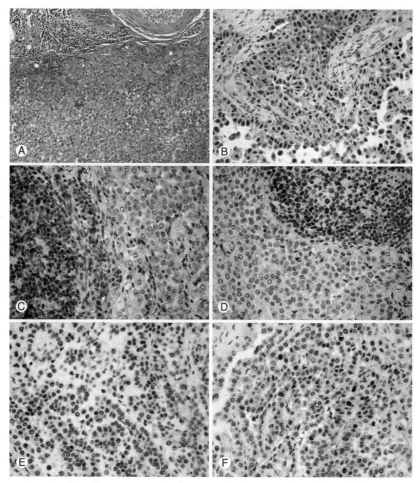

FIGURE 1.—A malignant mesothelioma showing an epithelioid morphology on hematoxylin and eosin stain (A) and positive expression of calretinin by IHC (B). Further immunohistochemical stains show the absence of nuclear staining for MLH1 (C) and PMS2 (D) but the presence of nuclear staining for MSH2 (E) and MSH6 (F) in the tumor. Note in parts C and D the positive nuclear staining in benign lymphoid cells, which serves as positive internal control. (Reprinted from Karamurzin Y, Zeng Z, Stadler ZK, et al. Unusual DNA mismatch repair—deficient tumors in Lynch syndrome: a report of new cases and review of the literature. *Hum Pathol.* 2012;43:1677-1687, Copyright 2012, with permission from Elsevier.)

have specific morphological and molecular phenotypes. For example, they display medullary growth pattern, intratumoral lymphocytes, high-frequency microsatellite instability (MSI), and loss of mismatch repair (MMR) genes proteins after immunostains (IHC). The recent use of screening tests for LS based on IHC and MSI has detected "atypical" tumor sites in LS patients, such as breast, prostate, lung, thyroid, adrenal cortex, and sarcomas and melanoma (Table 1). The authors add 4 additional unusual epithelial tumors with germline mutations of MMR (in 3 of the 4 tumors) but no MSI. The tumors were mesothelioma (depicted in Fig 1 showing loss of the 2 MMRs: MLH1 and PMS2 in

TABLE 1.—Unusual DNA MMR-Deficient Tumors in Patients with LS From Previous Reports and Current Study

Reference	Sex	Age (y)	Diagnosis	Unusual Tumor Lost Expression by IHC	MSI Status	Germ-Line Mutation
Multiple [17]	NA	NA	Breast carcinoma	Variable	MSI-H	Variable
Berends et al [21]	F	NA	Adrenal cortical carcinoma	None	MSS	MSH2
Sijmons et al [12]	M	45	MFH, leg	MSH2	MSI-H	MSH2
Soravia et al [18]	M	61	Prostate carcinoma	MSH2	MSI-H	MLH1
Broaddus et al [20]	M	34	Adrenal cortical carcinoma	MSH2	MSS	MSH2
	F	39	Anaplastic carcinoma of thyroid	MSH2	MSI-L	MSH2
Ponti et al [16]	M	43	Malignant melanoma	MSH2	MSI-H	MSH2
Clyne et al [13], Yu et al [14]	M	36	Leiomyosarcoma, thigh	MLH1	MSI-H	MLH1
Nilbert et al [15]	M	38	Liposarcoma, thigh	MSH2/MSH6	NA	MSH2
	M	32	Gliosarcoma, brain	MSH2/MSH6	NA	MSH2
	F	44	Leiomyosarcoma, uterus	MSH2/MSH6	MSI-H	NA
Nolan et al [19]	M	64	Lung adenocarcinoma	MSH2	MSI-H	MSH2
Petersen et al [24]	M	41	Pancreatic serous cystadenoma	MLH1	MSI-H	MLH1
Brieger et al [11]	M	43	MFH, left psoas muscle	MSH2	MSI-H	MSH2 c.2038C≥T
	M	50	MFH, Right upper leg	MSH2	MSI-H	MSH2 c.942 ± 3A ≥ T
Medina-Arana et al [22]	F	60	Adrenal cortical carcinoma	MSH2	MSS	MSH2
Our cases						
1	M	56	Peritoneal mesothelioma	MLH1/PMS2	MSS	MLH1*1456insT
2	F	65	Acinar cell carcinoma of pancreas	MSH6	MSS	MSH6*1312insA
3	F	50	Pancreatic endocrine neoplasm	MSH2/MSH6	MSS	NA
4	M	29	Adrenal cortical carcinoma	MSH2/MSH6	MSS	MSH2*1906GC

Abbreviations: MFH, malignant fibrous histiocytoma; NA, not available; F, female; M, male.
Editor's Note: Please refer to original journal article for full references.

C and D), pancreatic acinar carcinoma, well-differentiated pancreatic endocrine tumor, and adrenocortical carcinoma.

The report is interesting because the approach to the unusual tumors in LS is discussed in detail by leading experts on the topic.

The application of immunostains to assess mismatch repair genes (MMR) and MSI testing is not refined in unusual tumors (How do they stain for MMR products? Is MSI detectable? What antibodies for MMR are most useful in these cases? Is morphology typical in them too?). Of the 4 tumors reported, only the mesothelioma had numerous intratumoral lymphocytes; the other tumors retained their conventional morphology. It remains true that these tumors may provide another tissue source for the workup of family members at high risk of developing cancer. If the tests for LS are positive in the unusual tumors in individuals of LS families, the diagnosis of LS is achieved. This is especially useful to consider in young patients of LS families.

It must be remembered that patients with LS may very well develop sporadic "conventional" tumors: Those tumors will not have any MMR deficiency. It follows that an MMR-efficient and MSI-stable tumor does not rule out LS.

The authors carefully suggest that in unusual tumors in high-risk patients the loss of mismatch repair suggests LS and can guide further work-up, normal IHC for MMR does not exclude LS, interpretation of IHC has to be carefully optimized in terms of tissue processing, or a tumor may have lost a MMR protein but not be microsatellite instable. This may indicate that the loss of MMR gene is a secondary oncogenetic mechanism in that particular tumor or that not enough genetic mutations have occurred to incite MSI. Practically we cannot rely on MSI alone in assessing "unusual" tumors for LS: Both IHC to detect MMR deficiency and MSI are needed and the lack of MSI does not mean MMR germline mutation is absent.

Because we need to better understand the biologic significance and clinical implications of MMR deficiency in these tumors, the authors conclude that there is no evidence to recommend general surveillance and no suggestion is advanced that testing for mismatch repair deficiency of LS be performed in them.

G. De Petris, MD

The Lower Anogenital Squamous Terminology Standardization Project for HPV-Associated Lesions: Background and Consensus Recommendations from the College of American Pathologists and the American Society for Colposcopy and Cervical Pathology
Darragh TM, for members of the LAST Project Work Groups (Univ of California — San Francisco; et al)
Arch Pathol Lab Med 136:1266-1297, 2012

The terminology for human papillomavirus (HPV)—associated squamous lesions of the lower anogenital tract has a long history marked by disparate diagnostic terms derived from multiple specialties. It often does not reflect current knowledge of HPV biology and pathogenesis. A consensus process was convened to recommend terminology unified across lower anogenital

TABLE 3.—Summary of Recommendations

Recommendation	Comment
SQUAMOUS INTRAEPITHELIAL LESIONS, WG2 1. A unified histopathologic nomenclature with a single set of diagnostic terms is recommended for all HPV-associated preinvasive squamous lesions of the LAT.	
2. A 2-tiered nomenclature is recommended for noninvasive HPV-associated squamous proliferations of the LAT, which may be further qualified with the appropriate −IN terminology.	−IN refers to the generic intraepithelial neoplasia terminology, without specifying the location. For a specific location, the appropriate complete term should be used. Thus, for an −IN 3 lesion: cervix = CIN 3, vagina = VaIN 3, vulva = VIN 3, anus = AIN 3, perianus = PAIN 3, and penis = PeIN 3
3. The recommended terminology for HPV-associated squamous lesions of the LAT is LSIL and HSIL, which may be further classified by the applicable −IN subcategorization.	
SUPERFICIALLY INVASIVE SQUAMOUS CELL CARCINOMA, WG3 1. The term *superficially invasive squamous cell carcinoma (SISCCA)* is recommended for minimally invasive SCC of the LAT that has been completely excised and is potentially amenable to conservative surgical therapy.	Note: Lymph-vascular invasion (LVI) and pattern of invasion are not part of the definition of SISCCA, with the exception of penile carcinoma.

2. For cases of invasive squamous carcinoma *with positive biopsy/resection margins*, the pathology report should state whether:
    The examined invasive tumor exceeds the dimensions for a SISCCA (defined below) OR
    The examined invasive tumor component is less than or equal to the dimensions for a SISCCA and conclude that the tumor is "*At least a superficially invasive squamous carcinoma.*"	

3. In cases of SISCCA, the following parameters should be included in the pathology report:
    The presence or absence of LVI.
    The presence, number, and size of independent multifocal carcinomas (after excluding the possibility of a single carcinoma).	

4. CERVIX: SISCCA of the cervix is defined as an invasive squamous carcinoma that:
    Is not a grossly visible lesion, AND
    Has an invasive depth of ≤3 mm from the basement membrane of the point of origin, AND
    Has a horizontal spread of ≤7 mm in maximal extent, AND
    Has been completely excised.	

5. VAGINA: No recommendation is offered for early invasive squamous carcinoma of the vagina.	Owing to the rarity of primary SCC of the vagina, there are insufficient data to define early invasive squamous carcinoma in the vagina.

6. ANAL CANAL: The *suggested* definition of superficially invasive squamous cell carcinoma (SISCCA) of the anal canal is an invasive squamous carcinoma that:
    Has an invasive depth of ≤3 mm from the basement membrane of the point of origin, AND
    Has a horizontal spread of ≤7 mm in maximal extent, AND
    Has been completely excised.	

(Continued)

TABLE 3.—(*Continued*)

Recommendation	Comment
7. VULVA: Vulvar SISCCA is defined as an AJCC T1a (FIGO IA) vulvar cancer. No change in the current definition of T1a vulvar cancer is recommended.	Current AJCC definition of T1a vulvar carcinoma: Tumor ≤2 cm in size, confined to the vulva or perineum AND Stromal invasion ≤1 mm Note: The depth of invasion is defined as the measurement of the tumor from the epithelial-stromal junction of the adjacent most superficial dermal papilla to the deepest point of invasion.
8. PENIS: Penile SISCCA is defined as an AJCC T1a. No change in the current definition of T1a penile cancer is recommended.	Current AJCC definition of T1a penile carcinoma: Tumor that invades only the subepithelial connective tissue, AND No LVI AND Is not poorly differentiated (i.e., grade 3—4)
9. SCROTUM: No recommendation is offered for early invasive squamous carcinoma of the scrotum.	Owing to the rarity of primary SCC of the scrotum, there is insufficient literature to make a recommendation regarding the current AJCC staging of early scrotal cancers.
10. PERIANUS: The *suggested* definition for SISCCA of the perianus is an invasive squamous carcinoma that: Has an invasive depth of ≤3 mm from the basement membrane of the point of origin, AND Has a horizontal spread of ≤7 mm in maximal extent, AND Has been completely excised.	

BIOMARKERS IN HPV-ASSOCIATED LOWER ANOGENITAL SQUAMOUS LESIONS, WG4

1. p16 IHC is *recommended* when the H&E morphologic differential diagnosis is between precancer (−IN 2 or −IN 3) and a mimic of precancer (e.g., processes known to be not related to neoplastic risk such as immature squamous metaplasia, atrophy, reparative epithelial changes, tangential cutting).	Strong and diffuse block-positive p16 results support a categorization of precancerous disease.
2. If the pathologist is entertaining an H&E morphologic interpretation of −IN 2 (under the old terminology, which is a biologically equivocal lesion falling between the morphologic changes of HPV infection [low-grade lesion] and precancer), p16 IHC is *recommended* to help clarify the situation. Strong and diffuse block-positive p16 results support a categorization of precancer. Negative or non−block-positive staining strongly favors an interpretation of low-grade disease or a non−HPV-associated pathology.	
3. p16 is *recommended* for use as an adjudication tool for cases in which there is a professional disagreement in histologic specimen interpretation, with the caveat that the differential diagnosis includes a precancerous lesion (−IN 2 or −IN 3).	

(*Continued*)

TABLE 3.—(*Continued*)

Recommendation	Comment
4. WG4 *recommends against* the use of p16 IHC as a routine adjunct to histologic assessment of biopsy specimens with morphologic interpretations of negative, −IN 1, and −IN 3. a. SPECIAL CIRCUMSTANCE: p16 IHC is recommended as an adjunct to morphologic assessment for biopsy specimens interpreted as ≤ −IN 1 that are at high risk for missed high-grade disease, which is defined as a prior cytologic interpretation of HSIL, ASC-H, ASC-US/HPV-16+, or AGC (NOS).	Any identified p16-positive area must meet H&E morphologic criteria for a high-grade lesion to be reinterpreted as such.

sites. The goal was to create a histopathologic nomenclature system that reflects current knowledge of HPV biology, optimally uses available biomarkers, and facilitates clear communication across different medical specialties. The Lower Anogenital Squamous Terminology (LAST) Project was cosponsored by the College of American Pathologists and the American Society for Colposcopy and Cervical Pathology and included 5 working groups; 3 work groups performed comprehensive literature reviews and developed draft recommendations. Another work group provided the historical background and the fifth will continue to foster implementation of the LAST recommendations. After an open comment period, the draft recommendations were presented at a consensus conference attended by LAST work group members, advisors, and representatives from 35 stakeholder organizations including professional societies and government agencies. Recommendations were finalized and voted on at the consensus meeting. The final, approved recommendations standardize biologically relevant histopathologic terminology for HPV-associated squamous intraepithelial lesions and superficially invasive squamous carcinomas across all lower anogenital tract sites and detail the appropriate use of specific biomarkers to clarify histologic interpretations and enhance diagnostic accuracy. A plan for disseminating and monitoring recommendation implementation in the practicing community was also developed. The implemented recommendations will facilitate communication between pathologists and their clinical colleagues and improve accuracy of histologic diagnosis with the ultimate goal of providing optimal patient care (Table 3).

▶ The consensus recommendations for the Lower Anogenital Squamous Terminology (LAST) for human papilloma virus (HPV)—associated lesions is required reading for any practicing pathologist receiving specimens from the cervix, vagina, anal canal, vulva, penis, scrotum, or perianal area. The working groups, staffed by experts in the field for each organ system, have reviewed the pertinent evidence-based literature and provide standard terminology that is paralleled in each anatomic site, making the communication of intraepithelial neoplasia much more straightforward for pathologists to convey to the clinicians (Table 3).

Many of the recommendations are intuitive to pathologists; the document recommends using a 2-tiered system for grading of noninvasive squamous lesions (low-grade or high-grade squamous intraepithelial lesion), with a further option to use a 3-tiered system for grading of the appropriate intraepithelial neoplasia (−IN, graded as 1, 2, or 3). Most pathologists will find that this coincides with their practice patterns already. The article also addresses superficially invasive squamous cell carcinoma and use of p16 immunohistochemistry in a cost-effective and practical manner.

Perhaps understated in this recommendation is the slow movement toward the terminology of "intraepithelial neoplasia"—a designation that has been replacing the problematic terms "dysplasia" and "carcinoma in situ" that we have seen in other organ systems (ie, pancreas, biliary system). This is an important step forward for the field of pathology, and it is a joy to see the leaders in our field take the reins and clarify the nomenclature for both pathologists and clinicians such that we may better serve our patients. Hopefully, this trend will continue as we move through the next decade.

D. Lam-Himlin, MD

Consensus statement on the pathology of IgG4-related disease
Deshpande V, Zen Y, Chan JKC, et al (Massachusetts General Hosp, Boston; King's College Hosp, London, UK; Queen Elizabeth Hosp, Kowloon, Hong Kong; et al)
Mod Pathol 25:1181-1192, 2012

IgG4-related disease is a newly recognized fibro-inflammatory condition characterized by several features: a tendency to form tumefactive lesions in multiple sites; a characteristic histopathological appearance; and—often but not always—elevated serum IgG4 concentrations. An international symposium on IgG4-related disease was held in Boston, MA, on 4−7 October 2011. The organizing committee comprising 35 IgG4-related disease experts from Japan, Korea, Hong Kong, the United Kingdom, Germany, Italy, Holland, Canada, and the United States, including the clinicians, pathologists, radiologists, and basic scientists. This group represents broad subspecialty expertise in pathology, rheumatology, gastroenterology, allergy, immunology, nephrology, pulmonary medicine, oncology, ophthalmology, and surgery. The histopathology of IgG4-related disease was a specific focus of the international symposium. The primary purpose of this statement is to provide practicing pathologists with a set of guidelines for the diagnosis of IgG4-related disease. The diagnosis of IgG4-related disease rests on the combined presence of the characteristic histopathological appearance and increased numbers of IgG4+ plasma cells. The critical histopathological features are a dense lymphoplasmacytic infiltrate, a storiform pattern of fibrosis, and obliterative phlebitis. We propose a terminology scheme for the diagnosis of IgG4-related disease that is based primarily on the morphological appearance on biopsy. Tissue IgG4 counts and IgG4:IgG ratios are secondary in importance. The guidelines proposed in this statement do not supplant careful clinicopathological correlation and sound clinical judgment. As the spectrum of this disease continues to expand, we advocate the use of strict criteria for accepting newly proposed entities or sites as components of the IgG4-related disease spectrum.

▶ Immunoglobulin (Ig) G4-related disease (IgG4RD) was first recognized as an inflammatory process of the pancreas named autoimmune pancreatitis (AIP). In AIP a high number of IgG4-positive plasma cells are seen in the pancreas and a high serum levels of IgG4 is detected. IgG4RD has since been reported in numerous additional sites. With greater awareness of the disease and the involvement of numerous organs, the need for a consensus on the histopathology of Ig64D is keenly felt.

A group of experts from the United States, Europe, and Asia generated a consensus statement with the goal of providing histopathological criteria and diagnostic terminology for IgG4RD. It is suggested that IgG4RD diagnosis be based on 3 major histopathological findings: dense lymphoplasmacytic infiltrate, storiform fibrosis (not always present in every organ), and obliterative phlebitis (also not always present), and 2 minor criteria: nonobliterative phlebitis and increased number of eosinophils.

A terminology scheme based on histopathology is also proposed with 3 levels of "certainty" of the diagnosis (highly suggestive of, probable, and insufficient evidence of IgG4RD).

The handling of the issue of a cutoff number of IgG4-positive plasma cells/high-power field for the diagnosis could not be resolved, and rightly so in my opinion. The diagnosis of IgG4RD cannot rely only on the count of plasma cells positive for IgG4 but has to combine clinical and histopathological features. Variability in cutoff values according to the organ is acknowledged, as is the fact that the literature is not always abundant for IgG4RD of certain organs. In addition, several established diseases may have a high number of IgG4 cells (for example Rosai-Dorfman disease, Churg-Strauss disease, and, very importantly, some cancers).

Outstanding issues obviously remain (such as: Is IgG4RD a disease or is it an immunological marker common to various diseases?). Nonetheless, the consensus, by clarifying the spectrum of the disease and the problems in diagnosis, will further our understanding of it.

G. De Petris, MD

Developments in the Assessment of Venous Invasion in Colorectal Cancer: Implications for Future Practice and Patient Outcome
Messenger DE, Driman DK, Kirsch R (Royal United Hosp NHS Trust, Bath, UK; London Health Sciences Ctr and Univ of Western Ontario, Canada; Mount Sinai Hosp and Univ of Toronto, Ontario, Canada)
Hum Pathol 43:965-973, 2012

Venous invasion, or "large vessel" invasion, is a known independent prognostic indicator of distant recurrence and survival in colorectal cancer. Accurate assessment of venous invasion is of particular importance in stage

II disease because it may influence the decision to administer adjuvant therapy. Venous invasion is widely believed to be an underreported finding with significant variability in its reported incidence. In the most recent College of American Pathologists' cancer reporting protocol, venous invasion is not recorded separately from lymphovascular, or "small vessel" invasion, which may not be appropriate because these features confer differing prognostic information. The presence of extramural venous invasion is strongly predictive of adverse outcome, although the prognostic significance of intramural venous invasion remains unknown. There are no formal guidelines regarding the pathologic assessment of venous invasion or the application of specific reporting criteria. The routine use of an elastic stain results in an almost 3-fold increase in the venous invasion detection rate when compared with a standard hematoxylin and eosin stain and may be a cost-effective means of increasing the diagnostic yield of venous invasion. The development of high-resolution magnetic resonance imaging, where extramural venous invasion can be detected preoperatively, may also influence the manner in which pathologists process specimens. This review focuses on recent developments in the assessment of venous invasion and highlights their potential impact on future practice.

▶ This article was eye-opening because it detailed several methods of improving the detection of venous invasion in colorectal cancer, a finding that has significant prognostic value. Pathologists perform a routine examination of tumor slides for the presence of lymphovascular invasion, but adding any kind of special stain to this process frequently increases the turnaround time of a final report. As a result, if no definite venous invasion is identified in the original slides, the case may be released immediately in the interest of getting the information to the patients, surgeons, and oncologists expediently for the purposes of planning additional care, such as neoadjuvant therapy.

However, this article makes one reappraise whether this practice is truly in the best interests of the patient. Venous invasion is not only underreported, but it is also not a required element of the College of American Pathologists checklist for cancer reporting. However, given the likelihood that venous invasion confers different prognostic information from that of lymphatic or small vessel invasion, it would be prudent to search for and report this finding.

As a result, these authors have made me reappraise whether my evaluation for venous invasion is sufficient. Lately, more and more of my cases have been evaluated with the aid of an elastic stain, even if it results in additional delay of the final pathology. It will take some time to determine whether this results in improved detection in my practice, but the level of evidence presented by these authors is compelling. Follow-up studies of the efficacy of this practice will certainly be of interest.

The article also suggests that tangential tissue sections along the radial border of the tumor may increase the likelihood of capturing veins that pass at right angles across the bowel wall and into mesocolic tissues. This is not a common method of sampling at the grossing bench, because typical sections of colorectal cancer are taken perpendicular through the mucosa to the serosa. However, after conventional sections, taking a few additional sections in this manner does not compromise the specimen and is straightforward and quick enough to perform. It seems a worthwhile effort by pathologists and their assistants, and, when used in combination with an "up-front" elastic stain, this practice should yield increased detection without a slowed turnaround time.

D. Lam-Himlin, MD

Developments in the assessment of venous invasion in colorectal cancer: implications for future practice and patient outcome
Messenger DE, Driman DK, Kirsch R (Royal United Hosp NHS Trust, Bath, UK; London Health Sciences Centre and Univ of Western Ontario, London, Ontario, Canada; Mount Sinai Hosp and Univ of Toronto, Ontario, Canada)
Hum Pathol 43:965-973, 2012

Venous invasion, or "large vessel" invasion, is a known independent prognostic indicator of distant recurrence and survival in colorectal cancer. Accurate assessment of venous invasion is of particular importance in stage II disease because it may influence the decision to administer adjuvant therapy. Venous invasion is widely believed to be an underreported finding with significant variability in its reported incidence. In the most recent College of American Pathologists' cancer reporting protocol, venous invasion is not recorded separately from lymphovascular, or "small vessel" invasion, which may not be appropriate because these features confer differing prognostic information. The presence of extramural venous invasion is strongly predictive of adverse outcome, although the prognostic significance of intramural venous invasion remains unknown. There are no formal guidelines regarding the pathologic assessment of venous invasion or the application of specific reporting criteria. The routine use of an elastic stain results in an almost 3-fold increase in the venous invasion detection rate when compared with a standard hematoxylin and eosin stain and may be a cost-effective means of increasing the diagnostic yield of venous invasion. The development of high-resolution magnetic resonance imaging, where extramural venous invasion can be detected preoperatively, may also influence the manner in which pathologists process specimens. This review focuses on recent developments in the assessment of venous invasion and highlights their potential impact on future practice.

▶ The current practice of surgical pathology is rich of template-based reports of cancer resections. Colorectal cancer (CRC) reporting will benefit from this review. The current guidelines for CRC recording of the College of American Pathology leave venous/large vessel invasion (VI), defined as invasion of extramural muscularized vein, under the vastly more generic term of lymphovascular invasion. In addition, and perhaps consequently, pathologists do not report VI consistently. It is, however, well-documented that VI is an independent prognosticator of aggressive behavior. Stage II CRC with VI may benefit from chemotherapy because VI is such a powerful indicator of disease progression and CRC-related death. The authors' review of the surgical pathology issues related to VI highlights clearly why the pathology community needs to recognize and report VI. To that end, they provide practical guidelines (obtain at least 4 sections of tumor, sections be directed toward sampling the advancing front of the neoplasia or tangentional not perpendicular sectioning, use of elastic stain, correlation of gross exam with magnetic resonance imaging, and useful histological clues). These suggestions are applicable in the majority of pathology laboratories and are cost-effective. This article indicates how the venerable art of approaching and cutting surgical specimens in order to discover important histological variables is still and inevitably evolving.

S. S. Raab, MD

Serrated Polyposis Is an Underdiagnosed and Unclear Syndrome: The Surgical Pathologist has a Role in Improving Detection
Crowder CD, Sweet K, Lehman A, et al (The Ohio State Univ Med Ctr, Columbus; The Ohio State Univ, Columbus)
Am J Surg Pathol 36:1178-1185, 2012

Serrated polyposis syndrome (SPS) is poorly defined and patients have an increased but unspecified risk for colorectal carcinoma through the serrated pathway. Despite this association SPS remains relatively obscure and is therefore likely underrecognized. We determined the frequency of SPS among patients with any serrated polyps (SPs) over a 6-month "index" period, and in doing so we assessed the ability of surgical pathologists to improve SPS detection. Particular attention was given to the index procedure to assess the potential predictive value of the findings resulting from a single colonoscopy. A total of 929 patients with at least 1 SP were identified, 17 of whom (1.8%) were determined to meet World Health Organization criteria for SPS. Nine patients met the first criterion ($\geq$5 proximal SPs, 2 of which are >10 mm); 4 met the third criterion (>20 SPs of any size distributed throughout the colon); and 4 met both criteria. Although no specific SP size or number at the index procedure was clearly superior in its ability to predict SPS, >50% of cases would be detected if a cutoff of $\geq$3 SPs or a single SP $\geq$ 15 mm at the index procedure is used. In summary, SPS is rare but more likely underdiagnosed. Additional studies to address the underlying genetic basis for SPS are ongoing in order to shed further light on this syndrome. Surgical pathologists are in a unique position to assist in this endeavor by identifying those patients who either meet or seem to be at high risk of meeting World Health Organization criteria.

▶ Serrated polyposis syndrome (SPS), previously known as hyperplastic polyposis syndrome, is poorly understood for a variety of reasons. Crowder et al raise an important issue in this already confusing quagmire of serrated neoplasia—namely that identification of patients with serrated polyposis syndrome is an important task and the surgical pathologist can play a critical role in identifying these patients for the purposes of patient counseling and familial surveillance.

The article is important in raising awareness among pathologists and urging us to have a heightened vigilance for this entity, but a number of factors stand in the way for the general surgical pathologist. First, the serrated neoplasms have undergone recategorization, yielding an entirely new family of polyps with new terminology, as recently as 2010. Second, there are no good longitudinal studies or strong body evidence unequivocally showing the suspected short interval to carcinoma, despite the frequently cited molecular underpinnings of this so-called serrated pathway to neoplasia. In addition, the criteria for diagnosis of SPS, as outlined by the World Health Organization (WHO), are not entirely clear (ie, are the numbers of polyps intended to encompass only those identified at the index colonoscopy, or all colonoscopies for the lifetime of a patient). Finally, in light of the gray areas in the diagnosis of SPS, studies cited as showing a link between SPS and other neoplasias should be examined closely. The authors acknowledge some of these limitations, but I believe many general surgical pathologists are wary of overdiagnosis of the sessile serrated adenoma/polyp at routine sign-out, and as a result tend to lean toward under-diagnosis. It follows that most would also be hesitant to diagnose a syndrome such as SPS when such confusion around this topic persists.

Clearly, further study and education in this area is required, and I believe that future longitudinal studies will help clarify some of these issues. For the time being, however, it is likely worthwhile to flag patients meeting the WHO minimum criteria for SPS and to allow clinicians to make surveillance and genetic counseling decisions regarding these patients.

D. Lam-Himlin, MD

Lymphocytic Oesophagitis: Clinicopathological Aspects of an Emerging Condition

Haque S, Genta RM (Caris Res Inst, Irving, TX)
Gut 61:1108-1114, 2012

Objective.—Lymphocytic oesophagitis (LyE) has been reported in small series, but no consistent clinical correlations have emerged. The authors sought to determine the prevalence of LyE in a large population and define demographic, endoscopic and clinical findings associated with this condition.

Design.—In a pilot study, the authors established and disseminated criteria for the histopathological diagnosis of LyE to a group of gastrointestinal pathologists. Eighteen months later the authors reviewed cases with this diagnosis, collected demographic, clinical and endoscopic data, and compared them with patients with either eosinophilic oesophagitis (EoE) or normal oesophageal biopsies. The authors also determined the density of oesophageal lymphocytes in normal controls and in adults with established Crohn's disease.

Results.—There were 129 252 unique patients: 40 665 had normal mucosa (median age 55 years; 32% men); 3745 had EoE (median age 43 years; 66% men). A diagnosis of LyE was made in 119 patients (median age 63 years, 40% men). Dysphagia was as common in these patients as in those with EoE (53% vs 63%; ns); gastro-oesophageal reflux disease—the most common complaint in patients with normal biopsies (37%)—was low in both the LyE and the EoE groups (18% vs 19%, ns). EoE was suspected in one-third of the patients.

Conclusion.—LyE was detected in ~0.1% of patients with oesophageal biopsies. The clinical and endoscopic characteristics of LyE and EoE overlap considerably; however, LyE affects predominantly older women. Although the precise clinical significance of oesophageal lymphocytic infiltrates remains to be defined, their association with dysphagia and possibly motility disorders warrants further investigations.

▶ The presence of T-cell lymphocytes in the squamous epithelium of the esophagus is well known to the histopathologist. The clinical counterparts of an increase in lymphocytes in the epithelium of the esophagus have remained somewhat elusive, however. Intraepithelial lymphocytosis is seen in reflux, drug effect, and infections. Association with Crohn disease and celiac disease has been reported but not confirmed.

The article defines lymphocytic esophagitis (LE) as the presence of > 30 lymphocytes/high-power field (HPF) with an HPF of 0.23 mm^2. Normal controls in this study had an average of 5 + 4 lymphocytes/HPF. The distribution of lymphocytes was patchy, lymphocytes were mainly peripapillary, and necrotic keratinocytes were seen also providing a relatively nonspecific appearance for the histopathologist.

We learned that so defined LE is quite rare: Only 0.1% of patients suffered from it. The article is interesting because it shows that the clinical and endoscopic characteristics of LE overlap considerably but not completely with eosinophilic esophagitis (EE). It seems, therefore, that the histopathologist may offer new insight into those cases suspected of EE by the clinician but that prove not to have eosinophilia under the microscope. We are far away from understanding the disease or what to do in terms of therapy for LE, but we are seeing the start of the definition of a clinicopathological picture for LE. These observations should therefore increase the detection of LE. It seems likely that more will come from this area of esophagology.

G. De Petris, MD

European Society for Pediatric Gastroenterology, Hepatology, and Nutrition Guidelines for the Diagnosis of Coeliac Disease
Husby S, for the ESPGHAN Working Group on Coeliac Disease Diagnosis, on behalf of the ESPGHAN Gastroenterology Committee (Hans Christian Andersen Children's Hosp at Odense Univ Hosp, Denmark; et al)
J Pediatr Gastroenterol Nutr 54:136-160, 2012

Objective.—Diagnostic criteria for coeliac disease (CD) from the European Society for Paediatric Gastroenterology, Hepatology, and Nutrition (ESPGHAN) were published in 1990. Since then, the autoantigen in CD, tissue transglutaminase, has been identified; the perception of CD has changed from that of a rather uncommon enteropathy to a common multiorgan disease strongly dependent on the haplotypes human leukocyte antigen (HLA)-DQ2 and HLA-DQ8; and CD-specific antibody tests have improved.

Methods.—A panel of 17 experts defined CD and developed new diagnostic criteria based on the Delphi process. Two groups of patients were defined with different diagnostic approaches to diagnose CD: children with symptoms suggestive of CD (group 1) and asymptomatic children at increased risk for CD (group 2). The 2004 National Institutes of Health/Agency for Healthcare Research and Quality report and a systematic literature search on antibody tests for CD in paediatric patients covering the years 2004 to 2009 was the basis for the evidence-based recommendations on CD-specific antibody testing.

Results.—In group 1, the diagnosis of CD is based on symptoms, positive serology, and histology that is consistent with CD. If immunoglobulin A anti-tissue transglutaminase type 2 antibody titers are high (>10 times the upper limit of normal), then the option is to diagnose CD without duodenal biopsies by applying a strict protocol with further laboratory tests. In group 2, the diagnosis of CD is based on positive serology and histology. HLA-DQ2 and HLA-DQ8 testing is valuable because CD is unlikely if both haplotypes are negative.

Conclusions.—The aim of the new guidelines was to achieve a high diagnostic accuracy and to reduce the burden for patients and their families. The performance of these guidelines in clinical practice should be evaluated prospectively.

▶ Although this article represents clinical guidelines for the diagnosis of celiac disease, it is important for pathologists who review these biopsies to understand the clinical criteria and to have a working knowledge of the implications of their diagnostic reports in the setting of suspected celiac disease. These guidelines are timely and thoughtful, and they detail the evolution of our understanding of this disease.

The diagnosis of celiac disease has always remained a clinicopathologic diagnosis despite evolving guidelines.[1] However, with the development of highly accurate serologic testing and human leukocyte antigen (HLA) typing, the latest 2012 guidelines in this article suggest that, under the right conditions, the diagnosis of celiac disease can be made without biopsy support (a non-biopsy diagnosis of celiac disease). This is a significant deviation from the guidelines of years past, and, as noted by other experts in the field,[2,3] it remains to be seen whether we are ready to abandon biopsies in individuals who have strongly suggestive serologic findings. Further studies are clearly required.

The significance of this article for pathologists is in their understanding that the serologic findings play a heavily weighted role in the diagnosis of celiac disease. This should be taken into account during evaluation of small intestinal biopsies. For example, in the setting of equivocal histology (ie, mild intraepithelial lymphocytosis with mild villous blunting), the lack of a permissive HLA type essentially excludes the possibility of celiac disease. As such, it is important for pathologists to continue the tradition of a descriptive sign out, and to understand that a purely histologic diagnosis of celiac disease remains elusive. If anything, this article confirms that histology is playing a smaller role than ever in the diagnosis of celiac disease. It follows that pathologists can, review serologic findings in conjunction with histologic features in order to synthesize a more complete interpretation and integrated pathology report.

D. Lam-Himlin, MD

References

1. Hill I, Dirks M, Colletti R, et al. Guideline for the diagnosis and treatment of celiac disease in children: recommendations of the North American Society for Pediatric Gastroenterology, Hepatology and Nutrition. *J Pediatr Gastroenterol Nutr.* 2005;40:1-19.
2. Hill ID, Horvath K. Nonbiopsy diagnosis of celiac disease: are we nearly there yet? *J Pediatr Gastroenterol Nutr.* 2012;54:310-311.
3. Kurppa K, Salminiemi J, Ukkola A, et al. Utility of the new ESPGHAN criteria for the diagnosis of celiac disease in at-risk groups. *J Pediatr Gastroenterol Nutr.* 2012;54:387-391.

The molecular basis of EPCAM expression loss in Lynch syndrome-associated tumors
Huth C, Kloor M, Voigt AY, et al (Univ Hosp Heidelberg, Germany)
Mod Pathol 25:911-916, 2012

Germline deletions affecting the Epithelial cell adhesion molecule (*EPCAM*) gene lead to silencing of *MSH2* and cause Lynch syndrome. We have recently reported that lack of EPCAM expression occurs in many, but not all tumors from Lynch syndrome patients with *EPCAM* germline deletions. The differences in EPCAM expression were not related to the localization of *EPCAM* germline deletions. We therefore hypothesized that the type of the second somatic hit, which leads to *MSH2* inactivation during tumor development, determines EPCAM expression in the tumor cells. To test this hypothesis and to evaluate whether lack of EPCAM expression can already be detected in Lynch syndrome-associated adenomas, we analyzed four carcinomas and two adenomas from *EPCAM* germline deletion carriers for EPCAM protein expression and allelic deletion status of the *EPCAM* gene region by multiplex ligation-dependent probe amplification. In four out of six tumors we observed lack of EPCAM expression accompanied by biallelic deletions affecting the *EPCAM* gene. In contrast, monoallelic retention of the *EPCAM* gene was observed in the remaining two tumors with retained EPCAM protein expression. These results demonstrate that EPCAM expression in tumors from EPCAM deletion carriers depends on the localization of the second somatic hit that inactivates MSH2. Moreover, we report lack of EPCAM protein expression in a colorectal adenoma, suggesting that EPCAM immunohistochemistry may detect *EPCAM* germline deletions already at a precancerous stage.

▶ The algorithmic approaches to the diagnosis of Lynch syndrome (LS) are based on clinical observation, immunohistochemistry (IHC), and microsatellite instability testing followed by gene analysis. The understanding of the information provided by IHC in LS is inevitably evolving with the expanding knowledge of the molecular basis of LS. Mutation of the mismatch repair gene *MSH2* is one of causes of LS. Most commonly mutations in *MSH2* are protein-truncating and the IHC offers easy interpretation. It is indeed the experience of many that IHC for *MSH2* is clearer than the sometimes frustratingly weak positivity of IHC for *MLH1*, the most commonly implicated gene in the genesis of LS. *MSH2*, however, has its own surprises: 2% to 3% of the cases of LS show loss of expression of *MSH2* without detectable germline mutation of the gene. This discrepancy is due to germline deletions in the EPCAM gene located upstream of *MSH2* causing silencing of *MSH2*. It could follow that EPCAM antibody (BER-Ep4) be added into the IHC panels used to detect LS. Things are not so simple, however. The study shows that lack of expression of EPCAM does not occur in all cases of LS because of EPCAM germline mutation and explains why.

EPCAM expression in tumor cells depends on the localization of the second somatic hit that inactivates *MSH2*: Loss of EPCAM occurs only in cases of biallelic deletions of the EPCAM gene. When the second hit occurs in *MSH2*, there may be no loss of EPCAM staining on IHC.

The study is an example of how our knowledge of the molecular basis of LS can explain some apparently discrepant IHC findings. Things are getting more and more interesting for pathologists interested in LS, and they point to the need of a good knowledge of the molecular mechanisms of LS to understand the IHC results.

G. De Petris, MD

Loss of SDHA Expression Identifies SDHA Mutations in Succinate Dehydrogenase–deficient Gastrointestinal Stromal Tumors

Dwight T, Benn DE, Clarkson A, et al (Kolling Inst of Med Res, St Leonards, New South Wales, Australia; Royal North Shore Hosp, St Leonards, New South Wales, Australia; et al)
Am J Surg Pathol 2012 [Epub ahead of print]

Succinate dehydrogenase–deficient gastrointestinal stromal tumors (SDH-deficient GISTs) are a unique class of GIST defined by negative immunohistochemical staining for succinate dehydrogenase B (SDHB). SDH-deficient GISTs show distinctive clinical and pathologic features including absence of *KIT* and *PDGFRA* mutations, exclusive gastric location, common lymph node metastasis, a prognosis not predicted by size and mitotic rate, and indolent behavior of metastases. They may be syndromal with some being associated with the Carney Triad or germline *SDHA*, *SDHB*, *SDHC*, or *SDHD* mutations (Carney-Stratakis syndrome). It is normally recommended that genetic testing for *SDHA*, *SDHB*, *SDHC*, and *SDHD* be offered whenever an SDH-deficient GIST is encountered. However, testing for all 4 genes is burdensome and beyond the means of most centers. In this study we performed *SDHA* mutation and immunohistochemical analyses for SDHA on 10 SDH-deficient GISTs. Three showed negative staining for SDHA, and all of these were associated with germline *SDHA* mutations. In 2 tumors, 3 novel mutations were identified (p.Gln54X, p.Thr267Met, and c.1663 + 3G > C), none of which has previously been reported in GISTs or other SDH-associated tumors. Seven showed positive staining for SDHA and were not associated with *SDHA* mutation. In conclusion, 30% of SDH-deficient GISTs in this study were associated with germline *SDHA* mutation. Negative staining for SDHA can be used to triage formal genetic testing for *SDHA* when an SDH-deficient GIST is encountered.

▶ This article explores further the genetic underpinning of the recently described gastrointestinal stromal tumors due to succinate dehydrogenase deficiency (SDH-GISTs). These tumors display several distinctive features: They are the most common GISTS in young patients, are exclusively gastric, epithelioid and angioinvasive, with nodal metastases but good prognosis, and they may be associated with syndromes (hereditary Carney-Stratakis syndrome and sporadic Carney triad). It is interesting to know that SDH-deficient GISTs are often associated with germline mutations of the succinate dehydrogenase subunits genes (SDHA, SDHB, SDHC, SDHD) rather than being caused by purely double-hit somatic mutations of these genes.

The proteins of the subunits are assembled in the mitochondria to form the mitochondrial complex 2. Defects in any of these subunits genes are detected by immunohistochemical stain for SDHB that will be negative. It happens that when a double hit inactivates any of the components of the complex, SDHB is degraded. SDHB therefore marks a defect of any of the proteins subunits not simply of SDHB and is therefore not specific.

Because SDH-GISTS are often the result of a germline mutation, it is necessary to provide genetic testing all subunit genes, which is burdensome and costly.

The study demonstrates that SDHA germline mutation can be detected by an immunostain for SDHA. This simplifies considerably the evaluation of these patients. Starting with an immunostain for SDHB and SDHA may help triage the order of the gene testing if this strategy proves useful in practice.

This is another example of morphology detecting a specific subset of tumors that need genetic testing. The study is likely one step toward the development of a screening approach to these tumors by simple and inexpensive means such as immunohistochemistry. In this, and in every case of genetic diseases, the pathologist's approach and tests should be coordinated with a geneticist to provide the best information to the individual patient.

G. De Petris, MD

Tumor Budding in Colorectal Carcinoma: Time to Take Notice
Mitrovic B, Schaeffer DF, Riddell RH, et al (Mount Sinai Hosp, Toronto, Ontario, Canada)
Mod Pathol 25:1315-1325, 2012

Tumor "budding," loosely defined by the presence of individual cells and small clusters of tumor cells at the invasive front of carcinomas, has received much recent attention, particularly in the setting of colorectal carcinoma. It has been postulated to represent an epithelial—mesenchymal transition. Tumor budding is a well-established independent adverse prognostic factor in colorectal carcinoma that may allow for stratification of patients into risk categories more meaningful than those defined by TNM staging, and also potentially guide treatment decisions, especially in T1 and T3 N0 (Stage II, Dukes' B) colorectal carcinoma. Unfortunately, its universal acceptance as a reportable factor has been held back by a lack of definitional uniformity with respect to both qualitative and quantitative aspects of tumor budding. The purpose of this review is fourfold: (1) to describe the morphology of tumor budding and its relationship to other potentially important features of the invasive front; (2) to summarize current knowledge regarding the prognostic significance and potential clinical implications of this histomorphological feature; (3) to highlight the challenges posed by a lack of data to allow standardization with respect to the qualitative and quantitative criteria used to define budding; and (4) to present a practical approach to the assessment of tumor budding in everyday practice.

▶ The review article is necessary reading to appreciate the current understanding of tumor budding (TB), one of the most powerful predictors of the behavior of stage I and II colorectal cancer (CRC) that is missing from the College of American Pathologists (CAP) checklist of tumor features but that is required in routine reporting of CRC by the Association of Directors of Anatomic and Surgical Pathology and the Union for International Cancer Control. In keeping with this, TB has proved to be an invaluable prognosticator in malignant colorectal polyps. The predictive value of TB persists across various studies despite of several different definitions of what TB is.

The definition of Ueno et al[1] is the most widely used: TB is the presence of more than 10 groups of equal or less than 5 tumor cells in a 20× field[1] usually sought at the invasive front of the colorectal cancer.

In the literature, there have been changes in definition even by the same authors in different publications. In general, agreement on TB is considered fair among different institutions when criteria are provided, with, however, expertise in the area contributing to this level of agreement.[2] The analysis in the article of the various parameters used to define budding sheds a light on the issues: definition of buds (number of cells, linkage to a gland of tumor), size of the optical field, use of keratin immunostain and overall begs for a synthesis and an approach for practice. For the latter, the authors do an excellent job to provide help to the practicing pathologist.

The clues for TB detection (infiltrating tumor growth, blurred interface between tumor and stroma, irregularity of tumor front) are listed, as are suggestions on when to use cytokeratin (if prominent stromal and inflammatory responses at invasive front are present). Confounders that should not count as TB are indicated in tumor fragments in mucin pool and fragmented glands because of retraction artifact.

The terrain has been prepared by this review to understand that consensus on what level of budding is clinically relevant is clearly needed, and that authors of studies including TB will have to provide careful definitions of TB to allow comparisons.

G. De Petris, MD

References

1. Ueno H, Murphy J, Jass JR, Mochizuki H, Talbot IC. Tumour 'budding' as an index to estimate the potential of aggressiveness in rectal cancer. *Histopathology.* 2002; 40:127-132.
2. Puppa G, Senore C, Sheahan K, et al. Diagnostic reproducibility of tumour budding in colorectal cancer: a multicentre, multinational study using virtual microscopy. *Histopathology.* 2012;61:562-575.

Syphilitic and Lymphogranuloma Venereum (LGV) Proctocolitis: Clues to a Frequently Missed Diagnosis

Arnold CA, Limketkai BN, Illei PB, et al (Ohio State Univ, Columbus; Johns Hopkins School of Medicine, Baltimore, MD; et al)
Am J Surg Pathol 2012 [Epub ahead of print]

A rising incidence of syphilis and lymphogranuloma venereum (LGV) underscores the importance of recognizing these sexually transmitted infections (STI) in routine anocolonic biopsies. To increase awareness of their morphologic manifestations, we undertook a clinicopathologic study of our experience: syphilis (7 patients, 7 specimens), LGV (2 patients, 4 specimens), and syphilis/LGV (1 patient, 3 specimens). The diagnoses of all study specimens were confirmed with pertinent clinical studies. All study patients were human immunodeficiency virus positive, and all 9 with available history were men who have sex with men. The majority presented with bleeding (9), pain (6), and tenesmus (4). Ulcerations were the most common endoscopic abnormality (7), whereas mass lesions were confined to the syphilis group (4). None of the initial impressions included LGV, and syphilis was prospectively suggested only by pathologists (6 of 8) without the knowledge of clinical information and on the basis of morphology. Alternative impressions included condyloma acuminatum (3), inflammatory bowel disease (3), and malignancy (2), among others. All study specimens shared the following histologic core features: an intense lymphohistiocytic infiltrate with prominent plasma cells and lymphoid aggregates, only mild to moderate acute inflammation, minimal basal plasmacytosis and crypt distortion, and only rare granulomas and Paneth cell metaplasia. The spirochetes were focally demonstrated on a *Treponema pallidum* immunohistochemical stain (1) but not on silver stains (3). All patients with available follow-up data showed resolution of symptoms and imaging abnormalities after STI therapy (6). In summary, we report a unique pattern of STI proctocolitis consistently identified in patients with serologically confirmed syphilis and/or LGV infection; pertinent STI therapy leads to resolution of clinical abnormalities. This histologic pattern is important to recognize for timely treatment, for prevention of onward STI transmission, and to avoid the diagnostic pitfalls of inflammatory bowel disease or malignancy.

▶ The authors report the clinicopathologic features of sexually transmitted infection (STI) proctitis in a series of human immunodeficiency virus (HIV)-positive men who have sex with men (MSM). This article is particularly important in increasing pathologist and gastroenterologist awareness of this entity because the prevalence of this disease is on the rise. In the article, the authors share that histologic findings can appear similar to those seen in inflammatory bowel disease (IBD), including the presence of skip lesions, Paneth cell metaplasia, and even granulomas. In addition, biopsy samples can lack the diagnostic organisms, even on immunohistochemistry, and clinical testing for lymphogranuloma venereum (LGV) (caused by specific serovars of *Chlamydia trachomatis*) and syphilis is necessary to ensure proper diagnosis.

Of particular interest to pathologists, one must be aware of the histologic overlap with IBD, and, although the authors admit that IBD can be a pitfall in diagnosis, the authors do not explicitly address this very important topic. Clearly, a follow-up study showing the histologic features of IBD compared directly with STI proctitis would be critical in knowing whether STI proctitis represents a pure morphologic diagnosis, a clinicopathologic diagnosis, or simply another differential diagnosis that exists under the umbrella of a chronic colitis pattern of injury.

In the interim, we pathologists must have a heightened awareness that STIs may represent a diagnostic pitfall with enormous clinical implications. In particular, patients with STI proctitis will not be steroid-responsive and will not show clinical improvement on immunomodulator therapy. As a result, I would further suggest that serologic testing for LGV and syphilis be a requirement before labeling a patient as having "refractory IBD," a diagnosis that results in the potential for colectomy.

The take-home message is that infectious etiologies should always be excluded in the setting of suspected IBD. And, particularly among the HIV-positive MSM population, exclusion of STIs would be of particular interest. Furthermore, it would be important for clinicians to specifically ask about sexual practices in their office visit and document these findings for future reference. Further studies to determine whether LGV and syphilitic proctitis exist in the immunocompetent and anal-receptive sexually active patient are also warranted.

D. Lam-Himlin, MD

4 Hepatobiliary System and Pancreas

Pancreatic-type acinar cell carcinoma of the liver: a clinicopathologic study of four patients
Agaimy A, Kaiser A, Becker K, et al (Univ of Erlangen, Germany; Klinikum Nürnberg, Germany; Technical Univ of München, Germany; et al)
Mod Pathol 24:1620-1626, 2011

Acinar cell carcinoma of pancreatic type rarely occurs at extra-pancreatic sites. We report four primary liver tumors with features of pancreatic acinar cell carcinoma. The patients were two males and two females with a mean age of 65 years (range, 49–72 years). They had upper abdominal pain, weight loss and/or an incidentally discovered liver mass. None had evidence of a primary pancreatic tumor. Grossly, the tumors were large (mean size, 12 cm), well circumscribed and showed a lobulated cut surface. Histologically, they showed a predominantly microacinar pattern, with occasional trabecular, solid and microcystic areas. Cellular atypia and mitotic activity varied within the same tumor and from tumor to tumor. Immunohistochemically, the tumor cells were positive for cytokeratin 18 and at least one acinar cell marker (ie, trypsin, amylase or lipase), but were negative for cytokeratins 7, 19 and 20, HepPar-1, AFP, CD10, carcinoembryonic antigen, CD56, Islet-1 and CDX2. Two tumors stained focally for synaptophysin and chromogranin A. Adjacent liver parenchyma displayed no evidence of cirrhosis. During a mean follow-up of 22 months (range, 3–38 months) no metastases occurred, but one patient developed local recurrence. Our study demonstrates that acinar cell carcinoma of pancreatic type may also originate from the liver and can be readily distinguished from other primary liver neoplasms by its distinct histological and immunohistochemical features. Because our cases were observed within a rather short period, it is likely that this tumor type is so far underrecognized and has been mistaken as a variant of hepatocellular carcinoma, cholangiocarcinoma or any other liver tumor.

▶ The authors describe their recent series of 4 pancreatic-type acinar cell carcinomas of the liver in the past 4 years. They raise 3 key questions with regard to these rare tumors including: 1) Are these truly pancreatic in origin or do they represent a metaplastic form of hepatocellular/cholangiolar carcinoma? 2) Could these tumors be the result of an occult metastatic pancreatic primary?

3) If these are primary to the liver, how can the histogenesis be explained? Based on the frequency with which the authors encountered these tumors, their suggestion that these tumors are underrecognized and/or misclassified as hepatic or cholangiolar carcinomas is likely. At this point, with only a total of 5 cases of this type published, there are insufficient data to provide answers to the proposed questions. It is up to anatomic pathologists to increase their awareness of these tumors and investigate morphologic changes in liver mass lesions that are not typical for hepatocellular or cholangiolar carcinoma. Hepatic malignancies that are atypical and negative for Hep-Par 1 should be evaluated for acinar markers such as trypsin, amylase, and lipase. It would have been interesting if the authors had investigated other stains typically used for the diagnosis of hepatocellular carcinoma such as reticulin and CD34.

M. L. Smith, MD

Reticulin Loss in Benign Fatty Liver: An Important Diagnostic Pitfall When Considering a Diagnosis of Hepatocellular Carcinoma
Singhi AD, Jain D, Kakar S, et al (The Johns Hopkins Med Institutions, Baltimore, MD; Yale Univ School of Medicine, New Haven, CT; Univ of California, San Francisco; et al)
Am J Surg Pathol 36:710-715, 2012

Reticulin stains are commonly used in surgical pathology to assess mass lesions for the possibility of hepatocellular carcinoma. The loss of normal reticulin staining can help support a diagnosis of hepatocellular carcinoma, and this stain has proven to be particularly helpful on limited biopsies and fine-needle aspirates. However, an underappreciated diagnostic pitfall is that non-neoplastic liver tissue can also show reticulin loss when there is fatty change. To further characterize this important diagnostic pitfall, reticulin staining was studied in cases of nonalcoholic steatosis, nonalcoholic steatohepatitis, and hepatic adenomas with fatty change. A total of 112 cases with varying degrees of steatosis were collected from 4 academic centers, including 49 cases of steatosis, 49 cases of steatohepatitis, and 14 hepatic adenomas with fatty change. Steatosis was graded as mild (5% to 30% macrovesicular steatosis), moderate (31% to 60%), and marked (> 60%). Reticulin stains were scored as the number of foci with diminished reticulin staining in 10 hpf. A focus of diminished reticulin was scored when the extent of reticulin loss was similar to that seen in hepatocellular carcinomas. In the total study set, 28 cases showed mild steatosis, 40 cases showed moderate steatosis, and 44 cases showed marked steatosis. Interestingly, increasing amounts of fat were associated with decreased reticulin staining. For mild steatosis, reticulin loss was rare, with the number of foci of reticulin loss per 10 hpf averaging 0.8 (range, 0 to 3); however, this increased for moderate steatosis, which showed a mean of 3.0 foci per 10 hpf (range, 0 to 5), and was most prominent with marked steatosis, which showed an average of 5.8 foci of reticulin loss per 10 hpf (range, 5 to 8). An almost identical pattern was seen in cases of nonalcoholic steatohepatitis.

Overall, reticulin loss was not associated with the degree of inflammation or with the presence or absence of balloon cell change. Reticulin loss also did not correlate with fibrosis stage. In hepatic adenomas, reticulin loss was seen only in areas of fatty change, and decreased reticulin again paralleled the amount of steatosis, with more prominent reticulin loss in those cases with marked steatosis. In conclusion, reticulin loss that reaches levels seen in hepatocellular carcinoma can be seen focally in benign liver tissues with fatty change. Overall, loss of reticulin is more common and more extensive with marked fatty change and does not seem to be linked to inflammation or fibrosis stage. Loss of reticulin can also be seen in hepatic adenomas with fatty change. Increased awareness of this important diagnostic pitfall will help prevent overcalling of reticulin loss when evaluating biopsies and resections of hepatic neoplasms with fatty change.

▶ Pathologists who routinely review liver biopsy reticulin stains may very well have encountered the pitfall of decreased reticulin staining in areas of increased steatosis in their practice. This article helps to document and quantify this finding. As the authors note, the reticulin loss increases with increased steatosis and is not associated with features of steatohepatitis. This is a significant finding because many pathologists rely heavily on the loss of reticulin framework when distinguishing benign from malignant hepatocellular lesions. It is also significant because type-1 adenomas, which lack portal areas and have unpaired arteries (features of both adenoma and carcinoma), may also show increased steatosis. In the setting of unpaired arteries, absence of portal tracts, and decreased reticulin, an incorrect diagnosis of hepatocellular carcinoma is very easy to make. These findings emphasize the need for using other immunohistochemical findings to make a definitive diagnosis of hepatocellular carcinoma. There is an ever-growing list of markers in addition to reticulin to aid in distinguishing malignancy and also classifying other hepatic mass lesions. Among these are beta-catenin, C-reactive protein, glypican-3, HSP70, glutamine synthetase, and liver fatty-acid–binding protein.[1,2] Also, the key histologic features of carcinoma, including increased nuclear density and nuclear atypia, should not be overlooked. Finally, hepatocellular carcinoma is uncommon in patients without liver disease or significant fibrosis, and thus clinical history also plays an important role.

M. L. Smith, MD

References

1. Di Tommaso L, Destro A, Seok JY, et al. The application of markers (HSP70 GPC3 and GS) in liver biopsies is useful for detection of hepatocellular carcinoma. *J Hepatol.* 2009;50:746-754.
2. Shafizadeh N, Kakar S. Diagnosis of well-differentiated hepatocellular lesions: role of immunohistochemistry and other ancillary techniques. *Adv Anat Pathol.* 2011; 18:438-445.

Donor-Specific Human Leukocyte Antigen Antibodies of the Immunoglobulin G3 Subclass Are Associated With Chronic Rejection and Graft Loss After Liver Transplantation

Kaneku H, O'Leary JG, Taniguchi M, et al (Univ of California Los Angeles; Baylor Univ Med Ctr, Dallas, TX; One Lambda, Incorporated, Los Angeles, CA; et al)
Liver Transpl 18:984-992, 2012

In a previous study, we found that 92% of patients with chronic rejection had donor-specific human leukocyte antigen antibodies (DSAs), but surprisingly, 61% of comparator patients without rejection also had DSAs. We hypothesized that immunoglobulin G (IgG) subclasses were differentially distributed between the 2 groups. A modified single-antigen bead assay was used to detect the presence of individual IgG subclasses against human leukocyte antigen in 39 chronic rejection patients and 66 comparator patients. DSAs of the IgG1 subclass were most common and were found in 45% of all patients; they were followed by IgG3 DSAs (21%), IgG4 DSAs (14%), and IgG2 DSAs (13%). The percentage of patients with multiple IgG subclasses was significantly higher in the chronic rejection group versus the comparator group (50% versus 14%, $P < 0.001$). Patients with normal graft function in the presence of DSAs mostly had isolated IgG1, whereas patients with chronic rejection had a combination of IgG subclasses. Patients who developed DSAs of the IgG3 subclass showed an increased risk of graft loss (hazard ratio = 3.35, 95% confidence interval = 1.39-8.05) in comparison with patients with

TABLE 2.—HLA Antibody Characteristics

	Chronic Rejection Group (n = 39)	Comparator Group (n = 66)	P Value
IgG DSAs (%)			
Any DSAs ever	92	56	**<0.001**
Preformed DSAs	60	41	0.07
De novo DSAs	62	29	**0.001**
Post-OLT DSAs	79	48	**0.003**
DSA class I only	10	8	0.72
DSA class II only	39	27	0.23
DSA classes I and II	44	21	**0.02**
Post-OLT IgG subclass DSAs (%)			
IgG1	72	32	**<0.001**
IgG2	19	11	0.27
IgG3	38	14	**0.007**
IgG4	25	9	**0.04**
Post-OLT IgG subclass DSA profile (%)			
Single IgG subclass	25	24	0.94
Multiple IgG subclasses	50	14	**<0.001**

NOTE: Bolded values are significant.
- For preformed DSAs, chronic rejection (n = 35).
- For de novo and post-OLT DSAs, chronic rejection (n = 34).
- Post-OLT IgG subclass DSAs and DSA profile, chronic rejection (n = 32).

DSAs of other IgG subclasses or without DSAs. Although further study is needed, the determination of the IgG subclass in DSA-positive patients may help us to identify patients with a higher risk of chronic rejection and graft loss (Table 2).

▶ This is another article highlighting the increased interest in the possibility of compliment activation and liver allograft damage via donor-specific antibodies (DSA). Because many patients show positive DSA but no evidence of graft dysfunction, the goal was to identify elements of the DSA that could be used to distinguish pathologic versus nonpathologic DSA. The authors used a case-control study to investigate the role immunoglobulin G (IgG) subclassification may play in allograft injury. The results are shown in Table 2 and highlight the increase in IgG1 and IgG3 in the chronic rejection group. IgG3 and IgG1 have strong Fc receptors and are believed to be the strongest fixers of compliment. One of the challenges in this study was the ability to gather sufficient control cases because the study patients with chronic rejection were gathered from years ago. The chronic rejection cohort underwent transplant earlier and thus experienced different immunosuppression regimes (cyclosporine more likely than tacrolimus) and also had an increased risk of cytomegalovirus infection. Further study is needed in a more recent group of patients to determine if IgG subclassification is clinically relevant. It is interesting that in the more extensively studied kidney allograft population, subclassification does not seem relevant.

M. L. Smith, MD

Does Cytotechnician Training Influence the Accuracy of EUS-Guided Fine-needle Aspiration of Pancreatic Masses?
Petrone MC, Arcidiacono PG, Carrara S, et al (Vita-Salute San Raffaele Univ, Milan, Italy)
Dig Liver Dis 44:311-314, 2012

Background/Aim.—The presence of on-site cytopathologists improves the diagnostic yield of endoscopic ultrasound-guided fine needle aspiration (EUS-FNA) of pancreatic masses; however, on-site cytopathologists are not available to all endoscopic units. We hypothesized that experienced cyto-technicians can accurately assess whether an on-site pancreatic mass fine needle aspiration specimen is adequate. The aim of this study was to evaluate the effect of formal cytotechnician training on the diagnostic accuracy of EUS-FNA of pancreatic masses.

Methods.—Single-centre, prospective study. The cytotechnician made an on-site assessment of specimen adequacy with immediate evaluation of smears over a 12-month period (pre-training period) then over another 12-month period (post-training period), with a year's intermediate training when the cytopathologist and the cytotechnician worked together in the room. The gold standard used to establish the final diagnosis was based on a non-equivocal fine needle aspiration biopsy reviewed by the same expert

TABLE 4.—Diagnostic Value of Endoscopic Ultrasound-Fine Needle Aspiration in Pre- and Post-Training Periods

	Pre-Training Period $n = 107$ Mean (sd)	Post-Training Period $n = 95$ Mean (sd)	p Value
Sensitivity	71.4% (65/91)	89.2% (75/84)	0.003*
Specificity	93.7% (15/16)	100% (11/11)	0.39
PPV	98.4% (65/66)	100% (75/75)	0.28
NPV	36.5% (15/41)	57.1% (11/20)	0.17
Accuracy	74.8% (80/107)	90.5% (86/95)	0.003*

PPV, positive predictive value; NPV, negative predictive value.
*Statistically significant.

cytopathologist. The main outcome measurements were the cytotechnician diagnostic accuracy before and after the training period.

Results.—A total of 107 patients were enrolled in the pre-training period. Cytotechnician in-room adequacy was 68.2% (73/107). The diagnostic accuracy was 74.8%. The adequacy for the blind-review pathologist was 93.4% (100/107), significantly higher ($p = 0.008$) than the cytotechnician's results. During the posttraining period, 95 EUS-FNA were performed and reviewed. Cytotechnician in-room adequacy was 87.4% (83/95). The diagnostic accuracy was 90.5%. The adequacy for the blinded pathologist was 95.8% (91/95), not significantly different from the cytotechnician ($p = 0.23$).

Conclusions.—An adequate training period with an expert pathologist significantly improves the cytotechnician skill in terms of judging adequacy and diagnostic accuracy (Table 4).

▶ Over the past decade, the number of endoscopic ultrasound-guided fine-needle aspiration specimens has increased dramatically. Although many cytology services initially supplied a pathologist on site for the procedure, as the volumes increased, cytotechnologists have been widely used to confirm accuracy of the cytologic preparations before completing the procedure. This study shows how a year-long apprenticeship model of experiential learning can improve a cytotechnologist's skills in judging adequacy and determining diagnoses. Table 4 shows the pre- and posttraining improvements in sensitivity and accuracy. Perhaps even more significant is the statistically significant decrease in the mean number of passes required, from 3.7 down to 2.5 ($P = .01$). Fewer passes likely means less procedure time and fewer complications, although not specifically addressed in this study. This study highlights what most already inherently know: Teams working together in complex systems improve with experience. Our goal should be to create a simulated learning environment for cytopathologists and cytotechnologists to gain this type of experiential education without causing increasing patient risk with increased numbers of passes and decreased sensitivity and accuracy.

M. L. Smith, MD

Atypical hepatocellular adenoma—like neoplasms with β-catenin activation show cytogenetic alterations similar to well-differentiated hepatocellular carcinomas

Evason KJ, Grenert JP, Ferrell LD, et al (Univ of California, San Francisco)
Hum Pathol 2012 [Epub ahead of print]

The distinction of hepatocellular adenoma from well-differentiated hepatocellular carcinoma (HCC) arising in noncirrhotic liver can be challenging, particularly when tumors histologically resembling hepatocellular adenoma occur in unusual clinical settings such as in a man or an older woman or show focal atypical morphologic features. In this study, we examine the morphologic, immunohistochemical, and cytogenetic features of hepatocellular adenoma—like neoplasms occurring in men, women 50 years or older or younger than 15 years, and/or those with focal atypia (small cell change, pseudogland formation, and/or nuclear atypia), designated atypical hepatocellular neoplasms, where the distinction of hepatocellular adenoma versus HCC could not be clearly established. Immunohistochemistry was performed for β-catenin, glutamine synthetase, and serum amyloid A in 31 hepatocellular adenomas, 20 well-differentiated HCCs, and 40 atypical hepatocellular neoplasms. Chromosomal gains/losses had previously been determined in 37 cases using comparative genomic hybridization or fluorescence in situ hybridization. β-Catenin activation was observed in 35% of atypical hepatocellular neoplasms compared with 10% of typical hepatocellular adenomas ($P < .05$) and 55% of well-differentiated HCCs ($P = .14$). Cytogenetic changes typically observed in HCC were present in all atypical hepatocellular neoplasms with β-catenin activation. β-Catenin activation in atypical hepatocellular neoplasms was also associated with atypical morphologic features. Follow-up data were limited, but adverse outcome was observed in 2 atypical hepatocellular neoplasms with β-catenin activation (1 recurrence, 1 metastasis); transition to areas of HCC was observed in 1 case. The similarity in morphologic and cytogenetic features of β-catenin—activated hepatocellular adenoma—like tumors and HCC suggests that the former tumors represent an extremely well-differentiated variant of HCC (Table 3).

▶ It has become increasingly evident in recent years that hepatocellular carcinoma (HCC) is not relegated to patients with chronic liver disease and fibrosis. As the molecular classification of hepatocellular adenomas (HA) has undergone intensive study in the last 15 years, type II adenomas have been defined as having a β-catenin mutation and an increased risk of malignant transformation to HCC. This increase in risk has prompted more aggressive treatment suggestions for patients with type II HA and also raised the possibility of whether these lesions are actually extremely well-differentiated HCC. This study furthers the theory that these lesions actually represent early HCC and may require more aggressive treatment. In the study, an atypical HA was defined in 2 ways: (1) atypical age or sex (occurring in men or women older than 50 and younger than 15) and (2) atypical morphology (focal cytologic or architectural atypia involving less than 5% of the

TABLE 3.—Morphologic, Immunohistochemical, and Cytogenetic Features of AHNs and WD-HCCs

	AHN, % (n)	WD-HCC, % (n)	P
Age ≥50 y	40 (14/35)	71 (10/14)	.047*
Male sex	29 (10/35)	50 (7/14)	.15
Atypical morphologic features	70 (28/40)	100 (20/20)	.0062*
β-Catenin activated	35 (14/40)	55 (11/20)	.14
SAA positive	56 (20/36)	21 (4/19)	.014*
Chromosomal abnormalities typical of HCC	59 (10/17)	55 (6/11)	.82

*P < .05 was considered statistically significant.

tumor, including areas of small cell change, pseudogland formation, or nuclear atypia). Nuclear atypia was not further defined. Table 3 shows the similarities between these atypical HA and well-differentiated HCC. Note that only 35% and 55% of tumors showed β-catenin activation by immunohistochemistry in atypical HA and well-differentiated HCC, respectively. This suggests there may be other HA in addition to type II β-catenin—activated ones that have cytogenetic abnormalities and may represent low-grade HCC. Further molecular and genetic studies of all HA types is necessary.

M. L. Smith, MD

Diagnostic Utility of CD10 in Benign and Malignant Extrahepatic Bile Duct Lesions

Tretiakova M, Antic T, Westerhoff M, et al (Univ of Chicago Med Ctr, Chicago, IL; et al)
Am J Surg Pathol 36:101-108, 2012

CD10, a cell surface enzyme with neutral metalloendopeptidase activity, is a marker for intestinal epithelial brush border. It is also present in normal bile ducts and gallbladder epithelia but is absent in cholangiocarcinomas. However, the expression profile of CD10 in benign and malignant extrahepatic biliary lesions has not been studied. In this study, 69 biopsies, 9 resections, and 9 cell blocks prepared from fine-needle aspirations of the extrahepatic bile ducts from 86 patients were studied immunohistochemically for CD10 expression. The majority of cases contained normal biliary epithelium (NL, n = 64), along with foci of benign or malignant lesions in various combinations. Benign lesions included reactive atypia (n = 35), low-grade dysplasia of unknown significance (n = 21), and bile duct adenoma (BDA, n = 1). Malignant lesions included high-grade dysplasia (HGD, n = 45) and invasive adenocarcinoma (IC, n = 30). As expected, the NL showed strong continuous staining at the apical surface in all cases. Benign lesions were also CD10 positive in all but 3 cases; however, the staining pattern was discontinuous, with positive cells varying from 20% to 80%. None of the malignant lesions showed CD10 immunoreactivity, except for

TABLE 1.—Demographic Data of Studied Patients and CD10 Expression in Different Types of Lesions

Histologic Lesion	No. Cases	Mean Age	M:F Ratio	CD10 (+) Continuous*	CD10 (+) Discontinuous*	CD10 (−)
Normal biliary mucosa	64	67.1	1:1	60 (93.75%)	4 (6.25%)	0
RA	35	59.2	1.2:1	0	33 (94.3%)	2 (5.7%)
LGD and BDA	22	69.5	1.5:1	2 (9%)	19 (86.4%)	1 (4.6%)
HGD	45	69.1	0.7:1	0	2 (4%)	43 (96%)
Invasive carcinoma	30	68.7	1:1	0	1 (3%)	29 (97%)

F indicates female; M, male.
*All CD10-positive cases with both continuous and discontinuous staining patterns showed moderate-to-strong immunoreactivity. The difference in CD10 expression was strongly statistically significant between all studied lesions ($P < 0.001$).

2 HGD cases and 1 IC case, which exhibited focal staining. The Pearson χ^2 and Fisher exact tests showed significant statistical difference in CD10 expression among the study groups ($P < 0.001$). Our findings suggest that absence of CD10 expression in strips of atypical biliary epithelial cells may be a phenotype associated with malignant transformation and may serve as a useful marker to aid in the evaluation of bile duct biopsies, in which distinction between benign and malignant lesions on biopsies or cytology specimens can be extremely challenging because of limited sampling, crush artifact, and frequent inflammatory/reactive changes (Table 1).

▶ Small biopsy specimens from the biliary tree for the evaluation of dysplasia and malignancy can be extremely challenging cases, many of which show some atypical morphologic features. This article suggests CD10 may be a useful ancillary study in these cases to help support a benign or malignant interpretation. Table 1 shows the results, and, if the group of atypical cells is continuously positive for CD10 or completely negative, the results may be useful. However, in the areas in which the cytologic distinction may be most difficult (low- vs high-grade dysplasia) the staining results often are discontinuous and may be less useful. One of the criticisms of this article is the use of histologic morphology as the gold standard. While the article states 3 pathologists before inclusion reviewed each case, it is not clear if this was a blinded or group review and how diagnostic discrepancies among the reviewers were handled. Only 44% of the study cases had confirmation of the biopsy diagnosis in the form of a surgical resection. Therefore, although the trend is toward loss of CD10 during the transformative process from benign to malignant, the point at which the loss happens still remains unclear. These specimens may benefit from other methodologies to detect risk of malignancy and genetic alteration like florescence in situ hybridization.

M. L. Smith, MD

Immunohistochemical Markers on Needle Biopsies Are Helpful for the Diagnosis of Focal Nodular Hyperplasia and Hepatocellular Adenoma Subtypes

Bioulac-Sage P, Cubel G, Taouji S, et al (Hôpital Pellegrin, Bordeaux, France; Université Bordeaux Segalen, France; et al)
Am J Surg Pathol 36:1691-1699, 2012

Phenotypic identification of focal nodular hyperplasia (FNH) and hepatocellular adenoma (HCA) subtypes using immunohistochemical markers has been developed from their molecular characteristics. Our objective was to evaluate the sensitivity of these markers in the definitive diagnosis of these lesions by core needle biopsies. A total of 239 needle biopsies paired with their surgical resection specimen (group A) or without an associated

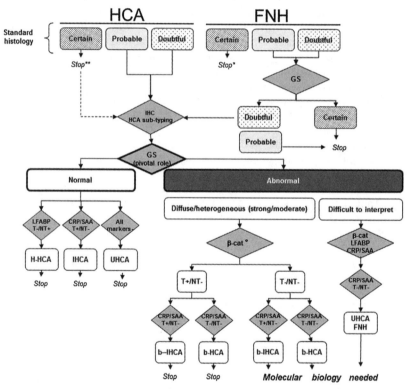

FIGURE 1.—Algorithm for IHC diagnosis of benign hepatocellular nodules: FNH and HCA. GS is not always mandatory for the diagnosis of FNH (*) or HCA (**) in routine practice, but was performed in this study. IHC is mandatory for HCA subtyping. IHC markers are presented in gray squares with their results positive (+) or negative (−) in tumor (T) and nontumoral liver (NT). °Aberrant β-catenin nuclear staining. Final diagnosis of HCA subtypes are: HNF1α inactivated (H-HCA), inflammatory (IHCA), β-catenin activated (b-HCA), β-catenin-activated inflammatory (b-IHCA), or unclassified (UHCA). (Reprinted from Bioulac-Sage P, Cubel G, Taouji S, et al. Immunohistochemical markers on needle biopsies are helpful for the diagnosis of focal nodular hyperplasia and hepatocellular adenoma subtypes. *Am J Surg Pathol.* 2012;36:1691-1699, with permission from Lippincott Williams & Wilkins.)

TABLE 2.—Degree of Confidence in the Diagnosis of HCA Subtypes

HCA Subtype	Markers	Certain	Diagnosis Probable	Doubtful
H-HCA	LFABP	Clear-cut difference between T negativity and NT positivity	Weak difference between T negativity and NT positivity	T negativity difficult to appreciate in the absence of NT tissue
IHCA	SAA/CRP	Clear-cut difference between T positivity and NT negativity	Difference between T positivity and NT negativity but some staining in the nontumoral liver	Very heterogenous staining and some staining in the NT liver
b-HCA	GS	Diffuse/heterogeneous (strong to moderate) staining	Diffuse/heterogeneous (strong to moderate) staining	Difficult to interpret (mostly focal)
b-IHCA	β-Catenin	Nuclear staining (few to numerous)	No nuclear staining	No nuclear staining
	—	See IHCA and b-HCA	See IHCA and b-HCA	See IHCA and b-HCA
UHCA	All markers	All negative	All negative but standard histology in favor of IHCA or FNH	All negative/GS difficult to interpret/standard histology in favor of IHCA or FNH

b-HCA indicates β-catenin-activated HCA; b-IHCA, β-catenin inflammatory HCA; H-HCA, HNF1α-inactivated HCA; IHCA, inflammatory HCA; NT, nontumoral liver; T, tumor; UHCA, unclassified HCA.

resection specimen (group B) were reviewed. Using a step-by-step algorithm after standard staining, appropriate immunostaining analyses were performed to determine the certainty of diagnosis of FNH, HNF1α-inactivated HCA, inflammatory HCA, β-catenin-activated HCA, or unclassified HCA. The diagnosis of FNH was certain or probable on routine stains in 53% of needle biopsies of group A, whereas after glutamine synthetase staining, the diagnosis was certain in 86.7% as compared with 100% on the corresponding surgical specimen ($P = 0.04$). In needle biopsies of group A, the diagnosis of HCA was certain on routine stains in 58.6% as compared with 94.3% on surgical specimens. After specific immunostaining, diagnosis was established on biopsies with 74.3% certainty, including all HCA subtypes, with similar distribution in surgical specimens. For each "certain diagnosis" paired diagnostic test (biopsy and surgical specimen), a positive correlation was observed ($P < 0.001$). No significant difference was observed between groups A and B for FNH ($P = 0.714$) or for HCA subtypes ($P = 0.750$). Compared with surgical specimens, immunohistochemical analysis performed on biopsies allowed the discrimination of FNH from HCA and the identification of HCA subtypes with good performance (Fig 1, Table 2).

▶ The classification of benign hepatocellular lesions has undergone many changes in the past decade and there are several new immunohistochemical (IHC) markers available. This article validates the use of IHC on needle core biopsy specimens from hepatic mass lesions and provides a nice algorithm for clinical use (Fig 1). As the algorithm demonstrates, glutamine synthetase (GS) plays a pivotal role in the classification process. GS may be a good candidate for anyone considering validating new antibodies in the immunohistochemistry laboratory. In addition to the use in classification of hepatocellular adenoma and the diagnosis of focal nodular hyperplasia, GS may also be used as a marker of malignancy in the diagnosis of hepatocellular carcinoma, along with glypican-3 and HSP70. It should be noted that the stains used in this study can be challenging to interpret and a table of "confidence levels" depending on the pattern of staining is provided (Table 2). Liver fatty acid binding protein can be a particularly challenging stain to optimize in the laboratory.

M. L. Smith, MD

Keratin 19 Demonstration of Canal of Hering Loss in Primary Biliary Cirrhosis: "Minimal Change PBC"?

Khan F, Komarla AR, Mendoza PG, et al (Beth Israel Med Ctr of Albert Einstein College of Medicine, NewYork)

Hepatology 2012 [Epub ahead of print]

Liver biopsy is important for diagnosing primary biliary cirrhosis (PBC). Prior investigations suggest that immunostaining for biliary keratin 19 (K19) may show the earliest changes suspicious for PBC, namely loss of the canals of Hering (CoH). We aimed to study the clinical outcomes of

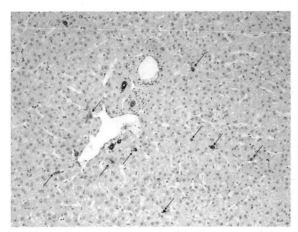

FIGURE 1.—Normal portal tract with immunostain for keratin 19. Numerous K19 positive canal of Hering cross-sections are arrayed in the periportal region surrounding this normal portal tract (arrows) (DAB, Hematoxylin counterstain, original magnification 10x). (Reprinted from Khan F, Komarla AR, Mendoza PG, et al. Keratin 19 demonstration of canal of Hering loss in primary biliary cirrhosis: "Minimal change PBC"? *Hepatology.* 2012, with permission from John Wiley and Sons.)

patients whose biopsy specimens appeared histologically near normal or with minimal inflammatory changes, but in which K19 staining revealed widespread periportal CoH loss, a finding we have termed "minimal change PBC."

Methods.—Ten patients were identified prospectively as having nearly normal or mildly inflamed biopsy specimens without diagnostic/suggestive histologic features of PBC, but with near complete CoH loss; 6 had available follow-up clinical data, one had follow-up biopsy. Controls for clinical and/ or K19 analysis included 6 normal livers and biopsy specimens from 10 patients with confirmed early PBC, 10 with early stage chronic hepatitis C (CHC), and 9 with resolving, self-limited hepatitis (RSLH).

Main Results.—Staining for K19 in normal controls, livers with "minimal change" PBC, CHC, and RSLH showed 9.2 + 6.0, 0.44 + 0.37 ($p < 0.0001$), 5.7 + 4.6 (n.s.), 4.1 + 2.1 ($p < 0.02$) CoH per portal tract, respectively. Patients with available clinical follow up, compared to patients with diagnostic early-stage PBC biopsies, showed identical treatment responses to ursodeoxycholic acid, similar rates and types of non-hepatic autoimmune diseases, and/or subsequent development of autoimmune hepatitis overlap syndrome.

Conclusion.—We suggest that CoH loss demonstrated by K19 immunostaining is an early feature in PBC. Clinical findings in years following biopsy, including response to ursodeoxycholic acid, show identical changes to patients with biopsy confirmed PBC. Thus, suggest that this "minimal change" feature that may be support a clinical diagnosis of PBC even in the absence of characteristic, granulomatous, duct destructive lesions (Fig 1).

▶ The diagnosis of early-stage primary biliary cirrhosis (PBC) can be challenging, as classic bile duct damage, including granulomatous damage, may be very focal and not seen on initial levels. Many hepatopathologists suggest obtaining multiple deeper hematoxylin and eosin—stained levels in an effort to search for these focal findings. Unfortunately, it is not uncommon to have a patient with a clinical suspicion of PBC and a normal biopsy without diagnostic findings. This article suggests the possibility of making the diagnosis of early-stage PBC based on the absence of canals of Hering. Fig 1 shows the canals of Hering in a normal portal tract. Based on the results, in appropriate clinical settings, it seems reasonable to perform biliary epithelial immunohistochemical stains and assess for canal of Hering density. Obviously, this finding needs further investigation with a larger sample size and then a prospectively designed study. It should be noted that the article used nonbiliary-type diseases for controls. It will be important and also interesting to see how the canal of Hering density in other biliary diseases compares with cases of PBC.

M. L. Smith, MD

Sinusoidal C4d Deposits in Liver Allografts Indicate an Antibody-Mediated Response: Diagnostic Considerations in the Evaluation of Liver Allografts

Kozlowski T, Andreoni K, Schmitz J, et al (Univ of North Carolina at Chapel Hill; Ohio State Univ, Columbus)
Liver Transpl 18:641-658, 2012

There is a paucity of data concerning the correlation of complement component 4d (C4d) staining in liver allografts and antibody-mediated rejection. Data about the location and character of C4d deposits in native and allograft liver tissues are inconsistent. We performed C4d immunofluorescence (IF) on 141 fresh-frozen liver allograft biopsy samples and native livers, documented the pattern of C4d IF staining, and correlated the findings with the presence of donor-specific alloantibodies (DSAs). A linear/granular sinusoidal pattern of C4d IF was noted in 18 of 28 biopsy samples obtained after transplantation from patients with positive crossmatch and detectable donor-specific alloantibody (pos-XM/DSA) findings. None of the 59 tested biopsy samples from patients with negative crossmatch and detectable donor-specific alloantibody (neg-XM/DSA) findings were C4d-positive ($P < 0.001$). No significant association was found between

TABLE 6.—Interlaboratory Variability: Selected Cases From Table 5

| | | | IHC Protocols | |
| | | | | UHB |
Case	IF Protocol: UNC	UNC	First	Second
2	Diffuse, strong, linear/granular	0	0	Focal, faint
5	Diffuse, moderate, granular	0	0	Focal, weak, linear/granular
4	Focal, weak, linear	0	0	Focal, faint
13	Focal, faint	0	0	NA
14	Diffuse, strong, linear	0	0	Focal, moderate, linear/granular
Control	0	0	NA	0
Control	0	0	0	0

pos-XM/DSA and C4d IF staining in other nonsinusoidal liver compartments. To compare the results of sinusoidal C4d staining with IF and 2 immunohistochemistry (IHC) techniques, C4d IHC was performed on 19 liver allograft biopsy samples in which a sinusoidal pattern of C4d IF had been noted. Sinusoidal C4d IHC findings were negative for 17 of the 19 biopsy samples; 2 showed weak and focal staining, and both patients had pos-XM/DSA findings. Portal vein endothelium staining was present in only 1 IF-stained biopsy sample (pos-XM/DSA) but in 11 IHC-stained biopsy samples (2 of the 11 samples had neg-XM/DSA findings). We conclude that sinusoidal C4d deposits detected by IF in frozen tissue samples from liver allograft recipients correlate with the presence of DSAs and an antibody-mediated alloresponse. These observations are similar to findings reported for other solid organ transplants and can provide relevant information for patient management. Further validation of IHC techniques for C4d detection in liver allograft tissue is required (Table 6).

▶ This is the most thorough study of C4d, donor-specific antibodies, and antibody-mediated rejection (AMR) in liver allograft specimens to date. AMR in the liver historically has been described as being exceedingly rare and not of significant clinical consequence. The majority of what we know about AMR comes of the renal transplant literature, where it has been extensively studied for years. Because of the lack of interest in C4d staining, most evaluations of C4d deposition in liver allografts have been based on immunohistochemistry (IHC) rather than immunofluoresence (IF) because of the lack of fresh frozen liver allograft tissue available. It is well established in the renal allograft literature that C4d staining by the IF method is more sensitive than that of the IHC method, and this study seems to confirm this finding in the liver (data shown in Table 6). Although AMR is still likely a rare cause of graft dysfunction, the data presented here suggest that AMR should be considered if there are no other obvious biopsy abnormalities. In the future, we may be setting aside a few millimeters of biopsy cores for IF C4d studies but likely only in selected patients. Finally, their data support only sinusoidal C4d reactivity as being suspicious for AMR.

M. L. Smith, MD

Beyond "Cirrhosis": A Proposal From the International Liver Pathology Study Group
Hytiroglou P, Snover DC, Alves V, et al (Aristotle Univ Med School, Thessaloniki, Greece; Fairview Southdale Hosp, Edina, MN; Univ of São Paulo School of Medicine, Brazil; et al)
Am J Clin Pathol 137:5-9, 2012

"Cirrhosis" is a morphologic term that has been used for almost 200 years to denote the end stage of a variety of chronic liver diseases. The term implies a condition with adverse prognosis due to the well-known complications of portal hypertension, hepatocellular carcinoma, and liver failure. However, recent advances in the diagnosis and treatment of chronic liver

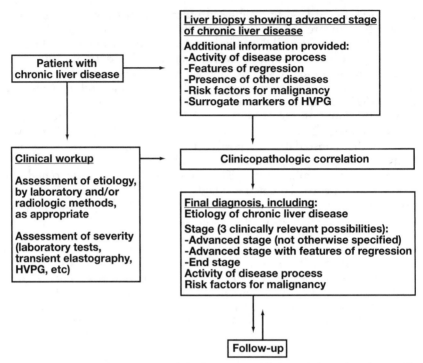

FIGURE 1.—A contemporary approach for the assessment of advanced chronic liver diseases. The stage is determined or confirmed by liver biopsy. The final diagnosis is derived from clinicopathologic correlation (assisted by follow-up, as needed), and includes the etiology, the stage, the activity of the disease process, and risk factors for malignancy. HVPG, hepatic venous pressure gradient. (Reprinted from Hytiroglou P, Snover DC, Alves V, et al. Beyond "cirrhosis": a proposal from the international liver pathology study group. *Am J Clin Pathol.* 2012;137:5-9, with permission from American Society for Clinical Pathology.)

diseases have changed the natural history of cirrhosis significantly. This consensus document by the International Liver Pathology Study Group challenges the usefulness of the word cirrhosis in modern medicine and suggests that this is an appropriate time to consider discontinuing the use of this term. The role of pathologists should evolve to the diagnosis of advanced stage of chronic liver disease, with emphasis on etiology, grade of activity, features suggestive of progression or regression, presence of other diseases, and risk factors for malignancy, within the perspective of an integrated clinico-pathologic assessment (Fig 1).

▶ Pathologists who routinely sign out liver biopsy specimens already recognize the clinical status spectrum of patients whose biopsies show so-called cirrhosis. Some are in multiorgan failure and are in dire need of a liver allograft for survival, whereas others are incidentally found to have elevated liver function tests and are completely asymptomatic. Within the article, the point is made that what is really needed is a staging system for patients with advanced liver disease that includes components of pathology (collagen proportionate area,[1] evidence of regression), hemodynamics (hepatic venous pressure gradient), and transient elastography. This potential staging system may help to further stratify advanced liver disease patients. Fig 1 is the recommendation from the International Study Group for the multidisciplinary approach to patients with advanced stage liver disease. From the pathologist perspective, an emphasis is put on retiring the use of the term "cirrhosis" in favor of "advanced stage" and reporting additional value added features such as the presence of regression,[2] disease activity, and malignant risk factors. Obviously, the term "cirrhosis" is firmly entrenched in our professions, and moving away from this will take time and evidence in increased usefulness of other proposals.

M. L. Smith, MD

References

1. Calvaruso V, Burroughs AK, Standish R, et al. Computer-assisted image analysis of liver collagen: relationship to Ishak scoring and hepatic venous pressure gradient. *Hepatology.* 2009;49:1236-1244.
2. Wanless IR, Nakashima E, Sherman M. Regression of human cirrhosis. Morphologic features and the genesis of incomplete septal cirrhosis. *Arch Pathol Lab Med.* 2000;124:1599-1607.

A Morphometric and Immunohistochemical Study to Assess the Benefit of a Sustained Virological Response in Hepatitis C Virus Patients With Cirrhosis

D'Ambrosio R, Aghemo A, Rumi MG, et al (Università degli Studi di Milano, Italy; et al)
Hepatology 56:532-543, 2012

Although annular fibrosis is the hallmark of cirrhosis, other microscopic changes that affect liver function such as sinusoid capillarization or loss of metabolic zonation are common. A sustained virological response (SVR) may halt fibrosis deposition in hepatitis C virus (HCV)-infected patients, but its impact on the other cirrhosis-associated lesions is unknown. The aim of this study was to assess the impact of an SVR on cirrhosis-related histopathological features. Paired pre- and posttreatment liver biopsies from 38 HCV patients with cirrhosis with an SVR were analyzed. Fibrosis was staged using the METAVIR scoring system, and the area of fibrosis was measured using morphometry. Ductular proliferation, metabolic zonation, sinusoid capillarization, and hepatic stellate cell activation were assessed by anti-cytokeratin-7, anti-glutamine synthetase (GS), anti-cytochrome P4502E1 (CYP2E1), anti-CD34, and anti a-smooth muscle actin (αSMA). After 61 months from an SVR, cirrhosis regression was observed in 61%, and the collagen content decreased in 89%. Although periportal and lobular necroinflammation vanished, portal inflammation persisted in 66%. Ductular proliferation decreased in 92%. Before treatment, metabolic zonation was lost, as shown by GS and CYP2E1, in 71% and 88%, respectively, with normalization in 79% and 73%, after an

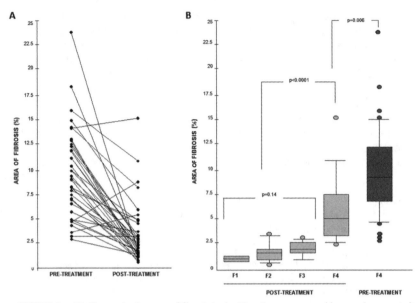

FIGURE 2.—(A) Changes in the areas of fibrosis in the 38 patients, as assessed by morphometry individually in pre- and posttreatment liver biopsies. (B) Distribution of the area of fibrosis as assessed by morphometry on the 38 pretreatment (right) and posttreatment (left) liver biopsies according to META-VIR fibrosis stage. (Reprinted from D'Ambrosio R, Aghemo A, Rumi MG, et al. A morphometric and immunohistochemical study to assess the benefit of a sustained virological response in hepatitis C virus patients with cirrhosis. *Hepatology.* 2012;56:532-543, with permission from Hepatology and John Wiley and Sons.)

SVR. Conversely, no changes in sinusoidal capillarization were observed after treatment, as assessed by CD34 ($P = 0.41$) and αSMA ($P = 0.95$). Finally, no differences in all the immunohistochemical scores emerged whether or not cirrhosis persisted.

Conclusion.—Cirrhosis regression and decreased fibrosis are frequently observed among HCV patients with cirrhosis with an SVR. Despite ductular proliferation vanishing and lobular zonation restoration, portal inflammation and sinusoidal capillarization may not regress after viral eradication (Fig 2).

▶ As more patients attain sustained viral responses (SVR) from treatment for hepatitis C virus infection, the pathology community will have increased opportunity to evaluate biopsies for regression of cirrhosis. This prospective study details a variety of post-SVR biopsy changes in addition to fibrosis. Subjects had at least 4 years of SVR, and the median biopsy length pretreatment was 18 mm, whereas the posttreatment length was 30 mm. Although the authors discuss the possibility that biopsy size may impact the fibrosis stage, they argue that the longer size posttreatment reduces the risk of staging error. Perhaps biopsy used for initial designation of cirrhosis would be more likely to have staging error. Fig 2 shows the changes in fibrosis between the pre- and posttreatment groups. Although there is certainly a trend to decreased fibrosis by morphometry, the pretreatment biopsy shows a large range of area of fibrosis by percentage. Further outcome-based studies are required to evaluate the prognosis of such regression. The findings from this study will help pathologists as they will be increasingly asked to evaluate liver biopsies in the setting of potential cirrhosis regression. For further reading, please see reference list.[1]

M. L. Smith, MD

Reference

1. Wanless IR, Nakashima E, Sherman M. Regression of human cirrhosis. Morphologic features and the genesis of incomplete septal cirrhosis. *Arch Pathol Lab Med.* 2000;124:1599-1607.

Accuracy and Disagreement of Computed Tomography and Magnetic Resonance Imaging for the Diagnosis of Small Hepatocellular Carcinoma and Dysplastic Nodules: Role of Biopsy
Sersté T, Barrau V, Ozenne V, et al (Hôpital Beaujon, Clichy, France)
Hepatology 55:800-806, 2012

Liver macronodules, ranging from benign to low-grade or high-grade dysplastic nodules (LGDNs/HGDNs) and hepatocellular carcinoma (HCC), may develop during chronic liver diseases (CLDs). Current guidelines were recently updated and the noninvasive criteria for the diagnosis of small HCC are based on a single typical radiological pattern and nonconclusive coincidental findings with two techniques. This study aimed to assess the accuracy and disagreements of noninvasive multiphasic examinations for the diagnosis of HCC and dysplastic nodules (DNs) and the role of biopsy. Seventy-four consecutive patients with CLD with ultrasound-detected 1-2-cm nodules underwent, within 1 month, multiphasic computed tomography (CT), magnetic resonance imaging (MRI), and biopsy of the nodule. Median age was 60 years; 33 patients (45%) had hepatitis C virus, 20 (27%) had hepatitis B virus, and 13 (18%) patients had no cirrhosis. Biopsy revealed 47 HCCs, 6 HGDNs, 1 LGDNs, 1 cholangiocarcinoma, and 1 epithelioid hemangioendothelioma. There were no tumors in the other 18 patients. All patients (31 of 31; 100%) who had conclusive coincidental findings (i.e., arterial enhancement and washout) on both examinations had HCC or HGDN (sensitivity, 57%; specificity, 100%). All patients (51 of 51; 100%) who had conclusive findings on at least one of the two examinations had HCC or HGDN (sensitivity, 96%; specificity, 100%). There was a disagreement regarding imaging findings between CT and MRI in 21 of 74 (28%) patients and no washout on both examinations in 23 of 74 patients (31%). In these 44 patients, liver biopsy provided an initial accurate diagnosis.

Conclusion.—The noninvasive diagnosis of HCC or HGDN can be obtained if arterial enhancement and washout are found in a single dynamic imaging examination. These findings are frequently discordant on both CT

TABLE 3.—Diagnostic Accuracy of CT and MRI for the Diagnosis of 1-2-cm Hepatocellular and HGDNs*

		Patient Number	Sensitivity (%)	Specificity (%)	Positive Predictive Value (%)	Negative Predictive Value (%)
CTscan	Suspicious[§]	51	43/53 (81)	13/21 (61)	43/51 (84)	13/23 (57)
	Conclusive[‖]	40	40/53 (75)	21/21 (100)	40/40 (100)	21/34 (59)
MRI	Suspicious	57	48/53 (90)	12/21 (57)	48/57 (84)	12/17 (70)
	Conclusive	42	42/53 (79)	21/21 (100)	42/42 (100)	21/32 (66)
Arterial uptake+washout at CT **and/or** MRI[†]	Criteria positive	51	51/53 (96)	21/21 (100)	51/51 (100)	21/23 (91)
Arterial uptake+washout at CT **and** MRI[‡]	Criteria positive	31	31/53 (57)	21/21 (100)	31/31 (100)	21/43 (49)

*N = 53. The patient with LGDN was not included.
[†]At least one typical vascular pattern on CT and/or MRI.
[‡]Coincidental typical vascular pattern on both CT and MRI.
[§]Suspicious refers arterial uptake of contrast medium.
[‖]Conclusive refers to arterial uptake of contrast medium and washout of contrast medium during portal or delayed phases.

and MRI, supporting the place of biopsy for the diagnosis of small HCCs (Table 3).

▶ Hepatocellular carcinoma (HCC) is being increasingly diagnosed on imaging studies such as computed tomography (CT) and magnetic resonance imaging (MRI) by demonstrating arterial enhancement and washout.[1,2] From a practical perspective, combining the cases confirmed as HCC and high-grade dysplastic nodules (HGDN) is reasonable because both lesions should be treated. In addition, the pathologic distinction between these 2 lesions on needle core biopsy alone can be very challenging. Indeed, 6 of the 7 cases initially diagnosed as HGDN progressed to HCC over time. It is not surprising that requiring 2 diagnostic modalities (CT and MRI) decreases the sensitivity (from 95% to 57%). Table 3 shows the accuracy of various imaging results with regard to sensitivity and specificity. On the surface this may seem concerning for pathologists; however, there are many other beneficial reasons to have biopsy material, including the ability to grade the tumor and the ability to evaluate the adjacent non-neoplastic hepatic parenchyma as well as the potential for individualized molecular testing on the tissue. One strength of this article is the inclusion of non-cirrhotic patients (18% of the total sample).

M. L. Smith, MD

References

1. International Consensus Group for Hepatocellular Neoplasia The International Consensus Group for Hepatocellular Neoplasia. Pathologic diagnosis of early hepatocellular carcinoma: a report of the international consensus group for hepatocellular neoplasia. *Hepatology.* 2009;49:658-664.
2. Bruix J, Sherman M. Management of hepatocellular carcinoma: an update. *Hepatology.* 2011;53:1020-1022.

Histopathology of De Novo Autoimmune Hepatitis

Pongpaibul A, Venick RS, McDiarmid SV, et al (Mahidol Univ, Nakhon Pathom, Thailand; Univ of California Los Angeles)
Liver Transpl 18:811-818, 2012

De novo autoimmune hepatitis (DAIH) is a well-recognized complication of pediatric liver transplantation (LT). The diagnosis is largely based on elevated liver function test results and the development of autoimmune antibodies. The histology of DAIH was first described in 1998. We present detailed histological data from the largest series to date of pretreatment and posttreatment biopsy samples from pediatric LT patients with DAIH. The histological evaluation included first an assessment of the predominant pattern of injury (hepatitis, rejection, or bile duct obstruction). Then, the necroinflammatory activity (interface, lobular, and perivenular), plasma cell density, rejection activity index, and fibrosis were scored. Seventy of 685 pediatric patients (10.2%) who underwent LT developed DAIH according to clinical and biopsy findings. Fifty-one pretreatment biopsy samples and 38 posttreatment biopsy samples were available for a retrospective review. The predominant pattern of injury (hepatitis, rejection, or bile duct obstruction) was determined, and biopsy samples were scored for the necroinflammatory activity (interface, lobular, and perivenular), plasma cell density, rejection activity index, and fibrosis. The most common pattern of injury was lobular hepatitis, which was frequently unaccompanied by interface necroinflammatory activity or prominent plasma cell infiltrates. Seven of the 51 cases had features strongly suggestive of acute rejection. Posttreatment biopsy samples showed a reduction in the degree of necroinflammatory activity and plasma cell infiltrates. In most patients, the degree of fibrosis was stable or had regressed. Because the histological features of DAIH are variable and nonspecific, a high index of suspicion and correlation with autoimmune antibodies are necessary to establish the diagnosis. In the majority of patients with DAIH, treatment appears to yield good clinical outcomes and histological improvements.

▶ Posttransplant de novo autoimmune hepatitis (DAIH) is increasingly described as a long-term complication after pediatric liver transplantation. DAIH is characterized by graft dysfunction, the development of autoimmune antibodies, and histologic evidence of hepatitis in liver transplant recipients without previous history of autoimmune liver disease. The article highlights the mild nature of the histological changes of DAIH. The predominant pattern of injury is, not surprisingly, hepatitic, but the hepatitis is lobular and mild, often with no evidence of plasma cell-rich infiltrate or of piecemeal/interface hepatitis. The latter is considered the hallmark of autoimmune hepatitis. A total of 18% of the samples had diagnosis of acute or chronic rejection in addition to DAIH.

The distinction of autoimmune hepatitis from rejection is histologically and conceptually difficult. As reviewed in previous work,[1] our criteria to distinguish the 2 may not be based on true pathogenetic mechanisms. Interface hepatitis is one of the criteria used for diagnosis of DAIH in the allograft,[1] and it is reported as absent in several cases in this report. The patients had histological response to treatment (less inflammation and no progression or regression of fibrosis at follow-up).

If the observations of the study are confirmed, it seems opportune to consider antibody testing in a larger spectrum of liver allograft patients manifesting without the classic features of autoimmune hepatitis in order to consider the possibility of DAIH.

S. S. Raab, MD

Reference

1. Banff working group, Demetris AJ, Adeyi O, Bellamy CO. Liver biopsy interpretation for causes of late liver allograft dysfunction. *Hepatology*. 2006;44:489-501.

5 Dermatopathology

Germline mutations in *BAP1* predispose to melanocytic tumors
Wiesner T, Obenauf AC, Murali R, et al (Med Univ of Graz, Austria; Memorial Sloan-Kettering Cancer Ctr, NY; et al)
Nat Genet 43:1018-1021, 2011

Common acquired melanocytic nevi are benign neoplasms that are composed of small, uniform melanocytes and are typically present as flat or slightly elevated pigmented lesions on the skin. We describe two families with a new autosomal dominant syndrome characterized by multiple, skin-colored, elevated melanocytic tumors. In contrast to common acquired nevi, the melanocytic neoplasms in affected family members ranged histopathologically from epithelioid nevi to atypical melanocytic proliferations that showed overlapping features with melanoma. Some affected individuals developed uveal or cutaneous melanomas. Segregating with this phenotype, we found inactivating germline mutations of *BAP1*, which encodes a ubiquitin carboxy-terminal hydrolase. The majority of melanocytic neoplasms lost the remaining wild-type allele of *BAP1* by various somatic alterations. In addition, we found *BAP1* mutations in a subset of sporadic melanocytic neoplasms showing histological similarities to the familial tumors. These findings suggest that loss of *BAP1* is associated with a clinically and morphologically distinct type of melanocytic neoplasm.

▶ This study reports the discovery of a genetic syndrome resulting from loss of function of BAP1, a protein likely involved in DNA damage repair. These families develop histologically and clinically distinct melanocytic tumors. They report several affected family members that also develop cutaneous and uveal melanomas. This syndrome is certainly important for pathologists who routinely read skin biopsies to understand because helping to identify affected individuals and families is significant, however rare. Another feature of their findings may have more widespread impact. They also found alterations of BAP1 genes in sporadic lesions without the autosomal dominantly inherited syndrome seen in the familial cases. In these latter instances, the lesions have the similar characteristic histopathologic features as the lesions discovered in familial cases. In doing so this report also proposes a nonfamilial clinicopathologic entity, or should we say a clinicopathologic and genetic entity? This is yet another instance where our nosology for melanocytic lesions is being refined by molecular techniques and improved genetic understating. Interestingly, 2 of these sporadic lesions discovered to have BAP1 alterations where originally classified as "atypical Spitz tumors." Spitzoid lesions, as many of us are all too well aware, are renowned

95

for being among the most challenging dermatopathology quandaries, and here we find more evidence that these are not a heterogeneous collection of lesions; more importantly, we now have the opportunity to bring a bit of diagnostic clarity to a subset of these cases. Possibly most significantly, this report brings us one step closer to a molecular understating of melanocytic lesions.

J. Wisell, MD

Cutaneous γδ T-cell Lymphomas: A Spectrum of Presentations With Overlap With Other Cytotoxic Lymphomas

Guitart J, Weisenburger DD, Subtil A, et al (Northwestern Univ Feinberg Med School, Chicago, IL; Univ of Nebraska Med Ctr, Omaha, Nebraska; Yale Univ, New Haven, CT; et al)

Am J Surg Pathol 36:1656-1665, 2012

We reviewed our multicenter experience with gamma-delta (γδ) T-cell lymphomas first presenting in the skin. Fifty-three subjects with a median age of 61 years (range, 25 to 91 y) were diagnosed with this disorder. The median duration of the skin lesions at presentation was 1.25 years (range, 1 mo to 20 y). The most common presentation was deep plaques (38 cases) often resembling a panniculitis, followed by patches resembling psoriasis or mycosis fungoides (10 cases). These lesions tended to ulcerate over time (27 cases). Single lesions or localized areas of involvement resembling cellulitis or pyoderma were reported in 8 cases. The most common anatomic site of involvement was the legs (40 cases), followed by the torso (30 cases) and arms (28 cases). Constitutional symptoms were reported in 54% (25/46) of the patients, including some with limited skin involvement. Significant comorbidities included autoimmunity (12 cases), other lymphoproliferative disorders (5 cases), internal carcinomas (4 cases), and viral hepatitis (2 cases). Lymphadenopathy (3/42 cases) and bone marrow involvement (5/28 cases) were uncommon, but serum lactose dehydrogenase (LDH) was elevated in 55% (22/39) of the patients. Abnormal positron emission tomography and/or computed tomography scans in 20/37 subjects mostly highlighted soft tissue or lymph nodes. Disease progression was associated with extensive ulcerated lesions resulting in 27 deaths including complications of hemophagocytic syndrome (4) and cerebral nervous system involvement (3). Median survival time from diagnosis was 31 months. Skin biopsies varied from a pagetoid pattern to purely dermal or panniculitic infiltrates composed of intermediate-sized lymphocytes with tissue evidence of cytotoxicity. The most common immunophenotype was $CD3^+/CD4^-/CD5^-/CD8^-/BF1^-/\gamma$-$M1^+/TIA\text{-}1^+/granzyme\text{-}B^+/CD45RA^-/CD7^-$, and 4 cases were Epstein-Barr virus positive. This is the largest study to date of cutaneous γδ T-cell lymphomas and demonstrates a variety of clinical and pathologic presentations with a predictable poor outcome.

▶ Gamma-delta T-cell lymphomas are uncommon tumors largely restricted to a set of specific sites, including liver, spleen, gastrointestinal tract, and skin.

Cutaneous γ-δ T-cell lymphomas have been incompletely described, likely because of their rarity as well as historic difficulties in directly identifying the γ-δ T-cell receptor from paraffin-embedded tissue. As such, this report of 53 affected patients adds significant understating to the character and definition of these lesions. The authors of this series present a bewildering array of clinical presentations, histologic appearances, phenotypic characteristics, and even survival, though most were lethal. It is no surprise that the World Health Organization has been slow to include cutaneous γ-δ T-cell lymphomas as an entity in their classification system for lymphomas. It seems likely that the taxonomy of these tumors will continue to undergo further refinement. Familiarity with the evolving understating of these lesions, including newly developed antibodies to the γ-δ T-cell receptor, will provide the astute pathologist with the best-available tools in dealing with these rare and often inconsistent tumors.

J. Wisell, MD

Fibroblastic Connective Tissue Nevus: A Rare Cutaneous Lesion Analyzed in a Series of 25 Cases

de Feraudy S, Fletcher CDM (Brigham and Women's Hosp, Boston, MA)
Am J Surg Pathol 36:1509-1515, 2012

Fibroblastic connective tissue nevus (FCTN) represents a rare and distinct benign cutaneous mesenchymal lesion of fibroblastic/myofibroblastic lineage, which broadens the spectrum of lesions presently recognized as connective tissue nevus. A series of 25 cases of FCTN has been analyzed to further characterize the clinicopathologic spectrum and immunohistochemical features of this entity. Sixteen patients were female (64%) and 9 were male (36%), with age at presentation ranging from 1.5 months to 58 years (median, 10 y). Most patients presented with a solitary, slowly growing, painless plaque-like or nodular skin lesion. Eleven cases (44%) arose on the trunk, 9 (36%) on the head and neck, and 5 (20%) on the limbs. The lesion was present for a median duration of 11.5 months (mean, 13.2 mo). Grossly, the lesions were tan-brown to tan-white, smooth, and firm. Their size ranged from 0.3 to 2.0 cm in greatest dimension (mean size, 0.67 cm; median, 0.6 cm). All tumors showed poor circumscription and were situated primarily in the reticular deep dermis, extending into the superficial subcutis in 13 cases (52%). The lesion was associated with papillomatous epidermis in 17 cases (70%) and the presence of adipose tissue in the reticular dermis in 14 cases (60.9%). All tumors were composed of a proliferation of bland intradermal fibroblastic/myofibroblastic cells with indistinct palely eosinophilic cytoplasm and tapering nuclei, with no significant cytologic atypia or pleomorphism, arranged in short-intersecting fascicles and entrapping appendages. No mitoses were identified. Immunostains showed positivity for CD34 in 20 of 23 cases (87%) and weak focal positivity for smooth muscle actin in 9 of 19 cases (47%). No case stained positively for desmin or S100 protein. Clinical follow-up was obtained for 14 patients (median duration, 4 y). No tumor recurred locally, even when surgical excision was incomplete. No lesion metastasized. FCTN occurs most commonly as a plaque on the trunk and head/neck of children, involves deep dermis and superficial subcutis, and stains mainly for CD34. FCTN most likely represents a localized developmental dermal anomaly; it is entirely benign and should not be confused with dermatofibrosarcoma protuberans or other neoplasms such as dermatomyofibroma.

▶ Dermal lesions with a spindle cell morphology that express CD34 include benign lesions, such as spindle cell lipoma, as well as more concerning lesions, chiefly dermatofibrosarcoma protuberans with its propensity for local recurrence and rare reports of metastasis. This group of tumors may display overlapping features and, given the different behaviors, accurate differentiation between them is important to ensure adequate management. This report proposes yet another entity to consider among these lesions. Although this does not make the differential diagnosis simpler, it does identify another potential pitfall, which, if taken, could lead to unnecessarily aggressive treatment. The authors detail their findings by identifying and following 25 "fibroblastic connective tissue nevi." After several years of follow-up, none have recurred, including at least 3 with grossly positive margins and likely many more with microscopically positive margins. The collection of CD34-positive dermal lesions will likely continue to see nosologic refinement; however, this report is a welcome addition for those of us who may have to identify which of these lesions requires aggressive treatment.

J. Wisell, MD

Chromosomal Aberrations by 4-Color Fluorescence In Situ Hybridization Not Detected in Spitz Nevi of Older Individuals

Horst BA, Fang Y, Silvers DN, et al (Columbia Univ Med Ctr, NY; Memorial Sloan-Kettering Cancer Ctr, NY)
Arch Dermatol 148:1152-1156, 2012

Objective.—To investigate whether Spitz nevi with typical histopathological features in older patients demonstrate chromosomal aberrations by 4-color fluorescence in situ hybridization (FISH).

Design.—Retrospective medical record review, with prospective masked histopathological and cytogenetic analyses.

Setting.—University-affiliated dermatology and dermatopathology setting.

Patients.—Twenty-five patients 50 years or older with melanocytic nevi showing histopathological features typical of Spitz nevi.

Main Outcome Measures.—Three dermatopathologists masked to the patients' ages reviewed histopathological sections of melanocytic lesions for features typical of Spitz nevi. FISH was performed on samples with typical histopathological features by a 4-color FISH probe set used for the evaluation of malignant melanocytic neoplasms.

Results.—None of the study cases showing histopathological features typical of Spitz nevi had detectable chromosomal abnormalities by FISH.

Conclusions.—Spitz nevi in older patients demonstrate molecular features similar to those of Spitz nevi in younger age groups. The findings of normal karyotypes in combination with typical histopathological features are reassuring of Spitz nevus diagnoses in older patients and suggest no correlation of increased malignant potential with advanced age per se.

▶ Fluorescence in situ hybridization (FISH) studies directed to specific chromosomal aberrations have been found to have value in separating benign from malignant melanocytic lesions; as such, these studies have been used increasingly in clinical practice. This study applies this technique to the not-so-uncommon and occasionally uncomfortable problem of diagnosing a Spitz nevus in an older person. Spitz nevi most often occur in the first 2 decades of life, and the use of the term *Spitz* in an older person often conjures skepticism as to absolute benignity of a lesion. This investigation adds further evidence that as long as the traditional features used to make the diagnosis of Spitz nevus are respected, the diagnosis of Spitz nevus remains valid in an older population, even though these patients have higher risk of melanoma. This study focused only on the presence of known FISH-detected abnormalities associated with malignancy and not clinical follow-up, so this study isn't as complete as one may like but still provides reassurance that making the diagnosis of Spitz nevus in this setting isn't impetuous. This study also broadens the experience for the use of these FISH probes in the diagnosis of melanoma.

J. Wisell, MD

2-cm versus 4-cm surgical excision margins for primary cutaneous melanoma thicker than 2 mm: a randomised, multicentre trial
Gillgren P, Drzewiecki KT, Niin M, et al (Karolinska Institutet, Stockholm, Sweden; Univ Hosp Rigshospitalet, Copenhagen, Denmark; North Estonian Regional Hosp, Tallin, Estonia; et al)
Lancet 378:1635-1642, 2011

Background.—Optimum surgical resection margins for patients with clinical stage IIA—C cutaneous melanoma thicker than 2 mm are controversial. The aim of the study was to test whether survival was different for a wide local excision margin of 2 cm compared with a 4-cm excision margin.

Methods.—We undertook a randomised controlled trial in nine European centres. Patients with cutaneous melanoma thicker than 2 mm, at clinical stage IIA—C, were allocated to have either a 2-cm or a 4-cm surgical resection margin. Patients were randomised in a 1:1 allocation to one of the two groups and stratified by geographic region. Randomisation was done by sealed envelope or by computer generated lists with permuted blocks. Our primary endpoint was overall survival. The trial was not masked at any stage. Analyses were by intention to treat. Adverse events were not systematically recorded. The study is registered with ClinicalTrials.gov, number NCT01183936.

Findings.—936 patients were enrolled from Jan 22, 1992, to May 19, 2004; 465 were randomly allocated to treatment with a 2-cm resection margin, and 471 to receive treatment with a 4-cm resection margin. One patient in each group was lost to follow-up but included in the analysis. After a median follow-up of 6.7 years (IQR 4.3—9.5) 181 patients in the 2-cm margin group and 177 in the 4-cm group had died (hazard ratio 1.05, 95% CI 0.85—1.29; $p = 0.64$). 5-year overall survival was 65% (95% CI 60—69) in the 2-cm group and 65% (60—70) in the 4-cm group ($p = 0.69$).

Interpretation.—Our findings suggest that a 2-cm resection margin is sufficient and safe for patients with cutaneous melanoma thicker than 2 mm.

▶ Famously, the original treatment for localized melanoma was determined from a single autopsy case in which a 2-inch (5-cm) margin was established. Unacceptable in the age of "evidence-based medicine," this standard survived for most of the 20th century. This report addresses the specific ongoing controversy of the appropriate margin for melanomas greater than 2 mm thick. Here they report no significant difference in overall survival or disease-specific survival between 2- and 4-cm margins. The trial fell short of their 2000-patient enrollment goal, somewhat diminishing the statistical power of their study. Still, their investigation adds significant evidence that a 2-cm margin is not clearly inferior to a 4-cm margin. Pathologists should be aware of these treatment issues, as we are frequently called on to clarify the margin status of wide local excision specimens; however, it should be made clear that these are clinically determined margins, not those measured microscopically. Moving forward, pathologists might be able to play an improved role in determining how far from the margin diseased melanocytes might extend. Methods newer than our 150-year-old hematoxylin and eosin staining, such as immunohistochemical studies for mutated B-RAF proteins and fluorescence in situ hybridization studies for specific chromosomal alterations, may provide greater insight into this issue.

J. Wisell, MD

Pityriasis Lichenoides et Varioliformis Acuta With Numerous CD30+ Cells: A Variant Mimicking Lymphomatoid Papulosis and Other Cutaneous Lymphomas. A Clinicopathologic, Immunohistochemical, and Molecular Biological Study of 13 Cases
Kempf W, Kazakov DV, Palmedo G, et al (Kempf und Pfaltz Histologische Diagnostik, Zurich, Switzerland; Charles Univ in Prague, Czech Republic; Dermatopathologie Bodensee, Friedrichshafen, Germany, et al)
Am J Surg Pathol 36:1021-1029, 2012

Pityriasis lichenoides comprises a clinicopathologic spectrum of cutaneous inflammatory disorders, with the 2 most common variants being pityriasis lichenoides et varioliformis acuta (PLEVA) and pityriasis lichenoides chronica. The aim of the study was to describe 13 cases of a unique PLEVA variant characterized in the conspicuous CD30$^+$ component and thus mimicking lymphomatoid papulosis (LyP), a condition currently classified in the spectrum of CD30$^+$ lymphoproliferative disorders. The cohort included 10 female and 3 male patients whose ages at diagnosis ranged from 7 to 89 years (mean 41 y; median 39 y). The clinical manifestation was that of PLEVA, with small erythematous macules quickly evolving into necrotic papules. No waxing and waning was seen on follow-up in any of the cases. Histopathologically, typical features of PLEVA were present, but an unusual finding was occurrence of a considerable number of CD30$^+$ small lymphocytes as detected immunohistochemically. Over half of the cases also displayed a large number of CD8$^+$ cells and showed coexpression of CD8 and CD30 in the intraepidermal and dermal component of the infiltrate. Of the 11 cases of PLEVA studied for T-cell receptor gene rearrangement, 6 evidenced a monoclonal T-cell population, and 5 were polyclonal. Parvovirus B19 (PVB19) DNA was identified in 4 of 10 cases investigated, and positive serology was observed for PVB19 in 2 patients, altogether suggesting that PVB19 is pathogenetically linked to PLEVA at least in a subset of cases. The presence of CD30$^+$ lymphocytes and CD8$^+$ lymphocytes would be consistent with an inflammatory antiviral response, as CD30$^+$, even atypically appearing lymphoid cells have been identified in some viral skin diseases. The main significance of the PLEVA variant is, however, its potential confusion with LyP or some cytotoxic lymphomas. Admittedly, the CD30$^+$ PLEVA variant described herein and LyP show considerable overlap if one takes into account all known variations of the 2 conditions recognized in recent years, thus suggesting that LyP and PLEVA may be much more biologically closely related entities than currently thought or can even occur on a clinicopathologic spectrum.

▶ Based solely on the histologic features, the confident diagnosis of pityriasis lichenoides et varioliformis acuta (PLEVA) can be difficult and other entities enter into the differential diagnosis. Combined with the appropriate clinical scenario including papules that quickly become ulcerative lesions, the diagnosis of PLEVA can typically be confirmed by the histologic appearance. This report describes a series of cases that express CD30 and takes up many of the contemporary issues that surround PLEVA. Some have proposed that PLEVA is a lymphoproliferative disorder—indeed, this report finds clonality in 6 of 11 cases. Many believe a "lymphocytic vasculitis" is the central pathogenic mechanism in the development of PLEVA lesions; this series found vascular changes in 8 cases. More recently, some have implicated parvovirus as the etiologic factor in PLEVA, and this series discovers parvovirus B19 DNA in 4 of 10 cases and positive serology in 2 more. Clearly a degree of heterogeneity appears to exist within the current PLEVA concept; this is only further complicated if we remember that PLEVA is considered by most to be part of a spectrum with pityriasis lichenoides chronica. Although this series reports the typical clinical setting for PLEVA in all of their cases, the presence of significant numbers of CD30 positive cells draws histologic similarity to lymphomatoid papulosis (LyP); it also broadens the immunoprofile that may accepted for cases of PLEVA. The concept of LyP has also been recently expanded with some including a "type D." The true relationship between the 2 disorders remains unclear. The evolution of our understanding of both conditions will likely continue to evolve, particularly with the widespread availability of molecular techniques as used by the authors in this report.

J. Wisell, MD

Specific Skin Lesions in Chronic Myelomonocytic Leukemia: A Spectrum of Myelomonocytic and Dendritic Cell Proliferations. A Study of 42 Cases
Vitte F, Fabiani B, Bénet C, et al (CHU Jean Minjoz, Besançon, France; Hôpital Saint-Antoine, Paris, France; Hôpital Saint-Louis, Paris, France; et al)
Am J Surg Pathol 36:1302-1316, 2012

Chronic myelomonocytic leukemia (CMML) is a rare clonal hematopoietic disorder that can also involve the skin. The histopathology of these skin lesions is not clearly defined, and few data are available in the literature. To better understand tumoral skin involvements in CMML we carried out an extensive, retrospective clinicopathologic study of 42 cases selected from the database of the French Study Group of Cutaneous Lymphomas. On the basis of clinical data, morphology, and phenotype we identified 4 clinicopathologic profiles representing 4 distinct groups. The first group comprised myelomonocytic cell tumors (n = 18), exhibiting a proliferation of granulocytic or monocytic blast cells, which were CD68 and/or MPO positive but negative for dendritic cell markers. The second group comprised mature plasmacytoid dendritic cell tumors (n = 16), denoted by a proliferation of mature plasmacytoid dendritic cells, which were CD123, TCL1, and CD303 positive but CD56, CD1a, and S100 negative. The third group comprised blastic plasmacytoid dendritic cell tumors (n = 4), characterized by a proliferation of monomorphous medium-sized blast cells, which were CD4, CD56, CD123, TCL1 positive but CD1a and S100 negative. The fourth group consisted of a putatively novel category of tumor that we named blastic indeterminate dendritic cell tumors (n = 4), distinguished by a proliferation of large blast cells that not only exhibited monocytic markers but also the dendritic markers CD1a and S100. These 4 groups showed distinctive outcomes. Finally, we showed, by fluorescence in situ hybridization analysis, a clonal link between bone marrow disease and skin lesions in 4 patients. Herein, we have described a novel scheme for pathologists and physicians to handle specific lesions in CMML, which correspond to a spectrum of myelomonocytic and dendritic cell proliferations with different outcomes. A minimal panel of immunohistochemical markers including CD68, CD1a, S100, Langerin, and CD123 is necessary to make the correct classification in this spectrum of cutaneous CMML tumors, in which dendritic cell lineage plays an important role.

▶ Uncommonly, chronic myelomonocytic leukemia (CMML) involves the skin. These tumors demonstrate differing phenotypes and the associated cutaneous lesions have not been well described, leading to inconsistent reporting and confusion over these cases. Building on their previous work, the authors of this study provide a broad description of cutaneous CMML lesions. Bringing some degree of clarity to the variable phenotypes one can see in CMML, they have identified 4 types of lesions and include clinical and morphologic correlates. Devising such a system is tremendously helpful for the practicing pathologist because it brings confidence to final diagnosis of such lesions. This system promises greater utility as it potentially has prognostic significance, though the numbers of cases in this series were likely still too small to clearly show if outcome differences exist among the different categories. These different subcategories also highlight the divergent differentiation that can be seen in these tumors, including the presence of a dendritic cell lineage. Additional investigations will be required to further develop and refine a classification scheme for CMML skin lesions with a special need to identify groups with significantly different outcomes and treatment needs. This report is a welcome initiation of such a process.

J. Wisell, MD

Increasing Tumor Thickness is Associated with Recurrence and Poorer Survival in Patients with Merkel Cell Carcinoma

Lim CS, Whalley D, Haydu LE, et al (Royal Prince Alfred Hosp, Camperdown, New South Wales, Australia; Royal Prince Alfred Hosp, Sydney, New South Wales, Australia; Melanoma Inst Australia, North Sydney, New South Wales, Australia; et al)
Ann Surg Oncol 19:3325-3334, 2012

Background.—Merkel cell carcinoma (MCC) is a rare, aggressive cutaneous neuroendocrine tumor usually occurring on sun-exposed skin in elderly patients. Clinical and pathologic factors associated with disease progression and mortality in patients with MCC are poorly defined. Recently, it has been reported that p63 expression in primary MCC is strongly associated with clinical outcome.

Methods.—MCC patients diagnosed between July 1, 1993 and July 31, 2009 were identified from the surgical pathology records of the Sydney South West Area Health Service. Clinical, pathologic, treatment, and survival data were obtained and immunohistochemical analyses for p53, p63, and Ki-67 were performed. The associations of clinical and pathologic features with disease-free and disease-specific survival were analyzed.

Results.—Ninety-five patients were identified (67 males, 28 females; median age at diagnosis of primary MCC 76 [range, 42—93] years). Increasing primary tumor thickness was significantly associated with poorer disease-free survival (5-year survival 18% in tumors > 10 mm thick compared with 69% for patients with tumors ≤ 10 mm thick, $p = 0.002$) and disease-specific survival (5-year survival 74% in tumors > 10 mm thick compared with 97% for patients with tumors ≤ 10 mm thick, $p = 0.006$). There was a strong positive correlation between the Ki-67 index (proportion of Ki-67-positive tumor nuclei) and tumor thickness ($r = 0.39, n = 45, p = 0.008$). Positive staining for p63 in MCC was infrequent (9% of primary MCC) and showed no significant association with disease outcome.

Conclusions.—Tumor thickness is significantly associated with disease-free survival in MCC. We recommend that primary tumor thickness be routinely recorded in the pathology reports of patients with primary MCC.

▶ Merkel cell carcinoma is a primary cutaneous neuroendocrine carcinoma that has been associated both with chronic sun exposure and more recently a polyomavirus. These tumors are infamously aggressive tumors with high mortality. Fortunately, they are uncommon, but this latter feature has made it difficult to collect large series of tumors in which prognostically helpful features can be delineated. This study found a prognostically significant feature recognizable to those of us who routinely encounter cutaneous tumors: thickness. They did not find lymphovascular invasion, sentinel lymph node status, Ki-67 positivity, p53 positivity, or p63 positivity to correlate with patient outcome. Though their series is relatively large for this tumor type including histopathologic review, the absolute number of patients may still be too small to detect differences for some of these latter features; this will likely require a similar study spanning several institutions for this rare tumor. Nevertheless, similar to previous studies they are able make a strong argument for pursuing tumor thickness as a meaningful and reportable histologic feature. This is immediately useful, as it is easily done with a well-developed and familiar methodology.

J. Wisell, MD

Improved Survival with MEK Inhibition in BRAF-Mutated Melanoma
Flaherty KT, for the METRIC Study Group (Massachusetts General Hosp Cancer Ctr, Boston; et al)
N Engl J Med 367:107-114, 2012

Background.—Activating mutations in serine—threonine protein kinase B-RAF (BRAF) are found in 50% of patients with advanced melanoma. Selective BRAF-inhibitor therapy improves survival, as compared with chemotherapy, but responses are often short-lived. In previous trials, MEK inhibition appeared to be promising in this population.

Methods.—In this phase 3 open-label trial, we randomly assigned 322 patients who had metastatic melanoma with a V600E or V600K BRAF mutation to receive either trametinib, an oral selective MEK inhibitor, or chemotherapy in a 2:1 ratio. Patients received trametinib (2 mg orally) once daily or intravenous dacarbazine (1000 mg per square meter of body-surface area) or paclitaxel (175 mg per square meter) every 3 weeks. Patients in the chemotherapy group who had disease progression were permitted to cross over to receive trametinib. Progression-free survival was the primary end point, and overall survival was a secondary end point.

Results.—Median progression-free survival was 4.8 months in the trametinib group and 1.5 months in the chemotherapy group (hazard ratio for disease progression or death in the trametinib group, 0.45; 95% confidence interval [CI], 0.33 to 0.63; $P < 0.001$). At 6 months, the rate of overall survival was 81% in the trametinib group and 67% in the chemotherapy group despite crossover (hazard ratio for death, 0.54; 95% CI, 0.32 to 0.92; $P = 0.01$). Rash, diarrhea, and peripheral edema were the most common toxic effects in the trametinib group and were managed with dose interruption and dose reduction; asymptomatic and reversible reduction in the cardiac ejection fraction and ocular toxic effects occurred infrequently. Secondary skin neoplasms were not observed.

Conclusions.—Trametinib, as compared with chemotherapy, improved rates of progression-free and overall survival among patients who had metastatic melanoma with a BRAF V600E or V600K mutation. (Funded by GlaxoSmithKline; METRIC ClinicalTrials.gov number, NCT01245062.)

▶ Within the past few years, the future for patients with metastatic melanoma has begun to look slightly more promising. Until recently, there had never been a therapy shown to improve survival in this group of patients. The advent of targeted molecular therapies has provided a focused and individualized approach to treating tumors. The first of these for melanoma, ipilimumab, targets CTLA-4 and disinhibits T cells responding to the tumor. The second, vemurafenib, targets the B-RAF protein, which is constitutively active via mutation in a proportion of melanomas. This report indicates a third agent, trametinib, also improves survival by inhibiting MEK1 and MEK2 proteins, which are typically activated by B-RAF. The impact reported by these investigators appears less than for direct B-RAF inhibition, but the side effect profile is different and the possibility for a variety of combinatorial therapies is promising. Pathologists, with our focus on making the diagnosis, have not always been as concerned about the specific therapeutic options, but targeted molecular therapy changes that. With a growing list of targeted therapies in melanoma, pathologists are increasingly being asked to assist in determining which agent will be most effective in a specific tumor. The first question we are now often asked following a diagnosis of metastatic melanoma is, "Does it have a BRAF mutation?" These drugs appear to impose their own classification system that pathologists must appreciate.

J. Wisell, MD

An immunohistochemical comparison of cytokeratin 7, cytokeratin 15, cytokeratin 19, CAM 5.2, carcinoembryonic antigen, and nestin in differentiating porocarcinoma from squamous cell carcinoma
Mahalingam M, Richards JE, Selim MA, et al (Boston Univ School of Medicine, MA; Duke Univ Med Ctr, Durham, NC; et al)
Hum Pathol 43:1265-1272, 2012

The distinction of porocarcinoma from squamous cell carcinoma is clinically relevant but can often be a diagnostic dilemma. Current markers reported to be helpful in diagnosing porocarcinoma include carcinoembryonic antigen and cytokeratin 7; however, their expression has been demonstrated in 30% to 80% and 13% to 22% of squamous cell carcinoma cases, respectively. In this study, we assessed immunohistochemical expression of cytokeratin 7, cytokeratin 15, cytokeratin 19, CAM 5.2, carcinoembryonic antigen, and nestin in 67 cases (39 porocarcinomas and 28 moderately differentiated squamous cell carcinomas) to determine their use as histologic adjuncts. Expression of carcinoembryonic antigen, cytokeratin 19, cytokeratin 7, CAM 5.2, cytokeratin 15, and nestin was seen in 77%, 67%, 64%, 51%, 49%, and 13% of porocarcinomas, respectively; and in 57%, 18%, 26%, 32%, 30%, and 37% of squamous cell carcinomas, respectively. Of these, cytokeratin 19 was the most specific (specificity, 82%) in detecting porocarcinomas, and carcinoembryonic antigen was the most sensitive (sensitivity, 77%). By χ^2 test, statistically significant P values ($<.05$) were observed for cytokeratin 7, cytokeratin 19, and nestin in the distinction of porocarcinoma from squamous cell carcinoma. However, in a logistic regression and stepwise selection for predicting a porocarcinoma, statistical significance was observed only for cytokeratin 19 ($P = .0003$). In conclusion, we found cytokeratin 19 to be a helpful marker in the distinction of porocarcinoma from squamous cell carcinoma, although a focal staining pattern can be seen in a third of cases. The diagnostic sensitivity and specificity appear to be significantly improved using a selected panel of immunohistochemical stains that include cytokeratin 7, cytokeratin 19, and nestin.

▶ Porocarcinomas may behave aggressively, but they are rare and pathologists risk misinterpreting them as a more frequently encountered squamous cell carcinoma (SCC) variant. Even if the astute pathologist is concerned that a tumor may be a porocarcinoma, this can be a difficult distinction. Porocarcinomas often have areas of squamous differentiation; SCCs have several ways of mimicking a glandular pattern, and a robust discriminatory immunohistochemical marker has not yet emerged. This investigation looks to the last of these for an opportunity to help in this setting. Carcinoembryonic antigen (CEA) has long been the diagnostic marker most closely associated with porocarcinoma, where staining of ductal lumina can be seen. However, the diagnostic utility of this marker is limited, as the closest histologic imitator (SCC) also expresses this marker, although less frequently. Some have touted the ductal pattern of labeling by CEA in porocarcinoma to help differentiate it from SCC, but, in practice, this can be undependable, as glandlike areas in SCC may also label. On the basis of their investigation, the authors also do not strongly promote the use of CEA as a differentiating marker, noting that more than half of SCCs in their series labeled with this marker. They found more success with CK7 and nestin, but these still have slightly better than marginal discriminating power. From their data, if one were to rely solely on nestin to differentiate SCC from porocarcinoma, it would be wrong 37% of the time (false-positive rate). CK7 does somewhat better with around a 25% false-positive rate. The most promising marker from their series is CK19, the only marker to significantly predict porocarcinoma in their multivariate analysis. This is a helpful finding and could be integrated with morphologic findings to augment one's assessment, possibly aided to a lesser degree with CK7 and nestin. It should be noted that CK19 still has an 18% false-positive rate, indicating that at least some hematoxylin and eosin—based consternation will still likely exist for some of us in these cases.

J. Wisell, MD

6 Lung and Mediastinum

Histologic Patterns and Molecular Characteristics of Lung Adenocarcinoma Associated With Clinical Outcome

Solis LM, Behrens C, Raso MG, et al (The Univ of Texas MD Anderson Cancer Ctr, Houston)

Cancer 118:2889-2899, 2012

Background.—Lung adenocarcinoma is histologically heterogeneous and has 5 distinct histologic growth patterns: lepidic, acinar, papillary, micropapillary, and solid. To date, there is no consensus regarding the clinical utility of these patterns.

Methods.—The authors performed a detailed semiquantitative assessment of histologic patterns of 240 lung adenocarcinomas and determined the association with patients' clinicopathologic features, including recurrence-free survival (RFS) and overall survival (OS) rates. In a subset of tumors,

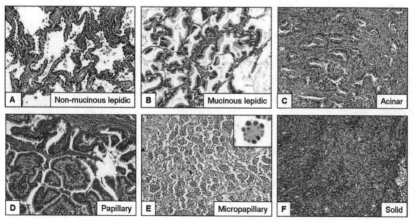

FIGURE 1.—These are photomicrographs of hematoxylin and eosin-stained sections of lung adenocarcinoma tumors with different growth patterns, including (A) lepidic (nonmucinous), (B) lepidic (mucinous), (C) acinar, (D) papillary, (E) micropapillary, and (F) solid (original magnification, ×100). (Reprinted from Solis LM, Behrens C, Raso MG, et al. Histologic patterns and molecular characteristics of lung adenocarcinoma associated with clinical outcome. *Cancer.* 2012;118:2889-2899, Copyright 2012, American Cancer Society. This material is reproduced with permission of Wiley-Liss, Inc., a subsidiary of John Wiley & Sons, Inc.)

expression levels of 2 prognostic molecular markers were evaluated: thyroid transcription factor-1 (TTF-1) (n = 218) and a panel of 5 proteins (referred as the FILM signature index) (n = 185).

Results.—Four mutually exclusive tumor histology pattern groups were identified: 1) any solid (38%), 2) any papillary but no solid (14%), 3) lepidic and acinar but no solid or papillary (30%), and 4) acinar only (18%). Patients in group 3 had a higher RFS rate than patients in group 1 (hazard ratio [HR], 0.4510; $P = .0165$) and group 2 (HR, 0.4253; $P = .0425$). Solid pattern tumors (group 1) were associated with a lower OS rate than nonsolid pattern tumors (all stages: HR; 1.665; $P = .0144$; stages I and II: HR, 2.157; $P = .008$). In the patients who had tumors with a nonsolid pattern, high TTF-1 expression was associated significantly with higher RFS (HR, 0.994; $P = .0017$) and OS (HR, 0.996; $P = .0276$) rates in all stages, and a high FILM signature index score was associated with lower

TABLE 1.—Clinical and Pathologic Characteristics of All 240 Primary Lung Adenocarcinoma Tumors Studied and Their Association with 4 Histologic Pattern Groups

		Histologic Pattern Group: No. of Patients (%)[a]				
Characteristic	All Tumors, N = 240	Group 1, N = 92	Group 2, N = 34	Group 3, N = 72	Group 4, N = 42	P
Age, y[b]						.00079
≤66.8	118	53 (45)	20 (17)	21 (18)	24 (20)	
>66.8	122	39 (32)	14 (11)	51 (42)	18 (15)	
Sex						.09314
Women	137	47 (34)	16 (12)	49 (36)	25 (18)	
Men	103	45 (44)	18 (17)	23 (22)	17 (17)	
Smoking status						.00010
Current	97	54 (56)	13 (13)	15 (15)	15 (15)	
Former	102	30 (29)	15 (15)	37 (36)	20 (20)	
Never	41	8 (20)	6 (15)	20 (49)	7 (17)	
IASLC stage[c]						.01377
I	167	54 (32)	23 (14)	60 (36)	30 (18)	
II	42	23 (55)	8 (19)	7 (17)	4 (10)	
III or IV	31	15 (48)	3 (10)	5 (16)	8 (26)	
TNM stage[d]						.00164
I	173	55 (32)	24 (14)	63 (36)	31 (18)	
II	36	22 (61)	7 (19)	4 (11)	3 (8)	
III or IV	31	15 (48)	3 (10)	5 (16)	8 (26)	
Adjuvant therapy[e]						.27792
No	163	57 (35)	26 (16)	53 (33)	27 (17)	
Yes	71	33 (47)	7 (10)	18 (25)	13 (18)	
Necrosis						<.0001
No	114	26 (23)	19 (17)	48 (42)	21 (18)	
Yes	126	66 (52)	15 (12)	24 (19)	21 (17)	
Lymphovascular invasion						.1398
No	200	74 (37)	26 (13)	66 (33)	34 (17)	
Yes	40	18 (45)	8 (20)	6 (15)	8 (20)	

Abbreviations: IASLC, International Association for the Study of Lung Cancer; TNM, tumor, lymph node, metastasis.
Editor's Note: Please refer to original journal article for full references.
[a]Histologic pattern groups were defined as follows: group 1, tumors with any solid pattern; group 2, any papillary pattern but no solid pattern; group 3, acinar and lepidic patterns but no solid or papillary patterns; and group 4, acinar pattern only.
[b]The median age of the entire population is indicated.
[c]See Detterbeck FC, Boffa DJ, Tanoue LT. The new lung cancer staging system. *Chest.* 2009;136:260-271.[38]
[d]See Mountain CF. The international system for staging lung cancer. *Semin Surg Oncol.* 2000;18:106-115.[37]
[e]Adjuvant treatment information was not available for 6 patients.

RFS and OS rates in all stages (RFS: HR, 1.343; $P = .0192$; OS: HR, 1.371; $P = .0156$) and in stages I and II (RFS: HR, 1.419; $P = .0095$; OS: HR, 1.315; $P = .0422$).

Conclusions.—The presence of a solid histologic pattern was identified as a marker of unfavorable prognosis in patients with primary lung adenocarcinoma. High TTF-1 expression and low FILM signature index scores were associated with a better prognosis for patients who had tumors with a nonsolid pattern (Fig 1, Table 1).

▶ The International Association for the Study of Lung Cancer/American Thoracic Society/European Respiratory Society for the Classification of Lung Cancer have suggested the adaptation of a detailed histologic assessment of lung adenocarcinomas. Previous studies have attempted to determine the clinical importance of subtyping but have been limited by sample size and varying methodologies. In this retrospective analysis, the authors looked at 240 lung adenocarcinomas (Table 1), their histologic growth patterns, and their clinicopathologic characteristics and compared them with the rates of recurrence-free survival and overall survival. All samples were primary lung adenocarcinomas with 1 tumor nodule and had been subject to extensive tumor sampling. A modification of the World Health Organization classification system was used to histologically subclassify the tumors, so practitioners will have to carefully follow the system derived by the authors to replicate their findings (Fig 1). It is of note that more than 80% of their tumors showed a mixed pattern on detailed histologic sampling. They recommend at least one block per centimeter of the tumor's greatest dimension, a sampling protocol that is readily acceptable to most pathology laboratories. The immunohistochemical panel recommended is extensive but does add to the power of the predictions. Many laboratories may choose to use TTF-1 only. For further reading, please see reference list.[1]

B. A. Carter, MD, FRCPC

Reference

1. Travis WD, Brambilla E, Noguchi M, et al. International association for the study of lung cancer/American thoracic society/European respiratory society international multidisciplinary classification of lung adenocarcinoma. *J Thorac Oncol.* 2011;6:244-285.

A grading system combining architectural features and mitotic count predicts recurrence in stage I lung adenocarcinoma
Kadota K, Suzuki K, Kachala SS, et al (Memorial Sloan-Kettering Cancer Ctr, NY)
Mod Pathol 25:1117-1127, 2012

The International Association for the Study of Lung Cancer (IASLC)/ American Thoracic Society (ATS)/European Respiratory Society (ERS) has recently proposed a new lung adenocarcinoma classification. We investigated whether nuclear features can stratify prognostic subsets. Slides of 485 stage I lung adenocarcinoma patients were reviewed. We evaluated

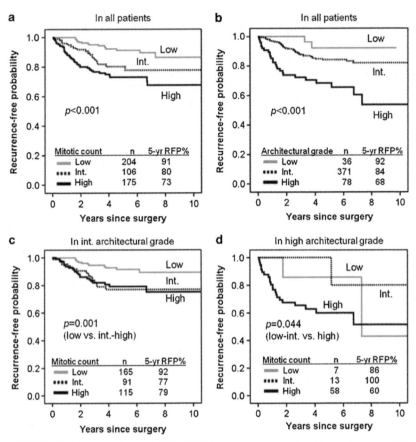

FIGURE 2.—Recurrence-free probability (RFP) by mitotic count and architectural grade. (a) The recurrence-free probability of patients with high mitotic count ($n = 175$) was the lowest (5-year recurrence-free probability = 73%), followed by intermediate ($n = 106$, 80%), and low ($n = 204$, 91%). (b) The RFP of patients with high architectural grade ($n = 78$) was the lowest (68%), followed by intermediate ($n = 371$, 84%), and low ($n = 36$, 92%). (c) Within the intermediate architectural grade, patients with low mitotic count ($n = 165$) had higher 5-year RFP (92%) compared with the intermediate ($n = 91$, 77%)—high mitotic count ($n = 115$, 79%). (d) Within the high architectural grade, patients with high mitotic count ($n = 58$) had lower 5-year RFP (60%) compared with the low ($n = 7$, 86%)—intermediate mitotic count ($n = 13$, 100%). (Reprinted from Kadota K, Suzuki K, Kachala SS, et al. A grading system combining architectural features and mitotic count predicts recurrence in stage I lung adenocarcinoma. *Mod Pathol.* 2012;25:1117-1127, with permission from USCAP, Inc.)

nuclear diameter, nuclear atypia, nuclear/cytoplasmic ratio, chromatin pattern, prominence of nucleoli, intranuclear inclusions, mitotic count/10 high-power fields (HPFs) or 2.4 mm², and atypical mitoses. Tumors were classified into histologic subtypes according to the IASLC/ATS/ERS classification and grouped by architectural grade into low (adenocarcinoma *in situ*, minimally invasive adenocarcinoma, or lepidic predominant), intermediate (papillary or acinar), and high (micropapillary or solid). Log-rank tests and Cox regression models evaluated the ability of clinicopathologic factors to predict recurrence-free probability. In univariate analyses, nuclear diameter

($P = 0.007$), nuclear atypia ($P = 0.006$), mitotic count ($P < 0.001$), and atypical mitoses ($P < 0.001$) were significant predictors of recurrence. The recurrence-free probability of patients with high mitotic count ($\geq 5/10$ HPF: $n = 175$) was the lowest (5-year recurrence-free probability $= 73\%$), followed by intermediate (2-4/10 HPF: $n = 106$, 80%), and low (0-1/10 HPF: $n = 204$, 91%, $P < 0.001$). Combined architectural/mitotic grading system stratified patient outcomes ($P < 0.001$): low grade (low architectural grade with any mitotic count and intermediate architectural grade with low mitotic count: $n = 201$, 5-year recurrence-free probability $= 92\%$), intermediate grade (intermediate architectural grade with intermediate–high mitotic counts: $n = 206$, 78%), and high grade (high architectural grade with any mitotic count: $n = 78$, 68%). The advantage of adding mitotic count to architectural grade is in stratifying patients with intermediate architectural grade into two prognostically distinct categories ($P = 0.001$). After adjusting for clinicopathologic factors including sex, stage, pleural/lymphovascular invasion, and necrosis, mitotic count was not an independent predictor of recurrence ($P = 0.178$). However, patients with the high architectural/mitotic grade remained at significantly increased risk of recurrence (high vs low: $P = 0.005$) after adjusting for clinical factors. We proposed this combined architectural/mitotic grade for lung adenocarcinoma as a practical method that can be applied in routine practice (Fig 2).

▶ Adenocarcinoma, the most frequent histologic type of lung cancer, has been subtyped recently in the International Association for the Study of Lung Cancer (IASLC)/American Thoracic Society (ATS)/European Respiratory Society (ERS) International Multidisciplinary Classification of Lung Adenocarcinoma in an effort to place patients in prognostic categories. The authors of this study sought to validate a grading system to identify patients at high risk of recurrence. The identification of patients at high risk for recurrence provides important information as traditionally chemotherapy is not offered. Kadota et al used relatively straightforward criteria to grade the lesions that can be easily applied by the practicing anatomic pathologist. As expected, the mitotic count was identified as the single most important criterion when predicting recurrence. Of interest, the Ki-67 proliferation index (< 10% or > 10%) correlated to the mitotic count, but offered no further useful information. The mitotic count also stratified intermediate architectural grade tumors with respect to their risk of recurrence. This easily adaptable grading system may aid in improved clinical decision making in patients with early-stage lung cancer. For further reading, please see reference list.[1]

B. A. Carter, MD, FRCPC

Reference

1. Travis WD, Brambilla E, Noguchi M, et al. International association for the study of lung cancer/American thoracic society/European respiratory society international multidisciplinary classification of lung adenocarcinoma. *J Thorac Oncol.* 2011;6:244-285.

Molecular Classification of Nonsmall Cell Lung Cancer Using a 4-Protein Quantitative Assay

Anagnostou VK, Dimou AT, Botsis T, et al (Yale Univ School of Medicine, New Haven, CT; Univ of Tromsø, Norway; et al)
Cancer 118:1607-1618, 2012

Background.—The importance of definitive histological subclassification has increased as drug trials have shown benefit associated with histology in nonsmall cell lung cancer (NSCLC). The acuity of this problem is further exacerbated by the use of minimally invasive cytology samples. Here we describe the development and validation of a 4-protein classifier that differentiates primary lung adenocarcinomas (AC) from squamous cell carcinomas (SCC).

Methods.—Quantitative immunofluorescence (AQUA) was employed to measure proteins differentially expressed between AC and SCC followed by logistic regression analysis. An objective 4-protein classifier was generated to define likelihood of AC in a training set of 343 patients followed by validation in 2 independent cohorts (n = 197 and n = 235). The assay was then tested on 11 cytology specimens.

Results.—Statistical modeling selected thyroid transcription factor 1 (TTF1), CK5, CK13, and epidermal growth factor receptor (EGFR) to generate a weighted classifier and to identify the optimal cutpoint for differentiating AC from SCC. Using the pathologist's final diagnosis as the criterion standard, the molecular test showed a sensitivity of 96% and specificity of 93%. Blinded analysis of the validation sets yielded sensitivity and specificity of 96% and 97%, respectively. Our assay classified the cytology specimens with a specificity of 100% and sensitivity of 87.5%.

Conclusions.—Molecular classification of NSCLC using an objective quantitative test can be highly accurate and could be translated into a diagnostic platform for broad clinical application (Table 4).

▶ Advances in targeted therapies for non-small-cell lung cancer (NSCLC) revealed that histology is predictive of clinical efficacy outcomes. Adenocarcinomas of the lung have shown, in multiple studies, increased response rates to the epidermal growth factor receptor tyrosine kinase inhibitors erlotinib and gefitinib, and absence of hemorrhagic complications with vascular endothelial growth factor inhibitors and the molecule tyrosine kinase inhibitors sorafenib and sunitinib. NSCLC histological subclassification is usually determined by surgical pathologists using light microscopic assessment of hematoxylin and eosin—stained sections as well as histochemical stains for mucin and immunohistochemical detection of TTF1 and P63. In this study quantitative immunofluorescence was performed on formalin-fixed, paraffin-embedded tissues or cytology samples. Subtyping showed high sensitivity and acceptable specificity in both minimal samples using the authors' 4-protein classifier (Table 4). Because reliable preoperative histologic subclassification of NSCLC on scant material has been found to be as low as 35%,[1] it was inevitable that a plethora

TABLE 4.—Classification for All NSCLC Specimens by the 4-Protein Test

| | Assay Classification | | | |
	Adenocarcinoma (Score ≥0.49)	Squamous Cell Carcinoma (Score <0.49)	PPV	NPV
Histologic diagnosis				
Training cohort			92.31%	96.55%
Adenocarcinoma	120	5		
SCC	10	140		
Validation cohort 1			98.88%	80.55%
Adenocarcinoma	86	7		
SCC	1	29		
Validation cohort 2			97.29%	95.16%
Adenocarcinoma	72	3		
SCC	2	59		

Abbreviations: NPV, negative predictive value; PPV, positive predictive value; SCC, squamous cell carcinoma.

of molecular tools would be studied. The study is limited by its sample size and its retrospective nature.

B. A. Carter, MD, FRCPC

Reference

1. Edwards SL, Roberts C, McKean ME, Cockburn JS, Jeffrey RR, Kerr KM. Preoperative histological classification of primary lung cancer: accuracy of diagnosis and use of the non-small cell category. *J Clin Pathol.* 2000;53:537-540.

Positive pre-resection pleural lavage cytology is associated with increased risk of lung cancer recurrence in patients undergoing surgical resection: a meta-analysis of 4450 patients
Saso S, Rao C, Ashrafian H, et al (Imperial College London, UK)
Thorax 67:526-532, 2012

Introduction.—The value of pleural lavage cytology (PLC) in assessing the prognosis of early stage lung cancer is still controversial. No systematic review has investigated the relationship between PLC and lung cancer recurrence. Our primary goal was to investigate the association between positive pre-resection PLC and pleural, distant and overall tumour recurrence in patients undergoing surgical resection.

Methods.—Medline, EMBASE and Google Scholar databases were searched up to 2011. All studies reporting relevant outcomes in both patient groups were included. Data were extracted for the following outcomes of interest: overall, local and distant recurrence; and freedom from death (survival-overall and patients with stage I disease only). Random effects meta-analysis was used to aggregate the data. Sensitivity and heterogeneity analysis were performed.

Results.—A meta-analysis of eight studies at maximum follow-up demonstrated a significant association between positive pre-resection PLC and increased risk of post-resection overall recurrence (OR 4.82, 95% CI 2.45 to 9.51), pleural recurrence (OR 9.89, 95% CI 5.95 to 16.44) and distant cancer recurrence (OR 3.18, 95% CI 1.57 to 6.46). Furthermore, a meta-analysis of 17 studies suggested that positive pre-resection PLC was also associated with unfavourable survival (HR 2.08, 95% CI 1.71 to 2.52). These findings were supported by sensitivity analysis.

Discussion.—Positive pre-resection PLC is associated with higher overall, distant and local tumour recurrence and unfavourable patient survival outcomes. This technique may therefore act as a predictor of tumour recurrence and adverse survival. Furthermore, its role in including adjuvant chemotherapy to the management protocol should be investigated within randomised controlled trials.

▶ In this meta-analysis, Saso et al looked at the literature up to and including 2011 on pleural lavage in the prognostication of early-stage lung cancer. Pleural lavage cytology (PLC) is the instillation of saline into the chest cavity during surgery for non-small-cell lung cancer with analysis of the fluid by a cytopathologist. Despite numerous supportive articles in the past few years, the prognostic significance of the findings of this procedure has yet to be widely accepted in the treatment of early-stage lung carcinoma. However, it is widely accepted that the detection of free cancer cells within the peritoneal cavity at the time of surgery influences prognosis in abdominal malignancies, especially in gastric, colorectal, and gynecological cancers, so it stands to reason that the same would apply to the pleural cavity. Saso and his group, in their analysis of multiple studies, found that a positive preresection PLC is associated with higher overall, distant, and local tumor recurrence. Positive PLC was also associated with other unfavorable patient survival outcomes. They conclude that this technique is helpful in predicting tumor recurrence and adverse survival.

B. A. Carter, MD, FRCPC

Histopathologic Response Criteria Predict Survival of Patients with Resected Lung Cancer After Neoadjuvant Chemotherapy
Pataer A, The University of Texas MD Anderson Lung Cancer Collaborative Research Group (Univ of Texas MD Anderson Cancer Ctr, Houston)
J Thorac Oncol 7:825-832, 2012

Introduction.—We evaluated the ability of histopathologic response criteria to predict overall survival (OS) and disease-free survival (DFS) in patients with surgically resected non-small cell lung cancer (NSCLC) treated with or without neoadjuvant chemotherapy.

Methods.—Tissue specimens from 358 patients with NSCLC were evaluated by pathologists blinded to the patient treatment and outcome. The surgical specimens were reviewed for various histopathologic features in the tumor including percentage of residual viable tumor cells, necrosis, and fibrosis. The relationship between the histopathologic findings and OS was assessed.

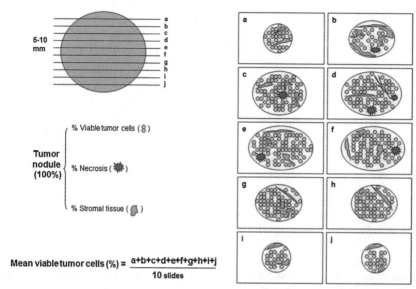

FIGURE 1.—Schematic diagram of histologic evaluation of lung cancer tissue resected from patients treated with neoadjuvant chemotherapy. (Reprinted from Pataer A, The University of Texas MD Anderson Lung Cancer Collaborative Research Group. Histopathologic response criteria predict survival of patients with resected lung cancer after neoadjuvant chemotherapy. *J Thorac Oncol.* 2012;7:825-832, with permission from the International Association for the Study of Lung Cancer.)

Results.—The percentage of residual viable tumor cells and surgical pathologic stage were associated with OS and DFS in 192 patients with NSCLC receiving neoadjuvant chemotherapy in multivariate analysis ($p = 0.005$ and $p = 0.01$, respectively). There was no association of OS or DFS with percentage of viable tumor cells in 166 patients with NSCLC who did not receive neoadjuvant chemotherapy ($p = 0.31$ and $p = 0.45$, respectively). Long-term OS and DFS were significantly prolonged in patients who had ≤10% viable tumor compared with patients with >10% viable tumor cells (5 years OS, 85% versus 40%, $p < 0.0001$ and 5 years DFS, 78% versus 35%, $p < 0.001$).

Conclusion.—The percentages of residual viable tumor cells predict OS and DFS in patients with resected NSCLC after neoadjuvant chemotherapy even when controlled for pathologic stage. Histopathologic assessment of resected specimens after neoadjuvant chemotherapy could potentially have a role in addition to pathologic stage in assessing prognosis, chemotherapy response, and the need for additional adjuvant therapies (Fig 1).

▶ This article emphasizes the expanding role of anatomic pathologists in the care of cancer patients. Most pathologists spend over 50% of their time diagnosing cancer or assessing cancer patients for residual or recurrent disease. This report deals with the role of histopathology in determining overall survival and disease-free survival rates after neoadjuvant therapy for lung cancer. The treatment of choice in patients with localized non-small-cell lung cancer (NSCLC) is resection of the lesion. Neoadjuvant chemotherapy followed by resection has been used in patients with locally advanced NSCLC to address the high rate of local and systemic failure. Although its use is controversial, neoadjuvant therapy has been shown in several studies to downstage NSCLC and improve overall survival.[1] This large study of 192 patients shows that an easily calculable (Fig 1) percentage of residual viable tumor is associated with overall survival and disease-free survival. The recommended sampling (minimum 1 block per centimeter of resected tumor) exceeds that of most laboratories' grossing protocols but is reasonable and likely would be readily accepted into the workflow of the practicing pathologist.

B. A. Carter, MD, FRCPC

Reference

1. Betticher DC, Hsu Schmitz SF, Tötsch M, et al. Mediastinal lymph node clearance after docetaxel-cisplatin neoadjuvant chemotherapy is prognostic of survival in patients with stage IIIA pN2 non-small-cell lung cancer: a multicenter phase II trial. *J Clin Oncol.* 2003;21:1752-1759.

Usefulness of imprint and brushing cytology in diagnosis of lung diseases with flexible bronchoscopy
Michels G, Topalidis T, Büttner R, et al (Univ of Cologne, Germany; Cytologic Inst, Hannover, Germany)
J Clin Pathol 65:649-653, 2012

Background.—To increase the diagnostic yield in pulmonary diseases, histopathology, imprint cytology and brushing cytology are assessed in combination during flexible bronchoscopy. However, the individual diagnostic discrimination of the three methods is unclear.

Methods.—The authors performed the three sampling techniques in 102 consecutive patients with suspected pulmonary pathologies and compared the definitive diagnosis with those of histopathology, imprint and brushing cytology for their diagnostic values regarding evidence of malignancy.

Results.—33.3% of all histopathological specimens, 31.4% of all imprints and 26.5% of brush biopsy specimens were positive for malignancy. The values for sensitivities were 94% for histopathology, 89% for imprint cytology and 75% for brushing cytology, respectively. Although brushing cytology had limited sensitivity, in two cases a malignant lung tumour was only diagnosed from cytological examination of brushing.

TABLE 1.—Diagnosis by Histopathology, Brushing Cytology and Imprint Cytology

	Histopathology (n = 102)	Imprint Cytology (n = 102)	Brushing Cytology (n = 102)
No malignancy	68 (66.7%)	70 (68.6%)	75 (73.5%)
Non-small-cell lung carcinoma	30 (29.4%)	28 (27.5%)	23 (22.5%)
Small-cell lung carcinoma	4 (3.92%)	3 (2.94%)	3 (2.94%)
Other carcinoma	0 (0%)	1 (0.98%)	1 (0.98%)

TABLE 2.—Correlation of *Imprint Results* with the Definitive Diagnosis

| | Definitive Diagnosis | | |
Imprint Diagnosis	Malignant	Benign	Total
Malignant	32	0	32
Benign	4	66	70
Total	36	66	102

TABLE 3.—Correlation of *Brushing Cytology* with the Definitive Diagnosis

| | Definitive Diagnosis | | |
Brush Diagnosis	Malignant	Benign	Total
Malignant	27	0	27
Benign	9	66	75
Total	36	66	102

TABLE 4.—Correlation of *Histopathology* with the Definitive Diagnosis

| | Definitive Diagnosis | | |
Histopathology Diagnosis	Malignant	Benign	Total
Malignant	34	0	34
Benign	2	66	68
Total	36	66	102

TABLE 5.—Statistical Analysis of Imprint/Brushing Cytology and Histopathology of all Cases (n = 102)

	Sensitivity (95% CI)	Specificity (95% CI)	PPV (95% CI)	NPV (95% CI)
Imprint cytology	88.9% (0.73% to 0.96%)	100% (0.93% to 1%)	100% (0.87% to 1%)	94.3% (0.85% to 0.98%)
Brushing cytology	75% (0.57% to 0.87%)	100% (0.93% to 1%)	100% (0.84% to 1%)	88% (0.78% to 0.94%)
Histopathology	94.4% (0.80% to 0.99%)	100% (0.93% to 1%)	100% (0.87% to 1%)	97.1% (0.89% to 0.99%)

NPV, negative predictive value; PPV, positive predictive value.

Conclusion.—In conclusion, routine imprint cytology does not increase the diagnostic sensitivity, whereas routine brushing cytology should be used in combination with histopathology to obtain the highest diagnostic rate of yield (Tables 1-5).

▶ This is a simply designed prospective study that takes imprint cytology of bronchoscopically derived tissue biopsies off the table in the diagnosis of lung lesions. Histopathology is the gold standard for the diagnosis of lung cancer but bronchoscopists perform multiple sampling techniques at the time of examination to improve the diagnostic yield and a recent[1] publication emphasized the role of multiple techniques. Very few studies have examined the role of imprint cytology, but most conclude that it is of value. In this report the authors, using a straightforward study design and solid statistical analysis (Tables 1-5), conclude that imprint cytology does not increase the diagnostic accuracy for detection of lung cancer when added to conventional forceps biopsies and brushings.

B. A. Carter, MD, FRCPC

Reference

1. Travis WD, Brambilla E, Noguchi M, et al. International association for the study of lung cancer/American Thoracic Society/European Respiratory Society international multidisciplinary classification of lung adenocarcinoma. *J Thorac Oncol.* 2011;6:244-285.

Prospective study of endobronchial ultrasound–guided transbronchial needle aspiration of lymph nodes versus transbronchial lung biopsy of lung tissue for diagnosis of sarcoidosis

Oki M, Saka H, Kitagawa C, et al (Nagoya Med Ctr, Japan)
J Thorac Cardiovasc Surg 143:1324-1329, 2012

Objective.—Endobronchial ultrasound–guided transbronchial needle aspiration (EBUS-TBNA) has been reported to be an accurate and safe method to confirm a pathologic diagnosis of sarcoidosis. However, only a few retrospective or small prospective studies have been published on EBUS-TBNA versus transbronchial lung biopsy (TBLB), which has been the standard method for making a pathologic diagnosis of sarcoidosis so far. The aim of this study was to compare the diagnostic yield of EBUS-TBNA and TBLB through a flexible bronchoscope in patients with stage I and II sarcoidosis.

Methods.—A total of 62 patients with suspected stage I and II sarcoidosis were included in this prospective study. EBUS-TBNA was performed (2 lymph nodes, 2 needle passes for each lymph node), followed by TBLB (5 biopsy specimens from multiple lung segments) in the same setting. The final diagnosis of sarcoidosis was based on clinicoradiologic compatibility and pathologic findings.

Results.—Of the 62 patients enrolled, 54 were given a final diagnosis of sarcoidosis. The diagnostic yield of EBUS-TBNA and TBLB for sarcoidois by showing noncaseating epithelioid cell granuloma was 94% (stage I, 97%; stage II, 88%) and 37% (stage I, 31%; stage II, 50%), respectively. The difference was statistically significant ($P < .001$). One case of pneumothorax and 3 cases of moderate bleeding (7%) resulted from TBLB, and 1 case of severe cough (2%) from EBUS-TBNA.

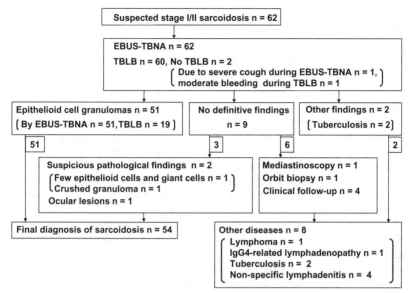

FIG. 1.—Diagnostic flow chart. *EBUS-TBNA*, Endobronchial ultrasound—guided transbronchial needle aspiration; *TBLB*, transbronchial lung biopsy; *IgG*, immunoglobulin G. (Oki M, Saka H, Kitagawa C, et al. Prospective study of endobronchial ultrasound—guided transbronchial needle aspiration of lymph nodes versus transbronchial lung biopsy of lung tissue for diagnosis of sarcoidosis. *J Thorac Cardiovasc Surg.* 2012;143:1324-1329, Copyright 2012, with permission from The American Association for Thoracic Surgery.)

Conclusions.—The diagnostic yield of EBUS-TBNA for stage I and II sarcoidosis is higher than for TBLB (Fig 1).

▶ Clinical and radiologic findings are very reliable in the diagnosis of sarcoidosis. Transbronchial lung biopsy has been the standard method for making a pathologic diagnosis of noncaseating epithelioid cell granulomas consistent with sarcoidosis. Endobronchial ultrasound—guided transbronchial needle aspiration (EBUS-TNBA) has begun to replace that standard on the basis of small retrospective studies. Oki et al, in their prospective study of 62 patients, show the significant advantage that EBUS-TBNA has over transbronchial lung biopsy (Fig 1). The diagnostic yield for transbronchial lung biopsy was surprisingly low, and this may be because of advances in imaging modalities and the identification of earlier-stage disease. Older literature shows a diagnostic yield of up to 70%, whereas more recent studies show a decrease to 40%—50%. The diagnostic yield of EBUS-TBNA was more than 90% in the authors' hands and showed a negligible complication rate. In short, pathologists will improve their diagnostic rate by supporting the use of EBUS-TBNA at their institutions.

B. A. Carter, MD, FRCPC

Suitability of EBUS-TBNA Specimens for Subtyping and Genotyping of NSCLC: A Multi-Centre Study of 774 Patients

Navani N, Brown JM, Nankivell M, et al (Univ College London, UK; MRC Clinical Trials Unit, London, UK; et al)

Am J Respir Crit Care Med 185:1316-1322, 2012

Rationale.—The current management of advanced non-small cell lung cancer (NSCLC) requires differentiation between squamous and non-squamous sub-types as well as epidermal growth factor receptor (EGFR) mutation status. Endobronchial ultrasound-guided transbronchial needle aspiration (EBUS-TBNA) is increasingly used for the diagnosis and staging of lung cancer. However, it is unclear whether cytology specimens obtained with EBUS-TBNA are suitable for the sub-classification and genotyping of NSCLC.

Objectives.—To determine whether cytology specimens obtained from EBUS-TBNA in routine practice are suitable for phenotyping and genotyping of NSCLC.

Methods.—Cytological diagnoses from EBUS-TBNA were recorded from 774 patients with known or suspected lung cancer across 5 centres in the United Kingdom between 2009 and 2011.

Measurements and Main Results.—The proportion of patients with a final diagnosis by EBUS-TBNA in whom subtype was classified was 77% (95% CI 73%−80%). The rate of NSCLC not otherwise specified (NSCLC-NOS) was significantly reduced in patients who underwent immunohistochemistry (adjusted OR 0.50 95% CI 0.28−0.82, $P = 0.016$). EGFR mutation analysis was possible in 107 (90%) of the 119 patients in whom mutation analysis was requested. The sensitivity, negative predictive value and diagnostic accuracy of EBUS-TBNA in patients with NSCLC was 88% (95% CI 86%−91%), 72% (95% CI 66%−77%) and 91% (95% CI 89%−93%) respectively.

Conclusions.—This large multi-centre pragmatic study demonstrates that cytology samples obtained from EBUS-TBNA in routine practice are suitable for sub-typing of NSCLC and EGFR mutation analysis and that use of immunohistochemistry reduces the rate of NSCLC-NOS.

▶ Long past are the days when pathologists could simply classify lung carcinomas into non-small-cell lung carcinomas (NSCLC) and small-cell carcinomas. Today's treatment modalities demand the further subclassification of non-small-cell carcinomas of the lung. Increasingly, our clinical colleagues are supplying pathologists with minimal samples for that classification. These small samples usually are the product of the relatively new technique, endobronchial ultrasound−guided transbronchial needle aspiration (EBUS-TBNA). The suitability of this sample type and size for the subtyping and genotyping of NSCLC has not been established. In this prospective study, 774 consecutive patients with suspected NSCLC underwent EBUS-TBNA, and local pathologists classified the lesions (Figs 1 and 2 in the original article). EBUS-TBNA was very sensitive for the detection of malignancy and allowed subtyping and genotyping in most of the patients, permitting increased use of personalized therapies. The study was limited by a lack of central review of pathology (although the authors make a convincing argument that this could be a strength). A new algorithm for the diagnosis of adenocarcinoma in small biopsies and cytologic samples has been proposed by an international consortium.[1] This study shows that samples from EBUS-TBNA obtained in routine practice fit well in this new diagnostic algorithm.

B. A. Carter, MD, FRCPC

Reference

1. Travis WD, Brambilla E, Noguchi M, et al. International association for the study of lung cancer/American thoracic society/European respiratory society international multidisciplinary classification of lung adenocarcinoma. *J Thorac Oncol.* 2011;6:244-285.

Limited role of Ki-67 proliferative index in predicting overall short-term survival in patients with typical and atypical pulmonary carcinoid tumors

Walts AE, Ines D, Marchevsky AM (Cedars-Sinai Med Ctr, Los Angeles, CA)
Mod Pathol 25:1258-1264, 2012

Pulmonary carcinoid tumors are currently classified as typical or atypical based on the mitotic index (2 per 10 hpf) and/or the presence of necrosis. Following incorporation of the Ki-67 index into the classification of GI carcinoid tumors, our oncologists have also been requesting this test as part of the work-up of pulmonary carcinoid tumors although there are currently no established criteria for interpreting Ki-67 index in these neoplasms. We utilized the Ariol® SL50 Image Analyzer system to measure the Ki-67 index in 101 pulmonary carcinoid tumors (78 typical and 23 atypical) and then correlated the Ki-67 index and the histological diagnoses in univariate and multivariable analysis with overall survival. The mean Ki-67 indices for the typical carcinoids (3.7 s.d ± .4.0) and the atypical carcinoids (18.8 s.d. ± 17.1) were significantly different ($P < 0.001$) although the frequency distributions of Ki-67 indices in the two groups overlapped considerably. Receiver operating characteristic curve analysis showed that a Ki-67 index cutoff value of 5% provided the best fit for specificity and sensitivity in predicting overall survival. Histological diagnosis and the Ki-67 index cutoff of 5% were each independently strong predictors of survival ($P < 0.001$ and $P = 0.003$, respectively). When considered together in multivariable analysis, histological diagnosis was the stronger predictor of overall survival and a Ki-67 index cutoff of 5% did not provide additional significant predictive survival information within either the typical carcinoid or the atypical carcinoid patient group. A few typical carcinoid patients with Ki-67 indices of 5% appeared to have worse survival after 5 years than those with Ki-67 indices <5%, but the data set was insufficiently powered to further analyze this. These findings do not provide best evidence for the routine use of Ki-67 index to prognosticate overall short-term survival in patients with pulmonary carcinoid tumors.

▶ The value of this study lies in its support of the unreliability of Ki-67 as a replacement for a surgical pathologist's mitotic count. The World Health Organization classification of lung tumors and the American Joint Commission on Cancer staging manual define pulmonary carcinoids as typical and atypical based on the mitotic index and the presence or absence of necrosis. Most recently, Ki-67 labeling has been incorporated into the assessment of neuroendocrine tumors of the gastrointestinal tract. Of course, medical oncologists are now requesting this assessment for their lung patients. Like many previous authors, Walts et al describe difficulties with automation versus naked eye examination, identification of hotspots for counting, appropriate cutoff values, and definition of adequate field size for accurate assessment. The authors conclude that the results of the study underscore the limitations in automatically assuming that "new data" are better or more informative than older data obtained with conventional histopathology, and I agree.

Histological diagnosis in lung carcinoids still provides the strongest prognostic value.

B. A. Carter, MD, FRCPC

Liposarcomas of the Mediastinum and Thorax: A Clinicopathologic and Molecular Cytogenetic Study of 24 Cases, Emphasizing Unusual and Diverse Histologic Features
Boland JM, Colby TV, Folpe AL (Mayo Clinic, Rochester, MN; Mayo Clinic, Scottsdale, AZ)
Am J Surg Pathol 36:1395-1403, 2012

Liposarcoma rarely occurs in the mediastinum, and most reports predate the current genetically based classification system. We report the clinicopathologic and molecular genetic features of a series of thoracic liposarcomas identified over a 60-year period. Twenty-four confirmed cases were reclassified using the most recent World Health Organization classification. Fluorescent in situ hybridization for *CPM* amplification and/or *DDIT3* rearrangement was performed on selected cases. The 24 cases occurred in 13 men and 11 women (mean age, 53 y; range, 15 to 73 y) and arose in all mediastinal compartments. All subtypes were encountered with 8 well-differentiated liposarcomas, 6 dedifferentiated liposarcomas (3 of 6 confirmed *CPM+*), 7 pleomorphic liposarcomas (2 of 7 confirmed *CPM−*, 1 of 7 confirmed *DDIT3−*), 2 myxoid liposarcomas, and 1 unclassifiable liposarcoma (*CPM−* and *DDIT3−*). Unusual histologic features included myxoid well-differentiated liposarcoma mimicking myxoid liposarcoma (2 cases), lipoleiomyosarcoma (1 case), dedifferentiated liposarcoma with "meningothelial"-like dedifferentiation, differentiated myxoid liposarcoma mimicking well-differentiated liposarcoma (*CPM−*), and pleomorphic liposarcoma with epithelioid and myxoid change. Follow-up information was

TABLE 1.—Clinicopathologic Features of 24 Cases of Mediastinal and Thoracic Liposarcoma

Cases	Age	Sex	Site	Year	Histology/Genetics	Recurrence	Metastasis	Status	Follow-up (mo)
1	68	F	SM	1958	WDL	1961, 1966	No	AWD	101
2	60	M	AM/SM	1990	WDL	No	No	Alive	252
3	73	F	MC	2004	WDL	Unresectable	No	DOD	11
4	52	F	PM	2007	WDL with hypercellular foci/CPM−	No	No	ANED	60
5	57	M	PM	2010	WDL	No	No	ANED	11
6	50	F	AM	2011	WDL, lipoleiomyosarcoma	NA	NA	NA	NA
7	16	M	PM	1965	WDL with myxoid change	No	No	ANED	123
8	32	M	MM	2005	WDL with myxoid change	No	No	ANED	60
9	68	M	PM	1987	DL, high grade	1991, 1992	No	AWD	72
10	63	F	AM	2003	DL with osteosarcomatous differentiation	2005, 2006	Lung, chest	DOD	34
11	47	F	MM	2006	DL with meningothelial-like whorls/CPM+	None	None	ANED	60
12	71	F	PM	2010	DL, high grade	Residual	None	AWD	12
13	69	M	MC	2011	DL, high grade/CPM+	NA	NA	NA	NA
14	76	F	AM	2011	DL, high grade/CPM+	NA	NA	NA	NA
15	51	M	AM	1972	PL	1972	None	DOD	14
16	31	M	PM	1994	PL/CPM−	1995	Bone, soft tissue	DOD	62
17	71	M	AM	2008	PL/CPM−	Residual	Lung	DOD	8
18	23	F	AM	1975	Myxoid PL	1977	Pleura	DOD	15
19	48	M	PS	2008	Myxoid PL/DDIT3−	Unknown	Unknown	Alive	36
20	62	M	MM	2011	Myxoid PL/EWS−, DDIT3−	No	No	ANED	9
21	69	F	MC	2010	Epithelioid PL	Unresectable	Liver	DOD	11
22	15	M	SM	1958	ML, low grade	1959, 1960, 1962	None	DOD	58
23	47	M	MC	1998	Differentiating ML/CPM−, DDIT3−	1998, 2000	None	DOD	72
24	57	F	MC	2008	Unclassifiable/CPM−, FUS−, DDIT3−	Unknown	Unknown	Alive	36

AM indicates anterior mediastinum; ANED, alive, no evidence of disease; AWD, alive with disease; DL, dedifferentiated liposarcoma; DOD, dead of disease; MC, multiple compartments; ML, myxoid liposarcoma; MM, middle mediastinum; NA, not applicable; PL, pleomorphic liposarcoma; PM, posterior mediastinum; PS, pleural space; SM, superior mediastinum; WDL, well-differentiated liposarcoma.

available for 19 patients (mean, 55 mo; range, 8 to 252 mo). Outcome was strongly associated with histologic subtype, with death from disease occurring in 1 of 6 well-differentiated, 1 of 4 dedifferentiated, 5 of 7 pleomorphic, and 2 of 2 myxoid liposarcomas. The mediastinum shows a preponderance of uncommon subtypes and unusual morphologic variants. Correct classification has important implications, with most patients with well-differentiated/dedifferentiated liposarcoma having a protracted clinical course, in contrast to the more rapid disease progression seen in patients with myxoid and pleomorphic liposarcoma (Table 1).

▶ Although liposarcomas are a common specimen for surgical pathologists, primary liposarcomas of the mediastinum and thorax are exceedingly rare, as demonstrated in this 60-year study at a large institution with only 24 patients (Table 1). When these lesions are found in the mediastinum/thorax, they most likely represent metastatic disease from a retroperitoneal location. Because of their paucity and advances in classification and genetic approaches to soft-tissue tumors, there are few literature sources that aid the pathologist when faced with a primary adipocytic lesion of the thorax/mediastinum. This study serves as a concise and up-to-date review of the topic. All cases were classified using the most recent World Health Organization classification and were genetically subtyped as per modern protocols. The materials and methods sections contain good information on genetic testing needed in these lesions. The pleomorphic and myxoid subtypes of liposarcoma were somewhat common in this study in counterdistinction from the subtypes found elsewhere in the body. Many of the tumors, despite subtype, had unusual morphologic features emphasizing the need for accurate criteria for diagnosis, given the varying outcomes. Ancillary molecular genetic testing is encouraged for any case in which correct classification is in doubt.

B. A. Carter, MD, FRCPC

7   Cardiovascular

Approach to the cardiac autopsy
Sheppard MN (Royal Brompton Hosp, London, UK)
J Clin Pathol 65:484-495, 2012

This article deals with a detailed analysis of the dissection of the heart at autopsy. Since most of causes of death are cardiac it is essential that all pathologists are familiar with the approach to dissection of the heart, taking of blocks for histology and possible analysis of the conduction tissue (Fig 15).

▶ This review article by Sheppard is a very detailed and up-to-date description of the way pathologists should approach heart dissection at an autopsy. Given that the cause of death (COD) for the vast majority of hospital autopsies is cardiovascular disease and that those with other COD show significant cardio-vascular disease, this review should be read by all pathologists and residents participating in autopsy service. The value of clinical history, communication with families and clinicians, and issues of consent (albeit from a UK point of view) are discussed. The author likens her stepwise approach and 10-block submission in cases of cardiac death (noncardiac deaths only require 2 blocks) to a minimal dataset for cancer reporting, stressing the lack of value of vague or incomplete reports. The article could have been improved by the inclusion of a reporting template.

B. A. Carter, MD, FRCPC

⩣ Mid-ventricular slice between AV junction and apex
ANTERIOR

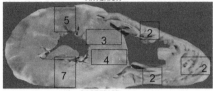

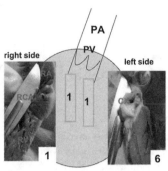

right side

left side

CX: circumflex, MV: mitral valve, LA: left atrium, LV: left ventricle, PA: pulmonary artery, PV: pulmonary valve, RCA: right coronary artery, RA: right atrium, RV: right ventricle

POSTERIOR

KEY: Blocks
- 1
  - − Right ventricular outflow tract (RVOT) (x2)
  - − RA & RCA & tricuspid valve leaflet & RV (x1)
- 2 Anterior, lateral, posterior RV (x3)
- 3 IVS anterior (x1)
- 4 IVS posterior (x1)
- 5 Anterior LV and LAD (x2)
- 6 LA & CX & Mitral valve leaflet & Lateral LV (x1)
- 7 Posterior LV and aorta (x2)
- 8 SA node (x2 - x4)
- 9 AV node (x2)
- 10 AV node (x2)

10 blocks of tissue

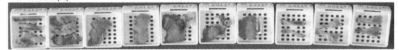

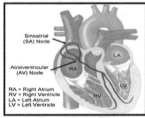

Sinoatrial (SA) Node

Atrioventricular (AV) Node

RA = Right Atrium
RV = Right Ventricle
LA = Left Atrium
LV = Left Ventricle

SA node at junction of SVC with
Right Atrial Appendage(RAA)

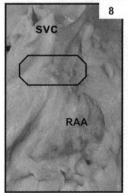

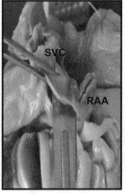

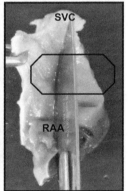

SVC

RAA

SVC

RAA

SVC

RAA

FIGURE 15.—Diagrams of heart dissection with 10 blocks taken from lateral cuts, right ventricular outflow tract and heart slice. (Reprinted from Sheppard MN. Approach to the cardiac autopsy. *J Clin Pathol.* 2012;65:484-495, with permission from the BMJ Publishing Group Ltd.)

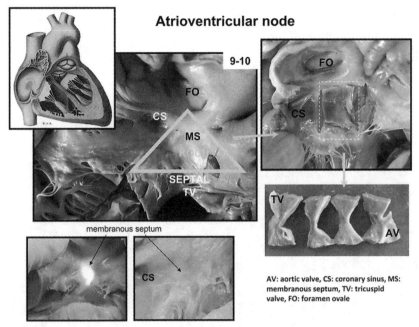

Atrioventricular node

9-10

FO

FO

CS

CS

MS

SEPTAL
TV

TV

AV

membranous septum

CS

AV: aortic valve, CS: coronary sinus, MS:
membranous septum, TV: tricuspid
valve, FO: foramen ovale

FIGURE 15.—(*Continued*).

2011 Consensus statement on endomyocardial biopsy from the Association for European Cardiovascular Pathology and the Society for Cardiovascular Pathology
Leone O, Veinot J P, Angelini A, et al (Azienda Ospedaliero-Universitaria S.Orsola-Malpighi, Bologna, Italy; The Ottawa Hosp, Ontario, Canada; Padua, Italy; et al)
Cardiovasc Pathol 21:245-274, 2012

The Association for European Cardiovascular Pathology and the Society for Cardiovascular Pathology have produced this position paper concerning the current role of endomyocardial biopsy (EMB) for the diagnosis of cardiac diseases and its contribution to patient management, focusing on pathological issues, with these aims:

- Determining appropriate EMB use in the context of current diagnostic strategies for cardiac diseases and providing recommendations for its rational utilization
- Providing standard criteria and guidance for appropriate tissue triage and pathological analysis
- Promoting a team approach to EMB use, integrating the competences of pathologists, clinicians, and imagers (Table 3).

▶ This article places great emphasis on the role of the pathologist in morphological tissue assessment for developing appropriate diagnostic strategies in

TABLE 3.—Endomyocardial Biopsy Diagnostic Potential in Cardiac Diseases with Grading of Recommendation

Clinically Suspected Disease	EMB Diagnostic Potential and Histological Notes	Technical Aspects and Tissue Triage	Grading of Recommendation
Myocarditis/inflammatory cardiomyopathy	Definite diagnosis: lymphocytic, granulocytic, polymorphous, eosinophil, necrotizing eosinophilic, giant cell, granulomatous myocarditis, with or without associated myocyte damage/necrosis. Histological findings alone or together with molecular techniques may be able to specify the etiology of the inflammatory disease.	Recommended: In addition to formalin fixation, two fragments (or one if greater than 3 mm^2) could be snap-frozen or preserved in RNA-later for virus molecular investigation. One peripheral blood sample (5–10 ml) collected in EDTA or sodium citrate tubes. NB: Timing and number of EMB and serial histological sections are important for sensitive detection of myocarditis.	S
Cardiac sarcoidosis	Definite diagnosis: noncaseous granulomatous myocarditis. Histological findings pathognomonic or highly suggestive of the disease.	Possible increased utility with guided biopsy procedure.	S
Myocardial diseases due to drugs and chemical/"toxic" substances	Probable/possible diagnosis: hypersensitivity myocarditis (histological findings suggestive of the disease), toxic damage.	Glutaraldehyde or Karnowsky solution fixed fragment for electron microscopy may be useful for cardiotoxicity evaluation of some drugs.	S: hypersensitivity myocarditis M: cardiotoxicity
Peripartum cardiomyopathy	Probable diagnosis: myocarditis/borderline myocarditis. Histological findings give some indications of probable disease.	Fresh sample may be useful for virus molecular biology. Important: EMB timing	M
Cardiac amyloidosis	Definite diagnosis: amyloid infiltration. Histological findings+histomorphological stains are pathognomonic.	Recommended: Congo red, modified sulfated alcian blue, or thioflavin T stains. IHC, IF, immunoelectron microscopy, protein sequencing, and/or mass spectrometry to establish the type of amyloid. Frozen tissue is required for IF and protein sequencing	S

Iron overload	Definite diagnosis: iron intracellular deposition. Histological findings+iron staining are pathognomonic.	Iron staining is advisable for all diagnostic EMBs from patients with unexplained DCM.	S
Glycogen storage diseases: Type II glycogenosis (Pompe disease) Type III glycogenosis (Cori disease) Type V glycogenosis (Andersen disease) Danon disease PRKAG2 mutations	Probable diagnosis: diffuse intracellular glycogen storage. Histological findings may be suggestive, but not specific, for the diagnosis.	Recommended: Fresh sample for histochemical stains and glutaraldehyde or Karnowsky solution fixed fragment for electron microscopy are useful to assess the nature of intracellular deposits.	S
Anderson–Fabry disease	Probable diagnosis: histology: hypertrophic vacuolated cells with dislocation of contractile elements to the periphery of myocytes. Histological findings may be suggestive, but not specific for diagnosis.	Recommended: Glutaraldehyde or Karnowsky solution fixed fragment may be useful for electron microscopy to assess electron dense concentric lamellar bodies.	S
Desmin cardiomyopathy	Definite diagnosis based on ultrastructural findings: abnormal granulofilamentous aggregates of desmin-type intermediate filaments in the cytoplasm of cardiomyocytes (interfibrillar areas) and at the Z band level. Nonspecific light histological findings.	Recommended: Glutaraldehyde or Karnowsky solution fixed fragment for electron microscopy necessary. Immunoelectron microscopy confirms that these aggregates are formed by desmin.	S
Dystrophin cardiomyopathy	Definite diagnosis in Duchenne muscular dystrophy: absence of dystrophin in myocyte sarcolemma. Probable diagnosis in Becker muscular dystrophy: extensive irregularities and discontinuities of dystrophin in myocyte sarcolemma. Nonspecific histological findings.	Recommended: dystrophin IHC or IF stain in which dystrophin is markedly diminished or absent in affected individuals. Fresh sample is required for IF and may be required for IHC.	M
Laminopathies (lamin A/C)	Nonspecific diagnosis: interstitial/replacement fibrosis, myocyte hypertrophy and vacuolization, enlarged and irregular-shaped nuclei. Nonspecific histological findings.	Data on diagnostic use of IHC staining for lamin A/C in human EMB are not available. In centers performing IF, fresh samples are required.	N

(Continued)

Table 3.—(*Continued*)

Clinically Suspected Disease	EMB Diagnostic Potential and Histological Notes	Technical Aspects and Tissue Triage	Grading of Recommendation
Mitichondrial cardiomyopathies	Probable/possible diagnosis: morphologically altered mitochondria by electron microscopy Nonspecific histological findings: enlarged myocytes with extensive cytoplasmic vacuolization	Recommended: Fresh sample is needed for histoenzymatic stainings. Glutaraldehyde or Karnowsky solution fixed fragment is needed for ultrastructural tests.	M (especially in isolated MIC)
Arrhythmogenic right ventricle cardiomyopathy	Probable diagnosis: fibrous or fibrofatty replacement and myocardial atrophy. Nonspecific histological findings.	IF or IHC for plakoglobin and other cellular junction proteins is promising test (being validated). EMB from the interventricular septum may not be informative. Diagnostic accuracy increases if EMB sampling site is guided by imaging (MRI) or electrophysiological (electroanatomic mapping) techniques.	S (in selected cases having no clear-cut diagnosis with noninvasive and other invasive procedures)
Loeffler fibroplastic endocarditis/ endomyocardial fibrosis	Definite diagnosis in the acute phase: endomyocardial infiltrates rich in degranulated eosinophils and endocardial thrombosis. Specific histological findings. Possible diagnosis in the chronic phase: evidence of endocardial fibrous thickening and subendocardial myocyte abnormalities. Nonspecific histological findings.	EMB timing is important as the utility of biopsy probably decreases with disease time course.	S in the acute–subacute phase
Cardiac tumors	Definite diagnosis	IHC useful for tumor typing	S

	Possible/Definite diagnosis	Comments	
Hypertrophic cariomyopathy (sarcomeric mutations)	Possible diagnosis: myocyte hypertrophy, interstitial and/or substitutive fibrosis, disarray, and possible small vessel disease. Nonspecific histological findings.	M: The clinical diagnosis of HCM usually relies on noninvasive diagnostic tools, and EMB is not recommended in the diagnostic workup. However, in selected cases, EMB may be helpful in excluding infiltrative or storage diseases with variable diagnostic degrees of certainty.	
Idiopathic restrictive cardiomyopathy	Possible diagnosis: normal myocardium, and/or fibrosis and/or disarray. No other identifiable diseases causing restrictive phenotype. Nonspecific histological findings.	M: EMB is unable to give a specific diagnosis. However, in selected cases, EMB may be helpful in excluding infiltrative or storage diseases. Useful in the workup of constriction versus restriction.	
Idiopathic dilated cardiomyopathy	Possible diagnosis: myocyte hypertrophy, nuclear alterations, perinuclear halo, with or without fibrosis. Nonspecific histological findings.	M: EMB is unable to give a diagnostic picture, but may be helpful in excluding other diseases.	
Heart transplantation	Definite diagnosis: acute cellular rejection, some infectious disease, PTLD, and nonrejection posttransplant findings. Specific histological findings.	Recommended: C4d IHC/IF staining for AMR. Fresh sample is required for IF staining.	S

DCM, dilated cardiomyopathy; EDTA, ethylenediaminetetraacetic acid; EMB, endomyocardial biopsy; IF, immunofluorescence; IHC, immunohistochemistry; MRI, magnetic resonance imaging; M, mixed; N, not supported; PTLD, posttransplant lymphoproliferative disorders; S, supported.

collaboration with clinicians, imagers, molecular biologists, and geneticists for endomyocardial biopsies (EMB). Using an evidenced-based approach the authors, internationally recognized experts in cardiovascular pathology, review the use of EMB for the evaluation of cardiac tissue for transplant monitoring, myocarditis, drug toxicity, cardiomyopathy, arrhythmia, and secondary cardiac involvement by systemic diseases, and for the diagnosis of cardiac masses. A concise, clear description of the pathologic handling of tissues and the use of special studies and procedures is included (Table 3). To minimize variability in reporting, a common standardized approach is recommended. For more common disorders such as myocarditis, an expanded detailed description of EMB handling and reporting is provided. Although the authors state that EMB should be performed only in centers that are fully equipped for pathological workup and where specifically trained and experienced pathologists are available, this article serves as a valuable resource for those pathologists who may be interpreting EMB in specific situations and those who act as the first pathologist in a consultative practice.

B. A. Carter, MD, FRCPC

Myocardial infarction with normal coronaries: an autopsy perspective
Silvanto A, de Noronha SV, Sheppard MN (Royal Brompton and Harefield Hosps NHS Trust, London, UK; NHLI Imperial College, London, UK)
J Clin Pathol 65:512-516, 2012

Aim.—To analyse postmortem cases of myocardial infarction (MI) with normal coronary arteries in terms of patient characteristics, features of the MI and risk factors.

Methods.—This retrospective non-case controlled study was carried out at a specialist cardiac pathology department at a tertiary cardiac referral centre. Cases of histologically confirmed MI and normal coronary arteries during the period 1996—2010 were identified and analysed for the presence of risk factors.

Results.—Nineteen cases of histologically confirmed MI and normal coronary arteries were identified with a similar gender ratio 1:1.1 (male:female) and mean age of 33 ± 12 years (range 14—58). All patients died suddenly. The location of the infarct was variable, with left anterior descending artery territory being the single most prevalent (47%). Risk factors were identified in the majority of cases (n = 14), with some cases experiencing more than one association, including alcohol and/or predominately class A drug use (n = 7), including cocaine, inflammation (n = 2), hypercoagulable state (n = 3) and exertion (n = 2).

Conclusions.—Current data regarding prognosis in MI with normal coronary arteries suggests a favourable outcome in the context of major cardiovascular events. No large series of fatal cases have been reported. This study highlights that this entity can be fatal and its prognosis may be less favourable than currently considered. This autopsy series also demonstrates that the causation of MI with normal coronary arteries is

TABLE.—Patient Demographics, Circumstances of SCD, Relevant Medical History, Location and Timing of Infarction

Case	Sex	Age (Years)	Circumstances of SCD	Medical History	LVH‡	Location of Acute Infarct LV Wall*	Timing of Infarct
1	M	44	Sitting/home	Heroin use, alcoholism and hepatitis C positive	0	Anterior, lateral, posterior	1–6 weeks
2	F	16	Home	Pregnancy, family history of HHT	0	Anterior, lateral, septal	24–48 h
3	F	42	Post-exertion (community)	On contraceptive pill. BMI 23.5	0	Antero and posteroseptal	1–6 weeks + lateroseptal fibrosis
4	M	58	N/A	Asthma and emphysema	1 (septal)	Anterolateral	24–48 h
5	M	32	Bed/home	Chest pain. BMI 27.0	1 (septal)	Anteroseptal	Fibrosis
6	M	37	N/A	Heroin use, on detoxification and chlorpromazine. Hepatitis C+. BMI 20.2. Toxicology positive for morphine.	0	Anteroseptal	24–48 h
7	M	45	Home	Alcohol and cannabis use, chest pain	1	Anteroseptal	1–6 weeks
8	F	35	Home	Alcoholism, ischaemic ECG and chest pain, toxicology positive for cocaine, BMI 20.7	0	Anteroseptal	24–48 h
9	F	39	N/A	N/A	0	Anteroseptal	24–48 h
10	F	49	Hospital	Hypertension, asthma, phaeochromocytoma†	0	Anteroseptal	24–48 h + LV fibrosis
11	M	17	Post-exertion (bed/home)	Dyspnoea and chest pain	1	Circumferential	24–48 h + posterior LV fibrosis
12	F	16	Bed/home	Consumption of alcohol before death	0	Lateral	24–48 h
13	M	38	Sitting/home	Gout. BMI 23.0	0	Posterior	Fibrosis
14	F	26	Bed/home	On contraceptive pill	0	Posterobasal	24–48 h + posterior LV fibrosis
15	M	14	Community	Epilepsy, consumption of cannabis before death, BMI 20.0	0	Posterolateral	24–48 h
16	M	32	Bed/home	Epilepsy, BMI 21.5	0	Posteroseptal	fibrosis
17	F	25	Bed/home	Palpitations, consumption of alcohol before death. Toxicology positive for alcohol	0	Subendocardial, inc. papillary muscle	1–6 weeks + papillary muscle fibrosis
18	F	36	Home	Bronchitis, chest pain	0	Subendocardial RV (and LV)	24–48 h
19	M	41	Community	Smoker	1	Subendocardial	1–6 weeks

BMI, body mass index; HHT, hereditary haemorrhagic telangiectasia; HTN, hypertension; LV, left ventricle(ular); N/A, not available; RV, right ventricle; SCD, sudden cardiac death.
*Unless otherwise specified.
†Diagnosed at autopsy.
‡Left ventricular hypertrophy was mild (16-18 mm).

complex and multifactorial, including a history of alcohol and/or drug use. It also highlights the importance of accurate epidemiological data from referring pathologists (Table).

▶ The value of this report is that it demonstrates, in a small, non-case-controlled autopsy study of sudden death, a small but definite risk of mortality associated with myocardial infarction (MI) and normal coronary arteries. Most articles on this subject suggest that prognosis in patients with MI and normal coronary arteries is favorable.[1] Thorough examination of the left mainstem, left anterior descending, left circumflex, and right coronary arteries ensured that they were entirely normal macroscopically and histologically, with no atherosclerotic plaque. The presence of other cardiovascular pathology was excluded with detailed examination of the heart and great vessels. Atherosclerotic plaque rupture is the leading cause of myocardial infarction in patients with coronary heart disease. As expected the patients were younger in age and many had a history of alcohol or drug abuse (Table). Because both alcohol and drug abuse are becoming more common and in a younger population, pathologists may be reporting this association more frequently in the future. The study is limited in that it is retrospective and relied on referring pathologists for patient demographics and history.

B. A. Carter, MD, FRCPC

Reference

1. Ong P, Athanasiadis A, Borgulya G, Voehringer M, Sechtem U. 3-year follow-up of patients with coronary artery spasm as cause of acute coronary syndrome: the CASPAR (coronary artery spasm in patients with acute coronary syndrome) study follow-up. *J Am Coll Cardiol.* 2011;57:147-152.

Sudden Death after Chest Pain: Feasibility of Virtual Autopsy with Postmortem CT Angiography and Biopsy
Ross SG, Thali MJ, Bolliger S, et al (Univ of Berne, Switzerland; Univ of Zurich, Switzerland)
Radiology 264:250-259, 2012

Purpose.—To determine the potential of minimally invasive postmortem computed tomographic (CT) angiography combined with image-guided tissue biopsy of the myocardium and lungs in decedents who were thought to have died of acute chest disease and to compare this method with conventional autopsy as the reference standard.

Materials and Methods.—The responsible justice department and ethics committee approved this study. Twenty corpses (four female corpses and 16 male corpses; age range, 15—80 years), all of whom were reported to have had antemortem acute chest pain, were imaged with postmortem whole-body CT angiography and underwent standardized image-guided biopsy. The standard included three biopsies of the myocardium and a single biopsy of bilateral central lung tissue. Additional biopsies of pulmonary clots for differentiation of pulmonary embolism and postmortem organized

TABLE 2.—Main Findings at Postmortem CT Angiography—Biopsy and Autopsy—Histopathologic Examination and Causes of Death

Cadaver No./ Age (y)/Sex	Findings at Postmortem CT Angiography	Findings at Autopsy	Histologic Findings after Autopsy	Histologic Findings at Biopsy	Cause of Death
1/48/M	Severe CAD (one stem), stent in LAD artery with contrast material void, MH, PC	Severe CAD (one stem), stent in LAD artery with fresh in-stent thrombosis, MH, PC	CMI, PC	CMI	Cardiac arrest (coronary thrombosis)
2/71/M	No or minimal CAD, PC, contrast material void in pulmonary trunk	No or minimal CAD, PC, thrombus in pulmonary trunk	Thrombotic material in pulmonary artery, PC	Thrombotic material in pulmonary artery, PC	PE (right heart failure)
3/53/M	No or minimal CAD, pericardial tamponade	No or minimal CAD, pericardial tamponade	CMI	CMI	Cardiac tamponade (ruptured atheroma in ascending aorta)
4/33/F	No or minimal CAD, MB	No or minimal CAD, MB	Myocarditis	Myocarditis	Cardiac arrest (myocarditis)
5/58/M	Severe CAD (two stems), MH, MB, PC	Severe CAD (two stems), MH, MB, PC	Postmortem clot in pulmonary artery, CMI, PC	Postmortem clot in pulmonary artery, CMI, PC	Cardiac arrest (obstructive CAD)
6/63/M	Severe CAD (two stems), MH, MB, PC, contrast material void in LCX artery	Severe CAD (two stems), MH, MB, PC, fresh thrombus in LCX artery	CMI, PC	CMI, PC	Cardiac arrest (coronary thrombosis)
7/72/M	Severe CAD (two stems), CABG, MH, unilateral stenosis of carotid bifurcation	Severe CAD (two stems), CABG, MH, unilateral stenosis of carotid bifurcation	Postmortem clot in pulmonary artery, CMI	Postmortem clot in pulmonary artery, CMI	Cardiac arrest (obstructive CAD)
8/48/M	No or minimal CAD, MH, MB, pericardial tamponade	No or minimal CAD, MH, MB, pericardial tamponade	No pathologic findings	No pathologic findings	Cardiac tamponade (Stanford type A)
9/53/F	No or minimal CAD, PC, contrast material void in pulmonary trunk, small berry aneurysm in intracranial ICA	No or minimal CAD, PC, thrombus in pulmonary trunk, small berry aneurysm in intracranial ICA	Thrombotic material in pulmonary artery, PC	Thrombotic material in pulmonary artery, PC	PE (right heart failure)
10/24/M	No or minimal CAD, MB, ruptured aneurysm in right subclavian artery, unilateral hemothorax	No or minimal CAD, MB, ruptured aneurysm in right subclavian artery, unilateral hemothorax	No pathologic findings	No pathologic findings	Exsanguination (ruptured aneurysm in subclavian artery)
11/61/F	Intermediate CAD (one stem), MH, pericardial tamponade	Intermediate CAD (one stem), MH, pericardial tamponade	No pathologic findings	No pathologic findings	Cardiac tamponade (Stanford type A)

(Continued)

TABLE 2.—(Continued)

Cadaver No./ Age (y)/Sex	Findings at Postmortem CT Angiography	Findings at Autopsy	Histologic Findings after Autopsy	Histologic Findings at Biopsy	Cause of Death
12/15/M	No or minimal CAD, PC, contrast material void in pulmonary trunk	No or minimal CAD, PC, thrombus in pulmonary trunk	Thrombotic material in pulmonary artery, PC	Thrombotic material in pulmonary artery, PC	PE (right heart failure)
13/82/M	Severe CAD (one stem), contrast material void in RCA	Severe CAD (one stem), thrombus in RCA	CMI	CMI	Cardiac arrest (coronary thrombosis)
14/45/M	Severe CAD (two stems), MH, MB	Severe CAD (two stems), MH, MB, pericardial tamponade	MI	MI	MI (obstructive CAD)
15/71/M	Severe CAD (two stems), MH, CABG, PC, unilateral stenosis of carotid bifurcation	Severe CAD (two stems), MH, CABG, PC	MI, PC	MI, PC	MI (obstructive CAD)
16/58/M	Intermediate CAD (one stem), pericardial tamponade	Intermediate CAD (one stem), pericardial tamponade	No pathologic findings	No pathologic findings	Cardiac tamponade (Stanford type A)
17/52/F	No or minimal CAD, PC, contrast material void in pulmonary trunk	No or minimal CAD, PC, thrombus in pulmonary trunk	Thrombotic material in pulmonary artery, PC	Thrombotic material in pulmonary artery, PC	PE (right heart failure)
18/80/M	Severe CAD (two stems), CABG, MH, unilateral stenosis of carotid bifurcation	Severe CAD (two stems), CABG, MH	CMI	CMI	Cardiac arrest (obstructive CAD)
19/69/M	Intermediate CAD (two stems), erosion of the left inferior pulmonary artery and the bronchial system	Intermediate CAD (two stems), erosion of the left inferior pulmonary artery and the bronchial system	SCLC	SCLC	Exsanguination (SCLC with erosion of pulmonary artery)
20/73/M	Severe CAD (two stems), CABG, MH, PC, unilateral stenosis of carotid bifurcation	Severe CAD (two stems), CABG, MH, PC, unilateral stenosis of carotid bifurcation	MI, PC	CMI, PC	MI (obstructive CAD)

Note.—CABG = coronary artery bypass graft, CAD = coronary artery disease, CMI = chronic myocardial ischemia, ICA = internal carotid artery, LAD = left anterior descending, LCX = left circumflex, MB = myocardial bridging, MH = myocardial hypertrophy, MI = myocardial infarction, PC = pulmonary congestion, RCA = right coronary artery, SCLC = small cell lung cancer. Coronary artery disease was graded as follows: no significant or minimal disease (<50% stenosis), intermediate or significant disease (50%–75% stenosis), or severe disease (>75% stenosis).

thrombus were performed after initial analysis of the cross-sectional images. Subsequent traditional autopsy with sampling of histologic specimens was performed in all cases. Thereafter, conventional histologic and autopsy reports were compared with postmortem CT angiography and CT-guided biopsy findings. A Cohen κ coefficient analysis was performed to explore the effect of the clustered nature of the data.

Results.—In 19 of the 20 cadavers, findings at postmortem CT angiography in combination with CT-guided biopsy validated the cause of death found at traditional autopsy. In one cadaver, early myocardial infarction of the papillary muscles had been missed. The Cohen κ coefficient was 0.94. There were four instances of pulmonary embolism, three aortic dissections (Stanford type A), three myocardial infarctions, three instances of fresh coronary thrombosis, three cases of obstructive coronary artery disease, one ruptured ulcer of the ascending aorta, one ruptured aneurysm of the right subclavian artery, one case of myocarditis, and one pulmonary malignancy with pulmonary artery erosion. In seven of 20 cadavers, CT-guided biopsy provided additional histopathologic information that substantiated the final diagnosis of the cause of death.

Conclusion.—Postmortem CT angiography combined with image-guided biopsy, because of their minimally invasive nature, have a potential role in the detection of the cause of death after acute chest pain (Table 2).

▶ The demise of the hospital autopsy is of concern to pathologists, resident educators, and patient safety and quality committees. At a time when patient safety and quality are at the top of everyone's agenda, the 1 tool that acts as a gold standard in the auditing of patient care is suffering a major decrease in use. Although the cause of this phenomenon has not been definitively identified, lack of acceptance (and understanding) of traditional autopsy techniques by bereaved families and religious and cultural objections have been postulated. Is it time for the development of the minimally invasive autopsy?[1] Certainly quality assurance measures can be addressed in this manner. In the interest of keeping our health care systems safe, perhaps pathologists and resident educators could be early adaptors of this change. The authors found excellent agreement (Table 2) in diagnosis between the conventional autopsy and an "autopsy" consisting of postmortem computed tomography angiography and biopsy in patients with sudden death after chest pain. Other authors have shown similar agreements in a variety of clinical situations.[2] The study is seriously limited by the fact that the pathologists performing both autopsies were not blinded.

B. A. Carter, MD, FRCPC

References

1. Weustink AC, Hunink MG, van Dijke CF, Renken NS, Krestin GP, Oosterhuis JW. Minimally invasive autopsy: an alternative to conventional autopsy? *Radiology.* 2009;250:897-904.
2. Patriquin L, Kassarjian A, Barish M, et al. Postmortem whole-body magnetic resonance imaging as an adjunct to autopsy: preliminary clinical experience. *J Magn Reson Imaging.* 2001;13:277-287.

Immunoglobulin G4—related coronary periarteritis in a patient presenting with myocardial ischemia

Tanigawa J, Daimon M, Murai M, et al (Osaka Med College, Japan)
Hum Pathol 43:1131-1134, 2012

Recent studies suggest that the cardiovascular system might be a possible target of immunoglobulin G4—related disease. Here we present a 66-year-old man who was admitted to our hospital because of chest symptoms suggestive of acute coronary syndrome. Besides luminal narrowing of the coronary arteries, marked periarterial thickening around the coronary artery was observed by computed tomography coronary angiography. Serum immunoglobulin G4 levels of this patient were elevated (564 mg/dL). The patient underwent coronary bypass surgery. After incision of the pericardium, a glittery white-yellowish, elastic-hard periarterial mass surrounding the left circumflex artery could be seen. Histologic analysis of the biopsy specimen showed the formation of lymphoid follicles and the presence of immunoglobulin G4—positive plasma cells; therefore, the diagnosis was immunoglobulin G4—related coronary periarteritis accompanied by physiologically significant myocardial ischemia (Fig 3).

▶ The plethora of articles about immunoglobulin (Ig)G4 disease has now reached the coronary arteries. Over the past 5 years, this entity has been widely reported in surgical pathology (largely gastrointestinal) literature but rarely in cardiovascular literature. IgG4-related sclerosing disease is a pathologic condition with increased IgG4 in serum, fibrosclerosis, and migration of IgG4-positive plasma cells. In this report, the author discusses a patient diagnosed with IgG4-related coronary periarteritis, familiarizing pathologists with the microscopic findings (Fig 3) of this relatively new disorder. As well as providing a concise description of IgG4 disease, this article briefly reviews the clinical and histologic findings of the significant inflammatory disorders that can affect the cardiovascular system. For additional reading, please see reference list.[1]

B. A. Carter, MD, FRCPC

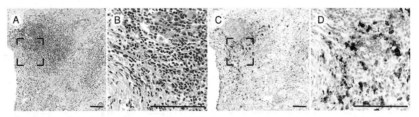

FIGURE 3.—Histologic and immunohistochemical analysis of the biopsy specimen obtained from the coronary periarterial lesion shown in Fig. 2. Hematoxylin-eosin staining of lower (A) and higher (B) magnification, and IgG4 staining of lower (C) and higher (D) magnification. Scale bars indicate 10 μm. Original magnifications: (A and C) ×100, (B and D) ×400. (Reprinted from Tanigawa J, Daimon M, Murai M, et al. Immunoglobulin G4-related coronary periarteritis in a patient presenting with myocardial ischemia. *Hum Pathol.* 2012;43:1131-1134, Copyright 2012, with permission from Elsevier.)

Reference

1. Smyrk TC. Pathological features of IgG4-related sclerosing disease. *Curr Opin Rheumatol.* 2011;23:74-79.

8 Soft Tissue and Bone

Loss of succinate dehydrogenase subunit B (SDHB) expression is limited to a distinctive subset of gastric wild-type gastrointestinal stromal tumours: a comprehensive genotype–phenotype correlation study
Doyle LA, Nelson D, Heinrich MC, et al (Brigham and Women's Hosp, Boston, MA; Oregon Health and Science Univ, Portland)
Histopathology 2012 [Epub ahead of print]

Aims.—Gastrointestinal stromal tumours (GISTs) typically harbour *KIT* or *PDGFRA* mutations; 15% of adult GISTs and >90% in children lack such mutations ('wild-type' GISTs). Paediatric and occasional adult GISTs show similar, distinctive features: multinodular architecture and epithelioid morphology, indolent behaviour with metastases, and imatinib resistance. Recent studies have suggested that these tumours can be identified by loss of succinate dehydrogenase subunit B (SDHB) expression. The aim of this study was to validate the predictive value of SDHB immunohistochemistry in a large genotyped cohort.

Methods and Results.—SDHB expression was examined in GISTs with known genotypes: 179 with *KIT* mutations, 32 with *PDGFRA* mutations, and 53 wild type. Histological features were recorded without knowledge of genotype or SDHB status. SDHB was deficient in 22 (42%) wild-type GISTs. All other tumours showed intact SDHB expression. All SDHB-deficient GISTs with known primary sites arose in the stomach, and had multinodular architecture and epithelioid or mixed morphology. None of the wild-type GISTs with intact SDHB showed multinodular architecture, and only four (13%) had epithelioid morphology.

Conclusions.—SDHB-deficient GISTs are wild-type gastric tumours with distinctive histology. Immunohistochemistry for SDHB can be used to confirm the diagnosis of this tumour class. SDHB expression is retained in all GISTs with *KIT* and *PDGFRA* mutations.

▶ Activating mutations of *c-Kit* and *PDGFRA* genes account for the development of the majority but not all gastrointestinal stromal tumors (GISTs). GISTs lacking *KIT* and *PDGFRA* mutations are called wild-type GISTs (WTGs). WTGs results from mutations in succinate dehydrogenase (SDH).

Germline mutations of SDH were reported in the past decade in paragangliomas of the head and neck, in thoracoabdominal paragangliomas in hereditary paraganglioma-pheochromocytoma, and in GISTs. They constitute 15% of GISTs in the adult and more than 90% of those in children, occur only in the stomach, respond poorly to imatinib treatment, can metastasize to lymph nodes, have a nodular and plexiform pattern of growth, and are epithelioid; criteria to predict biologic behavior are not yet available.[1]

The article is relevant because it determines how many of the adults with GIST are SDH-deficient in a large genotyped cohort in which mutations of *c-KIT* and *PDGFRA* mutations were absent.

In the study by Doyle et al, the focus is on adult WTGs. They found that, as expected, SDH-deficient GISTs are uncommon in this age group; however, they account for a significant subset of WTGs (42% of the adult WTGs are SDH-deficient).

To recognize these tumors is important: prognosis, therapy, and syndromic groups are different from "conventional" GISTs.

In practice, GISTs that appear epithelioid, multinodular, and plexiform, with lymphovascular invasion and nodal metastases, and GISTs arising in families with paraganglioma-pheochromocytoma history should be assessed for loss of SDH. Doyle's article suggests that because the frequency of SDH-deficient tumors is high among WTGs, it may be reasonable to test all WTGs for loss of SDH expression with immunohistochemistry.

S. S. Raab, MD

Reference

1. Miettinen M, Wang ZF, Sarlomo-Rikala M, Osuch C, Rutkowski P, Lasota J. Succinate dehydrogenase-deficient GISTs: a clinicopathologic, immunohistochemical, and molecular genetic study of 66 gastric GISTs with predilection to young age. *Am J Surg Pathol.* 2011;35:1750-1752.

NY-ESO-1 expression in synovial sarcoma and other mesenchymal tumors: significance for NY-ESO-1-based targeted therapy and differential diagnosis
Lai J-P, Robbins PF, Raffeld M, et al (Natl Cancer Inst, Bethesda, MD)
Mod Pathol 25:854-858, 2012

A promising targeted therapy against NY-ESO-1 (CTAG 1B) using genetically modified T-cells in synovial sarcomas was recently demonstrated in a clinical trial at the NCI. To investigate the role of NY-ESO-1 immunohistochemistry in patient selection and gain better insight into the incidence of NY-ESO-1 expression in synovial sarcomas and other mesenchymal tumors, we evaluated NY-ESO-1 expression by immunohistochemistry in 417 tumors. This collection of samples included: 50 SS18/SSX1/2 fusion positive synovial sarcomas, 155 gastrointestinal stromal tumors (GIST), 135 other spindle cell sarcomas as well as 77 other sarcomas (chondrosarcoma, osteosarcoma, dedifferentiated liposarcoma, alveolar soft part sarcoma, rhabdomyosarcoma, angiosarcoma, malignant mesothelioma, and Ewing's sarcoma). We report that 76% of synovial sarcomas expressed NY-ESO-1 in a strong and diffuse pattern (2−3+, >50−70% of tumor cells). In contrast, only rare cases of other spindle cell mesenchymal tumor expressed NY-ESO-1 (GIST (2/155), malignant peripheral nerve sheath tumors (1/34), and dermatofibrosarcoma protuberans (2/20)). Individual cases of other sarcomas (angiosarcoma, malignant mesothelioma, chondrosarcoma, osteosarcoma, dedifferentiated liposarcoma, alveolar soft part sarcoma, and Ewing's sarcoma) were positive for NY-ESO-1. However, no positive cases were identified amongst our cohort of leiomyosarcomas (0/24), hemangiopericytoma/solitary fibrous tumors (0/40), and cellular schwannomas (0/17). In summary, we find that NY-ESO-1 is strongly and diffusely expressed in a majority of synovial sarcomas, but only rarely in other mesenchymal lesions. Beyond its role in patient selection for targeted therapy, immunohistochemistry for NY-ESO-1 may be diagnostically useful for the distinction of synovial sarcoma from other spindle cell neoplasms.

▶ New York esophageal squamous cell carcinoma-1 (NY-ESO-1) is a cancer or testis antigen encoded by the *CTAG-1B* gene, which is aberrantly expressed in synovial sarcoma and in a variety of other neoplasms. A small clinical trial conducted at the National Cancer Institute has shown promising results with T-cell receptor—based gene therapy directed against NY-ESO-1, which was effective in mediating tumor regression in metastatic synovial sarcomas. Assessment of NY-ESO-1 expression before instituting the targeted therapy is critical to predict the response and in selecting the patients with synovial sarcomas who will most likely benefit from the treatment. In addition, studies have found that the rate of expression of NY-ESO-1 is quite high in synovial sarcomas in 80% of the reported cases. These observations prompted these authors to undertake a study using immunohistochemical methods by comparing the expression of NY-ESO-1 in synovial sarcomas with other mesenchymal tumors in 417 cases. Their goal was to determine the diagnostic utility of this marker and possible extension of the treatment benefit to nonsynovial sarcoma patients who harbor this antigen. Of the cases studied, 55 were synovial sarcomas that harbored the *SS18/SSX1/2* gene rearrangement, 155 were cases of gastrointestinal stromal tumors (GIST), 135 were cases of other spindle cell sarcomas, and 77 were cases of sarcomas of various other kinds. The study found 76% of synovial sarcomas showed strong and diffuse cytoplasmic and nuclear staining, but the staining rate was significantly lower for all other types of sarcomas (2 of 155 for GIST, 1 of 34 for malignant peripheral nerve sheath tumors, 2 of 20 for dermatofibrosarcoma protuberans). The results were even more striking for leiomyosarcoma, solitary fibrous tumors, and cellular schwannoma, which showed no staining for all cases examined. In rare instances, where nonsynovial sarcomas expressed the NY-ESO-1 antigen, the same T-cell receptor—based targeted therapy could be used, although its efficacy remains to be examined in clinical trails.

S. Mortuza, MD

Clinicopathologic correlation of vitamin D receptor expression with retinoid X receptor and MIB-1 expression in primary and metastatic osteosarcoma
Gallagher R, Keighley J, Tancabelic J, et al (Kansas Univ Med Ctr, Kansas City)
Ann Diagn Pathol 16:323-329, 2012

Vitamin D, in addition to its effects on bone, is important in cell cycle regulation. Vitamin D receptor (VDR) has been identified in breast, prostate, and colon cancers, as well as in canine and human osteosarcoma (OS) cell lines; however, it has not been well investigated in human OS-archived specimens. We correlated VDR, retinoid X receptor (RXR), and MIB-1 (Ki-67) expression in 110 archived OS cases with several clinicopathologic parameters including patient's age, sex, tumor location, tumor grade, and type and metastatic status. The expression of VDR and RXR was identified in human OS tissue obtained from primary and metastatic OS archival tissue. No statistically significant difference was found in VDR expression in relation with tumor grade, type, age, sex, or location. The expression of RXR was highest in higher-grade ($P = .0006$) and metastatic tumors but remained unchanged when correlated with tumor type, age, sex, or location. The expression of MIB-1 was statistically elevated in higher-grade tumors ($P = .001$), patients 25 years or younger ($P = .04$), tumors located in extremities ($P = .005$), and metastatic lesions, but was not impacted by tumor type or patient's sex. Proliferative activity was significantly reduced after treatment, as the mean MIB-1 expression dropped from 11% in primary biopsy samples to 6% in resection specimens. There appears to be a relationship between proliferative tumor activity and tumor grade, location, and metastasis. Additional studies on the analysis of the effects of vitamin D and RXR on OS proliferation, apoptosis, and differentiation are critical to further evaluate their potential role in OS treatment.

▶ Vitamin D has recently been described as having both in vivo and in vitro antitumor activity in various kinds of human malignancies. It may also enhance the effects of chemotherapy agents. Vitamin D decreases tumor cell proliferation by cell cycle arrest at G0/G1; then it may induce apoptosis and phenotypic differentiation of tumor cells. The reduced rate of proliferation of tumor cells treated with vitamin D therapy can be seen in tissue by Ki-67 (MIB-1) staining. Vitamin D is a steroid hormone that binds with a very high specificity with vitamin D receptor (VDR), which is a nuclear phosphoprotein. Binding of the active form of vitamin D with its receptor forms a heterodimer with retinoid X receptors (RXR), enabling the complex to bind various kinds of retinoids. The end result is the formation of $1,25(OH)_2D_3$-VDR-RXR complex that ultimately modulates the transcription of vitamin D—promoted gene products. Gallagher et al undertook a retrospective review study of patients treated for osteosarcomas over a period of 2 decades and collected 110 samples from 65 patients along with a rich array of demographic and clinical data. The tumor samples were primary biopsies (48), resection specimens after therapy (35), and metastatic lesions (27). The mean patient age was 27 years and ranged from 6 to 83. The tumors were distributed throughout the skeletal system, with the femur being the most common site (36 cases), followed by tibia (13 cases). Only grade II or III osteosarcomas were included in the study. Of the 27 cases of metastasis, all showed high-grade histomorphology with lung metastasis. Immunohistochemical stains were performed on tumors with VDR, RXR, and MIB-1. The results showed 86.4% immunoreactivity for VDR and 95.4% for RXR. The intensity and percentage of staining did not differ significantly among primary biopsies, resection specimens after therapy, and metastatic osteosarcomas. In addition, there was no statistically significant difference in the expression of VDR and RXR based on tumor grade, type, patient age and sex, and the anatomic location of the tumor—a finding that points to the role of vitamin D in osteosarcomas of all kinds. Metastatic osteosarcomas were most highly expressing RXR compared with primary, and there were no differences with regard to patients' demographic data and anatomic location. On the other hand, Ki-67 proliferation index was higher in higher-grade osteosarcomas, patients who were 25 years of age or younger, tumors in the extremities, and metastatic lesions. Most significantly, the proliferation index was reduced from 11% to 6% in osteosarcomas after treatment. The authors conclude that VDR is expressed in most osteosarcomas. They postulate that tumor grade, location, and metastatic status influence the proliferation activity, and vitamin D plays a key role in this. Better understanding of the role of vitamin D in tumor proliferation and differentiation can be exploited in "differentiation therapy" for controlling tumor growth and spread in various types of human malignancies.

S. Mortuza, MD

Liposarcomas of the Mediastinum and Thorax: A Clinicopathologic and Molecular Cytogenetic Study of 24 Cases, Emphasizing Unusual and Diverse Histologic Features
Boland JM, Colby TV, Folpe AL (Mayo Clinic, Rochester, MN; Mayo Clinic, Scottsdale, AZ)
Am J Surg Pathol 36:1395-1403, 2012

Liposarcoma rarely occurs in the mediastinum, and most reports predate the current genetically based classification system. We report the clinicopathologic and molecular genetic features of a series of thoracic liposarcomas identified over a 60-year period. Twenty-four confirmed cases were reclassified using the most recent World Health Organization classification. Fluorescent in situ hybridization for *CPM* amplification and/or *DDIT3* rearrangement was performed on selected cases. The 24 cases occurred in 13 men and 11 women (mean age, 53 y; range, 15 to 73 y) and arose in all mediastinal compartments. All subtypes were encountered with 8 well-differentiated liposarcomas, 6 dedifferentiated liposarcomas (3 of 6 confirmed *CPM+*), 7 pleomorphic liposarcomas (2 of 7 confirmed *CPM−*, 1 of 7 confirmed *DDIT3−*), 2 myxoid liposarcomas, and 1 unclassifiable liposarcoma (*CPM−* and *DDIT3−*). Unusual histologic features included myxoid well-differentiated liposarcoma mimicking myxoid liposarcoma (2 cases), lipoleiomyosarcoma (1 case), dedifferentiated liposarcoma with "meningothelial"-like dedifferentiation, differentiated myxoid liposarcoma mimicking well-differentiated liposarcoma (*CPM−*), and pleomorphic liposarcoma with epithelioid and myxoid change. Follow-up information was available for 19 patients (mean, 55 mo; range, 8 to 252 mo). Outcome was strongly associated with histologic subtype, with death from disease occurring in 1 of 6 well-differentiated, 1 of 4 dedifferentiated, 5 of 7 pleomorphic, and 2 of 2 myxoid liposarcomas. The mediastinum shows a preponderance of uncommon subtypes and unusual morphologic variants.

Correct classification has important implications, with most patients with well-differentiated/dedifferentiated liposarcoma having a protracted clinical course, in contrast to the more rapid disease progression seen in patients with myxoid and pleomorphic liposarcoma.

▶ Although liposarcoma is one of the most common soft tissue malignancies, mediastinal liposarcomas are very rare neoplasms. Boland et al reviewed the archived materials of the Mayo Clinic and reported 24 confirmed cases over a period of 60 years. The mean patient age was 53 years and ranged from 15 to 73 years. Because most of these tumors were originally diagnosed before the advent of current genetically based World Health Organization classification system, the authors undertook the task of reclassifying them using the latest molecular techniques, such as fluorescence in situ hybridization for *CPM* amplification, *DDIT3* rearrangements, *MDM2* amplification, and characteristic translocation on selected cases and detailed the clinicopathologic and molecular genetic features of theses liposarcomas that arose in the mediastinal compartment. Of the 24 cases studied, well-differentiated liposarcomas were the most common (8 cases), followed by pleomorphic liposarcoma (7 cases), dedifferentiated liposarcomas (6 cases), myxoid liposarcoma (2 cases), and unclassifiable liposarcoma (1 case). Interestingly, the mediastinal liposarcomas showed an unusual preponderance of uncommon subtypes and unusual histomorphologic features, such as myxoid well-differentiated liposarcoma mimicking myxoid liposarcoma, lipoleiomyosarcoma, and dedifferentiated liposarcoma that showed meningothelial-like dedifferentiation. A total of 19 patients had follow-up information of 8–252 months. There was strong correlation between histomorphologic subtype and survival. Both patients with the diagnosis of myxoid liposarcoma died of the disease and 5 of 7 patients with pleomorphic liposarcoma died of the disease, all of which showed rapid clinical deterioration. On the other hand, the well-differentiated/dedifferentiated liposarcoma group showed protracted clinical course and low rate of disease-related mortality with only 1 of 6 patients with well-differentiated liposarcoma and 1 of 4 patients with dedifferentiated liposarcoma dying of the disease. With this outcome analysis, the authors emphasize the significance of accurate classification of these rare tumors and illustrate the usefulness of molecular genetic techniques for this challenging task. The authors leave the question open of why there is striking overrepresentation of myxoid and pleomorphic liposarcoma and absence of high-grade round cell myxoid liposarcomas in mediastinum that was observed during their study of 24 cases spanning 6 decades.

S. Mortuza, MD

Expression of ERG, an Ets family transcription factor, identifies *ERG*-rearranged Ewing sarcoma

Wang W-L, Patel NR, Caragea M, et al (The Univ of Texas MD Anderson Cancer Ctr, Houston; Texas Children's Hosp and Baylor College of Medicine, Houston; Univ of Western Ontario, London, Canada; et al)
Mod Pathol 25:1378-1383, 2012

ERG gene encodes for an Ets family regulatory transcription factor and is involved in recurrent chromosomal translocations found in a subset of acute myeloid leukemias, prostate carcinomas and Ewing sarcomas. The purpose of this study was to examine the utility of an ERG antibody to detect *EWSR1-ERG*—rearranged Ewing sarcomas. A formalin-fixed paraffin-embedded tissue microarray and whole-tissue sections from 32 genetically characterized Ewing sarcomas were examined: 22 with *EWSR1-FLI1*, 8 with *EWSR1-ERG* and 2 with *EWSR1-NFATC2*. Immunohistochemistry was performed using a rabbit anti-ERG monoclonal antibody directed against the C-terminus of the protein and a mouse anti-FLI1 monoclonal antibody against a FLI1 Ets domain (C-terminus) fusion protein. Immunoreactivity was graded for extent and intensity of positive tumor cell nuclei. ERG labeling was seen in 7/8 *EWSR1-ERG* cases (predominantly diffuse (5+), moderate to strong), while only 3/24 non-*EWR1-ERG* cases showed labeling (very weak). FLI1 labeling was observed in 29/31 cases regardless of fusion variant; 23 displayed diffuse (5+) strong/moderate labeling (5/7 *EWSR1-ERG*, 18/22 *EWSR1-FLI1*). Both *EWSR1-NFATC2* cases had weak reactivity with FLI1 and weak or no reactivity for ERG. In conclusion, strong nuclear ERG immunoreactivity is specific for Ewing sarcomas with *EWSR1-ERG* rearrangement. In contrast, FLI1 was not specific to rearrangement type, likely because of cross reactivity with the highly homologous Ets DNA-binding domain present in the C-terminus of both ERG and FLI1.

▶ The most common translocation partner of EWSR1 (22q12) in Ewing sarcoma is FLI1 (11q12), found in approximately 85% of the cases; the remaining cases show translocation involving an alternating partner, most commonly ERG (21q12). The result of these translocations is the constitutive expression of a potent chimeric transcription factor. ERG is a member of the Ets family of transcription factors that is expressed in normal endothelial cells, where it plays an important role in angiogenesis and endothelial apoptosis. ERG expression is also found in other tissue types; up to 70% of prostate cancer has been shown to harbor translocation involving this ERG and TMPRSS2—a finding that is being increasingly used for the diagnosis of primary and metastatic prostate cancers by immunohistochemical methods. Wang et al at the MD Anderson Cancer Center used a rabbit anti-ERG monoclonal antibody to detect the EWSR1-ERG—rearranged Ewing sarcomas. Formalin-fixed, paraffin-embedded tissue microarray and whole tissue sections were obtained from 32 cases of Ewing sarcomas with known fusion transcript using reverse transcriptase polymerase chain reaction and verified with sequencing. The anti-ERG antibody was directed against the last 30 amino acids of the C-terminus of the protein. Of the 32 cases studied, the translocation partner of EWSR1 was FLI1 in 22 cases, ERG in 8 cases, and NFATC2 in 2 cases. An excellent correlation was observed between the molecular methods and IHC method in ERG-translocated Ewing sarcomas, in which 7 of the 8 cases studied showed diffuse, moderate-to-strong nuclear immunoreactivity (about 88% sensitivity, 88% specificity, 100% positive predictive value). This specificity of ERG staining using antibodies was much higher for EWSR1-ERG—translocated tumors compared with EWSR1-FLI1—translocated ones, when an anti-FLI1 antibody was used, which showed nonspecific immunostaining regardless of the translocation partner in 29 out of the 32 cases studied. In particular, 5 out of the 7 cases of known EWSR1-ERG—translocated sarcomas stained with FLI1 in a diffuse moderate-to-strong nuclear staining pattern. The authors postulate that this nonspecific staining of FLI1 is likely caused by cross reactivity of the C-terminus of both ERG and FLI1, which is a highly homologous Ets-binding domain present in both.

S. Mortuza, MD

***FUS* rearrangements are rare in 'pure' sclerosing epithelioid fibrosarcoma**
Wang W-L, Evans HL, Meis JM, et al (The Univ of Texas MD Anderson Cancer Ctr, Houston; et al)
Mod Pathol 25:846-853, 2012

Several recent reports have described low-grade fibromyxoid sarcoma with sclerosing epithelioid fibrosarcoma-like areas. We evaluated cases of pure sclerosing epithelioid fibrosarcoma lacking areas of low-grade fibromyxoid sarcoma for *FUS* rearrangement to determine whether this entity could be related to low-grade fibromyxoid sarcoma. Available formalin-fixed paraffin-embedded tissue of 27 sclerosing epithelioid fibrosarcoma from 25 patients was retrieved and tabulated with clinical information. Unstained slides from formalin-fixed paraffin-embedded blocks were prepared and fluorescence *in-situ* hybridization was performed using a commercial *FUS* break-apart probe. The median patient age at presentation was 50 (range, 14—78) years, with 14 males and 10 females. Sclerosing epithelioid fibrosarcoma most commonly involved the extremities ($n = 8$) or chest ($n = 6$). Sixteen patients had a median follow-up of 17 (range, 1—99) months; seven were alive and well at 12 (range, 5—30) months; three alive with disease at 28 (range, 9—99) months; five dead of disease at a median of 22 (range, 1—36) months and one was dead of unknown causes. Twelve patients were known to have metastases; the most common site was lung ($n = 7$), followed by bone ($n = 3$), lymph nodes ($n = 2$) and peritoneum ($n = 1$). Only 2 of 22 (9%) analyzable cases of sclerosing epithelioid fibrosarcoma showed rearrangement in the *FUS* locus by fluorescence *in-situ* hybridization. Although cytogenetically confirmed low-grade fibromyxoid sarcoma can have sclerosing epithelioid fibrosarcoma-like areas, *FUS* rearrangement, which is characteristic of low-grade fibromyxoid sarcoma, appears to be relatively rare in pure sclerosing epithelioid fibrosarcoma.

▶ Is there any relationship between pure sclerosing epithelioid fibrosarcoma and low-grade fibromyxoid sarcoma with sclerosing epithelioid fibrosarcoma-like areas? Several recent reports have described sclerosing epithelioid fibrosarcoma-like areas in low-grade fibromyxoid sarcomas. Some authors have even reported that pure sclerosing epithelioid sarcoma, which can mimic infiltrating carcinoma or sclerosing lymphoma, harbors the same molecular alterations found in low-grade fibromyxoid sarcoma. Knowing that low-grade fibromyxoid sarcoma can show morphologic variation, including hyalinizing spindle cell tumor with giant rosettes and sclerosing epithelioid fibromyxoid sarcoma-like areas, Wang et al from the MD Anderson Cancer Center undertook a fluorescent in situ hybridization study of 16q11 to detect *FUS* rearrangement using the LSI *FUS* dual-color, break-apart probe in pure sclerosing epithelioid fibrosarcomas that lacked areas of low-grade fibromyxoid sarcoma in an attempt to answer this question. Their goal was to determine if this pure entity is related to low-grade fibromyxoid sarcoma, such as being part of a morphologic spectrum, by examining the rate of translocation of the *FUS* gene, which is the most characteristic molecular feature of low-grade fibromyxoid sarcomas. Using archived materials, 27 cases of pure sclerosing epithelioid fibrosarcoma from 25 patients were retrieved along with clinical follow-up data. A fluorescent in situ hybridization study of unstained formalin-fixed, paraffin-embedded tissue using the *FUS* break-apart probe showed very low rate of rearrangement in only 2 of 22 cases (9%) in pure sclerosing epithelioid sarcomas. In contrast, *FUS* rearrangement is the characteristic molecular feature of low-grade fibromyxoid sarcoma found in almost all cases. By using molecular technique, the authors clarify that although cytogenetically confirmed low-grade fibromyxoid sarcoma can have sclerosing epithelioid sarcoma-like areas, pure sclerosing epithelioid fibrosarcoma lacks the characteristic *FUS* rearrangement most of the time, implying that genetically most cases of pure epithelioid fibrosarcomas are distinct entities. The authors' opinion is that focal sclerosing epithelioid fibrosarcoma-like areas in low-grade fibromyxoid sarcomas are still within the morphologic spectrum of low-grade fibromyxoid sarcoma, whereas pure sclerosing epithelioid fibrosarcoma is most likely a distinct entity. However, the natural history of tumors depicting the combined morphologic features of both low-grade fibromyxoid sarcoma and sclerosing epithelioid fibrosarcoma is uncertain and further studies are needed to better understand the clinical significance of this enigmatic entity.

S. Mortuza, MD

9 Female Genital Tract

The Lower Anogenital Squamous Terminology Standardization Project for HPV-Associated Lesions: Background and Consensus Recommendations from the College of American Pathologists and the American Society for Colposcopy and Cervical Pathology
Darragh TM, for members of the LAST Project Work Groups (Univ of California – San Francisco; et al)
Arch Pathol Lab Med 136:1266-1297, 2012

The terminology for human papillomavirus (HPV)—associated squamous lesions of the lower anogenital tract has a long history marked by disparate diagnostic terms derived from multiple specialties. It often does not reflect current knowledge of HPV biology and pathogenesis. A consensus process was convened to recommend terminology unified across lower anogenital sites. The goal was to create a histopathologic nomenclature system that reflects current knowledge of HPV biology, optimally uses available biomarkers, and facilitates clear communication across different medical specialties. The Lower Anogenital Squamous Terminology (LAST) Project was cosponsored by the College of American Pathologists and the American Society for Colposcopy and Cervical Pathology and included 5 working groups; three work groups performed comprehensive literature reviews and developed draft recommendations. Another work group provided the historical background and the fifth will continue to foster implementation of the LAST recommendations. After an open comment period, the draft recommendations were presented at a consensus conference attended by LAST work group members, advisors, and representatives from 35 stakeholder organizations including professional societies and government agencies. Recommendations were finalized and voted on at the consensus meeting. The final, approved recommendations standardize biologically-relevant histopathologic terminology for HPV-associated squamous intraepithelial lesions and superficially invasive squamous carcinomas across all lower anogenital tract sites and detail the appropriate use of specific biomarkers to clarify histologic interpretations and enhance diagnostic accuracy. A plan for disseminating and monitoring recommendation implementation in the practicing community was also developed. The implemented recommendations will facilitate communication between

TABLE 3.—Summary of Recommendations

Recommendation	Comment

Squamous intraepithelial lesions, WG2

1. A unified histopathologic nomenclature with a single set of diagnostic terms is recommended for all HPV-associated preinvasive squamous lesions of the LAT.

2. A 2-tiered nomenclature is recommended for noninvasive HPV-associated squamous proliferations of the LAT, which may be further qualified with the appropriate −IN terminology.

—IN refers to the generic intraepithelial neoplasia terminology, without specifying the location. For a specific location, the appropriate complete term should be used. Thus, for an −IN 3 lesion: cervix = CIN 3, vagina = VaIN 3, vulva = VIN 3, anus = AIN 3, perianus = PAIN 3, and penis = PeIN 3

3. The recommended terminology for HPV-associated squamous lesions of the LAT is LSIL and HSIL, which may be further classified by the applicable −IN subcategorization.

Superficially invasive squamous cell carcinoma, WG3

1. The term *superficially invasive squamous cell carcinoma (SISCCA)* is recommended for minimally invasive SCC of the LAT that has been completely excised and is potentially amenable to conservative surgical therapy.

Note: Lymph-vascular invasion (LVI) and pattern of invasion are not part of the definition of SISCCA, with the exception of penile carcinoma.

2. For cases of invasive squamous carcinoma *with positive biopsy/resection margins*, the pathology report should state whether:

   The examined invasive tumor exceeds the dimensions for a SISCCA (defined below)
   OR
   The examined invasive tumor component is less than or equal to the dimensions for a SISCCA and conclude that the tumor is *"At least a superficially invasive squamous carcinoma."*

3. In cases of SISCCA, the following parameters should be included in the pathology report:

   The presence or absence of LVI.
   The presence, number, and size of independent multifocal carcinomas (after excluding the possibility of a single carcinoma).

4. CERVIX: SISCCA of the cervix is defined as an invasive squamous carcinoma that:

   Is not a grossly visible lesion, AND
   Has an invasive depth of ≤3 mm from the basement membrane of the point of origin, AND
   Has a horizontal spread of ≤7 mm in maximal extent, AND
   Has been completely excised.

5. VAGINA: No recommendation is offered for early invasive squamous carcinoma of the vagina.

Owing to the rarity of primary SCC of the vagina, there are insufficient data to define early invasive squamous carcinoma in the vagina.

6. ANAL CANAL: The *suggested* definition of superficially invasive squamous cell carcinoma (SISCCA) of the anal canal is an invasive squamous carcinoma that:

   Has an invasive depth of ≤3 mm from the basement membrane of the point of origin, AND
   Has a horizontal spread of ≤7 mm in maximal extent, AND
   Has been completely excised.

(Continued)

TABLE 3.—(*Continued*)

Recommendation	Comment
7. VULVA: Vulvar SISCCA is defined as an AJCC T1a (FIGO IA) vulvar cancer. No change in the current definition of T1a vulvar cancer is recommended.	Current AJCC definition of T1a vulvar carcinoma: Tumor ≤ 2 cm in size, confined to the vulva or perineum AND Stromal invasion ≤ 1 mm Note: The depth of invasion is defined as the measurement of the tumor from the epithelial-stromal junction of the adjacent most superficial dermal papilla to the deepest point of invasion.
8. PENIS: Penile SISCCA is defined as an AJCC T1a. No change in the current definition of T1a penile cancer is recommended.	Current AJCC definition of T1a penile carcinoma: Tumor that invades only the subepithelial connective tissue, AND No LVI AND Is not poorly differentiated (i.e., grade 3–4)
9. SCROTUM: No recommendation is offered for early invasive squamous carcinoma of the scrotum.	Owing to the rarity of primary SCC of the scrotum, there is insufficient literature to make a recommendation regarding the current AJCC staging of early scrotal cancers.
10. PERIANUS: The *suggested* definition for SISCCA of the perianus is an invasive squamous carcinoma that: Has an invasive depth of ≤ 3 mm from the basement membrane of the point of origin, AND Has a horizontal spread of ≤ 7 mm in maximal extent, AND Has been completely excised.	
Biomarkers in HPV-associated lower anogenital squamous lesions, WG4	
1. p16 IHC is *recommended* when the H&E morphologic differential diagnosis is between precancer (−IN 2 or −IN 3) and a mimic of precancer (e.g., processes known to be not related to neoplastic risk such as immature squamous metaplasia, atrophy, reparative epithelial changes, tangential cutting).	Strong and diffuse block-positive p16 results support a categorization of precancerous disease.
2. If the pathologist is entertaining an H&E morphologic interpretation of −IN 2 (under the old terminology, which is a biologically equivocal lesion falling between the morphologic changes of HPV infection [low-grade lesion] and precancer), p16 IHC is *recommended* to help clarify the situation. Strong and diffuse block-positive p16 results support a categorization of precancer. Negative or non−block-positive staining strongly favors an interpretation of low-grade disease or a non−HPV-associated pathology.	
3. p16 is *recommended* for use as an adjudication tool for cases in which there is a professional disagreement in histologic specimen interpretation, with the caveat that the differential diagnosis includes a precancerous lesion (−IN 2 or −IN 3).	
4. WG4 *recommends against* the use of p16 IHC as a routine adjunct to histologic assessment of biopsy specimens with morphologic interpretations of negative, −IN 1, and −IN 3.	

(*Continued*)

TABLE 3.—(*Continued*)

Recommendation	Comment
a. SPECIAL CIRCUMSTANCE: p16 IHC is recommended as an adjunct to morphologic assessment for biopsy specimens interpreted as ≤ —IN 1 that are at high risk for missed high-grade disease, which is defined as a prior cytologic interpretation of HSIL, ASC-H, ASC-US/HPV-16+, or AGC (NOS).	Any identified p16-positive area must meet H&E morphologic criteria for a high-grade lesion to be reinterpreted as such.

pathologists and their clinical colleagues and improve accuracy of histologic diagnosis with the ultimate goal of providing optimal patient care (Table 3).

▶ Human papillomavirus (HPV)—associated lesions are commonly encountered in the anogenital tracts of both men and women; however, depending on the site of the lesion and local terminology preference, there have been many names assigned to morphologically similar lesions without regard to their biologic underpinnings. In an attempt to achieve a more reproducible system based on disease pathogenesis, the LAST (lower anogenital squamous terminology) project was developed and their consensus recommendations regarding terminology recently published (Table 3). Perhaps the most notable change as it relates to the female genital tract is the shift away from cervical intraepithelial neoplasia (CIN 1/2/3) terminology toward a 2-tiered system of low-grade squamous intraepithelial lesion (LSIL) and high-grade squamous intraepithelial lesion (HSIL). The authors acknowledge that many clinicians are more familiar with the intraepithelial neoplasia nomenclature and allow that the SIL terminology can be further described with the -IN designation, but found through a comprehensive literature review that current understanding of HPV biology does not support a 3-tiered system. They also argue for an expanded role for p16 immunohistochemistry to be used when deciding between a precancerous lesion (HSIL) and a benign mimic, between LSIL and HSIL, when there is disagreement among pathologists, and in cases in which there is a high likelihood of missing a precancerous lesion. Many useful figures in the article aid in stain interpretation. The ultimate goal of these recommendations is to generate a unified and scientifically based terminology that will optimize clinical management via improved communication between pathologists and our clinical colleagues. Although adoption of all recommendations may be slow, pathologists should be encouraged to utilize the new terminology and biomarkers.

M. D. Post, MD

Negative Loop Electrosurgical Cone Biopsy Finding Following a Biopsy Diagnosis of High-Grade Squamous Intraepithelial Lesion: Frequency and Clinical Significance
Witt BL, Factor RE, Jarboe EA, et al (Univ of Utah School of Medicine and ARUP Laboratories, Salt Lake City)
Arch Pathol Lab Med 136:1259-1261, 2012

Context.—Loop electrosurgical excision procedure (LEEP) is a therapeutic option following biopsy diagnosis of high-grade squamous intraepithelial lesion (HSIL). Most LEEPs will confirm the HSIL biopsy diagnosis but a number of them will not. Such negative findings suggest the possibility of an incorrect biopsy diagnosis, removal of the lesion by biopsy, or insufficient LEEP sampling.

Objective.—To determine the frequency of negative LEEP findings following HSIL biopsies and better understand the clinical significance of negative LEEP findings.

Design.—The Department of Pathology's records were searched for all patients undergoing LEEP excision who had prior cervical biopsies and subsequent clinical follow-up.

Results.—Three hundred seventy-eight women were found who had index biopsies, subsequent LEEPs, and clinical follow-up averaging 25.8 months. Three hundred six women had HSIL on biopsy with 223 (73%) showing HSIL on LEEP. Seventy-three (24%) LEEPs in women with HSIL index biopsy results yielded negative findings or disclosed low-grade squamous intraepithelial lesion (LSIL). Twenty-nine of 223 patients (13%) with an HSIL result both on biopsies and LEEPs had HSIL on biopsy and/or excisional clinical follow-up. Seven of 73 patients (10%) with positive (HSIL) biopsy results but negative LEEP findings or LSIL had HSIL on biopsy and/or excisional follow-up.

Conclusions.—Twenty-four percent of patients with HSIL on biopsy had negative findings or LSIL on LEEP. There is no statistical difference in development of HSIL after LEEP for those with positive biopsy and positive LEEP results (13%) versus positive biopsy and negative LEEP results (10%). The occurrence of a negative LEEP finding following a positive biopsy finding was frequent (24%) and does not portend a different clinical follow-up from a positive biopsy and positive LEEP result.

▶ This article explores the experience at one institution with the situation in which a high-grade squamous intraepithelial lesion biopsy is followed by a negative or low-grade squamous intraepithelial lesion loop electrosurgical excision procedure (LEEP) specimen. Because all cases in this situation should trigger an intradepartmental QA/QI investigation, it is a relevant issue for all pathologists. Further, although the morbidity for LEEPs is relatively low, there are documented complications regarding future ability to carry pregnancy to full term. Lastly, it has been shown that up to 10% of patients with a negative LEEP after a high-grade squamous intraepithelial lesion biopsy will have a persistent high-grade squamous intraepithelial lesion on subsequent biopsy. The authors point out that several reasons may account for the discrepancy between biopsy and resection diagnoses, including missampling at the time of resection, destruction or removal of the entire lesion during the biopsy and after the biopsy healing process, or diagnostic errors of the biopsy specimen. Via review of their cases in which both biopsy and resection specimens were available and correlation with clinical follow-up, they determined that misdiagnosis was the least likely explanation for the discordance. This should be reassuring to pathologists. Of further interest was the finding that there was no statistically significant difference in rates of follow-up high-grade squamous intraepithelial lesions between those populations with negative LEEP specimens versus LEEP specimens with high-grade squamous intraepithelial lesion. Overall, this makes the case for close clinical follow-up of all patients with a high-grade squamous intraepithelial lesion diagnosis on biopsy, irrespective of the findings at the time of resection.

M. D. Post, MD

Paired-box gene 2 is down-regulated in endometriosis and correlates with low epidermal growth factor receptor expression
de Graaff AA, Delvoux B, Van de Vijver KK, et al (Maastricht Univ Med Centre, The Netherlands; et al)
Hum Reprod 27:1676-1684, 2012

Background.—Paired-box 2 (Pax2) is involved in the development of the female genital tract and has been associated with endometrial pathologies. The expression of Pax2 is induced by epidermal growth factor (EGF) and estrogens. In the present study, Pax2 expression and regulation were investigated in endometriosis.

Methods and Results.—Pax2 protein expression was assessed by immunohistochemistry in the eutopic (i.e. inside the uterus) and ectopic tissue (endometriosis) from 11 patients. Immunoreactivity was high in the endometrium, with strong epithelial and weaker stromal staining. Similar expression patterns of Pax2 were observed in the endometrium of women without endometriosis ($n = 12$). The mRNA level of Pax2 was assessed by real-time PCR in the eutopic and ectopic endometria of 14 patients and in the endometrium from women without endometriosis ($n = 20$). Pax2 expression was lower in endometriotic lesions than that in the eutopic endometrium of patients ($P < 0.001$) and controls ($P = 0.007$). Three possible mechanisms determining low Pax2 expression were investigated: EGF signalling, CpG DNA methylation of the Pax2 promoter and steroid response. The mRNA level of the EGF receptor (EGFR1) was assessed in the samples used for Pax2 mRNA assessment. A significant correlation between EGFR1 and Pax2 in both eutopic and ectopic tissues was observed ($R = 0.58$; slope regression line, 0.81; 95% CI: 0.09—1.52 and $R = 0.54$; slope regression line, 2.51; 95% CI: 0.02—4.99, respectively). CpG DNA methylation was analyzed by methyl-specific PCR in two regions of the Pax2 promoter but they were unmethylated in all samples. Steroid responsiveness was assessed

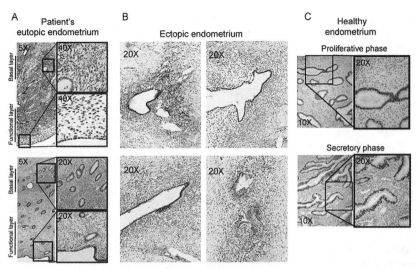

FIGURE 1.—Pax2 protein expression and localization in the normal endometrium and in endometriosis. (A) Representative pictures of Pax2 staining in eutopic tissue in two different women with endometriosis. For both images, the myometrium is at the top (basal layer) and the functional layer is at the bottom. (B) Representative images of Pax2 staining in endometriotic lesions. Three images are from the same patient (right top and both images at the bottom) and indicate that the percentage of Pax2 stromal positivity varies widely between distinct locations in the same sample. (C) Representative immunostainings of Pax2 in proliferative and secretory phase endometrial tissues from women without endometriosis. (Reprinted from de Graaff AA, Delvoux B, Van de Vijver KK, et al. Paired-box gene 2 is down-regulated in endometriosis and correlates with low epidermal growth factor receptor expression. *Hum Reprod.* 2012;27:1676-1684, by permission of The Author [2012] on behalf of the European Society of Human Reproduction and Embryology.)

using endometrial explant cultures and Pax2 was not regulated by either 17β-estradiol or progesterone.

Conclusions.—In endometriosis patients, Pax2 is down-regulated in the lesions compared with the eutopic tissue, possibly due to low EGF signalling (Fig 1).

▶ Endometriosis is among the most common diseases in benign gynecology and a significant cause of infertility, although its exact pathogenesis remains unknown. Recently, there has been investigation into the role Paired-box 2 (Pax2), a transcription factor involved in cell programming, differentiation, apoptosis, and migration, which is expressed in Müllerian duct—derived tissue, plays in endometrial carcinomas. This study hypothesized that Pax2 might also have a role in endometriosis. The authors analyzed paired sets of eutopic (intra-uterine) and ectopic (extrauterine) endometrial tissue for the immunohisto-chemical expression of Pax2 as well as RNA and DNA methylation analyses. Unfortunately, the samples used for immunohistochemical analysis were different than those used for RNA and DNA analysis, limiting to some extent the conclusions one can draw. Further, the control group of patients without endometriosis was randomly selected from an existing tissue bank, rather than being matched to the test subjects by age, parity, or other factors. They found that both eutopic and ectopic endometrial tissue were strongly positive for nuclear Pax2 expression by immunohistochemistry (Fig 1), although there was marked heterogeneity of staining within individual samples. The gene expression analysis showed, however, that Pax2 transcript levels were significantly lower in ectopic tissue. Further, there was significant correlation between levels of Pax2 and epidermal growth factor receptor 1 (EGFR1) expression, supporting the idea that Pax2 is regulated by EGFR. This study argues against one current theory regarding the origin of endometriosis, namely, that the lesions are induced via metaplasia of ovarian or peritoneal serosal epithelium and raises interesting questions about the possible transcriptional regulation of Pax2 by EGF. It clearly highlights the need for additional studies focused on teasing out the unique characteristics of endometriotic lesions and the possible link between endometriosis and endometrial neoplasia.

M. D. Post, MD

PAX2 Loss by Immunohistochemistry Occurs Early and Often in Endometrial Hyperplasia
Allison KH, Upson K, Reed SD, et al (Univ of Washington Med Ctr, Seattle; et al)
Int J Gynecol Pathol 31:151-159, 2012

Immunohistochemical markers to assist in the diagnosis and classification of hyperplastic endometrial epithelial proliferations would be of diagnostic use. To examine the possible use of PAX2 as a marker of hyperplastic endometrium, cases of normal endometrium, simple and complex hyperplasia without atypia, atypical hyperplasia, and International Federation of Gynecology and Obstetrics (FIGO) grade 1 endometrioid carcinomas were stained for PAX2. Two hundred and six endometrial samples were available for interpretation of PAX2 staining. The percentage of cases with complete PAX2 loss (0% of cells staining) increased with increasing severity of hyperplasia: 0% of normal proliferative and secretory endometrium (n = 28), 17.4% of simple hyperplasia (n = 23), 59.0% of complex hyperplasia (n = 83), 74.1% of atypical hyperplasia (n = 54), and 73.3% of FIGO grade 1 endometrioid cancers (n = 15). Partial loss of PAX2 expression did occur in normal endometrium (17.9%) but in smaller proportions of tissue and was less frequent than in simple hyperplasia (47.8% with partial loss), complex hyperplasia (32.5%), atypical hyperplasia (22.2%), and FIGO grade 1 carcinomas (20.0%). Uniform PAX2 expression was rare in complex (8.4%) and atypical hyperplasia (3.7%) and carcinoma (6.7%). When evaluating loss of PAX2 in histologically normal endometrium adjacent to lesional endometrium in a given case, statistically significant differences in staining were observed for simple hyperplasia ($P = 0.011$), complex hyperplasia ($P < 0.001$), atypical hyperplasia ($P < 0.001$), and FIGO grade 1 endometrioid cancer ($P = 0.003$). In summary, PAX2 loss seems to occur early in the development of endometrial precancers and may prove useful in some settings as a diagnostic

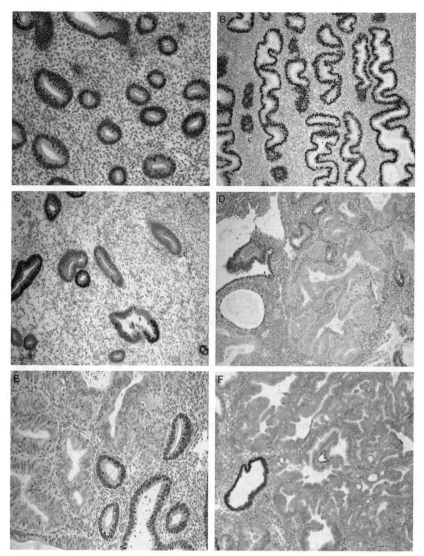

FIGURE 2.—Strong and uniform nuclear PAX2 expression was characteristic of normal proliferative endometrium (**A**) and secretory endometrium (**B**). Occasional partial loss of PAX2 expression did occur in background histologically normal endometrium (**C**). Complete loss of nuclear PAX2 expression was much more characteristic of complex hyperplasia (**D**) atypical hyperplasia (**E**) and International Federation of Gynecology and Obstetrics grade 1 endometrioid carcinoma (**F**). (Reprinted from Allison KH, Upson K, Reed SD, et al. PAX2 loss by immunohistochemistry occurs early and often in endometrial hyperplasia. *Int J Gynecol Pathol.* 2012;31:151-159, with permission from International Society of Gynecological Pathologists.)

marker in determining normal endometrium from complex and atypical hyperplasia and low-grade carcinomas. However, it is not useful in distinguishing between these diagnostic categories (Fig 2).

▶ These authors studied PAX2 expression in a spectrum of endometrial lesions (classified according the World Health Organization system). It has been shown previously that there is poor interobserver reproducibility in the hematoxylin and eosin (H&E) diagnosis of endometrial hyperplasia and that there are no good, readily available markers (with the possible exception of PTEN) to distinguish among the various lesions. They nicely show a difference in PAX2 staining between normal versus precancerous or cancerous lesions (Fig 2), although this distinction is, in this study, usually accompanied by a relatively straightforward H&E diagnosis. There was no evidence of utility in using PAX2 to differentiate between precancerous lesions and carcinoma. Advantages of the study include its utilization of a reproducible system (simply divided into complete, partial, or minimal loss), a well-characterized study population, and robust statistical findings (even with various groups excluded, they encountered similar findings). Disadvantages are that this may have limited clinical utility in routine practice, as most cases examined here were benchmark diagnostic entities, and the authors did not state how frequently (if at all) the immunohistochemical staining was in discordance with the H&E diagnosis. This study may provide insight into the evolving understanding of the role PAX2 plays in endometrial carcinogenesis and offers a preliminary tool to resolve selected dilemmas in endometrial pathology.

M. D. Post, MD

The Diagnosis of Endometrial Carcinomas With Clear Cells by Gynecologic Pathologists: An Assessment of Interobserver Variability and Associated Morphologic Features
Fadare O, Parkash V, Dupont WD, et al (Vanderbilt Univ School of Medicine, Nashville, TN; Vanderbilt Univ Med Ctr, Nashville, TN; Yale Univ School of Medicine, New Haven, CT; et al)
Am J Surg Pathol 36:1107-1118, 2012

The purposes of this study are to assess the level of interobserver variability in the diagnosis of endometrial carcinomas with clear cells by gynecologic pathologists based purely on their morphologic features and to comparatively describe the cases of putative clear cell carcinoma (CCC) with and without significant interobserver variability. A total of 35 endometrial carcinomas (1 slide per case) were reviewed by 11 gynecologic pathologists (median experience: 10 y) from 11 North American institutions. The cases were selected from the files of 3 institutions on the basis of the presence of at least focal clear cells and had previously been classified as a variety of histotypes at these institutions. Diagnoses were rendered in a blinded manner and without predetermined diagnostic criteria or categories. The κ values between any pair of observers ranged from 0.18 to

TABLE 1.—Diagnostic Frequencies for the Various Histotypes

	CCC	Endometrioid Carcinoma	No. Diagnoses (%, Approximated) Serous Carcinoma	UC	Carcinosarcoma	Mixed Carcinoma	Diagnosis Deferred
Case #1	0 (0)	**11 (100)**	0 (0)	0 (0)	0 (0)	0 (0)	0 (0)
Case #2	**10 (91)**	0 (0)	0 (0)	0 (0)	0 (0)	1 (9)	0 (0)
Case #3	**4 (36)**	**4 (36)**	0 (0)	1 (9)	0 (0)	1 (9)	1 (9)
Case #4	0 (0)	**10 (91)**	0 (0)	0 (0)	0 (0)	1 (9)	0 (0)
Case #5	**10 (91)**	0 (0)	0 (0)	0 (0)	0 (0)	1 (9)	0 (0)
Case #6	2 (18)	1 (9)	2 (18)	1 (9)	0 (0)	**4 (36)**	1 (9)
Case #7	**9 (82)**	2 (18)	0 (0)	0 (0)	0 (0)	0 (0)	0 (0)
Case #8	0 (0)	**10 (91)**	0 (0)	0 (0)	1 (9)	0 (0)	0 (0)
Case #9	2 (18)	**4 (36)**	2 (18)	1 (9)	0 (0)	2 (18)	0 (0)
Case #10	**11 (100)**	0 (0)	0 (0)	0 (0)	0 (0)	0 (0)	0 (0)
Case #11	0 (0)	**4 (36)**	0 (0)	0 (0)	0 (0)	7 (64)	0 (0)
Case #12	0 (0)	**11 (100)**	0 (0)	0 (0)	0 (0)	0 (0)	0 (0)
Case #13	**4 (36)**	3 (27)	2 (18)	1 (9)	0 (0)	1 (9)	0 (0)
Case #14	0 (0)	**11 (100)**	0 (0)	0 (0)	0 (0)	0 (0)	0 (0)
Case #15	0 (0)	**7 (64)**	0 (0)	0 (0)	0 (0)	3 (27)	1 (9)
Case #16	1 (9)	**4 (36)**	0 (0)	1 (9)	2 (18)	0 (0)	3 (27)
Case #17	0 (0)	0 (0)	**9 (82)**	0 (0)	0 (0)	0 (0)	2 (18)
Case #18	0 (0)	**11 (100)**	0 (0)	0 (0)	0 (0)	0 (0)	0 (0)
Case #19	**11 (100)**	0 (0)	0 (0)	0 (0)	0 (0)	0 (0)	0 (0)
Case #20	**8 (73)**	0 (0)	2 (18)	0 (0)	0 (0)	0 (0)	1 (9)
Case #21	2 (18)	1 (9)	**6 (54)**	1 (9)	0 (0)	0 (0)	1 (9)
Case #22	0 (0)	**11 (100)**	0 (0)	0 (0)	0 (0)	0 (0)	0 (0)
Case #23	**9 (82)**	1 (9)	0 (0)	1 (9)	0 (0)	0 (0)	0 (0)
Case #24	**11 (100)**	0 (0)	0 (0)	0 (0)	0 (0)	0 (0)	0 (0)
Case #25	1 (9)	**4 (36)**	0 (0)	0 (0)	0 (0)	6 (54)	0 (0)
Case #26	1 (9)	**5 (45)**	0 (0)	0 (0)	0 (0)	5 (45)	0 (0)
Case #27	**10 (91)**	0 (0)	0 (0)	1 (9)	0 (0)	0 (0)	0 (0)
Case #28	**8 (73)**	0 (0)	2 (18)	0 (0)	0 (0)	1 (9)	0 (0)
Case #29	3 (27)	1 (9)	0 (0)	**6 (54)**	0 (0)	0 (0)	1 (9)
Case #30	1 (9)	1 (9)	**4 (36)**	1 (9)	0 (0)	3 (27)	1 (9)
Case #31	**9 (82)**	1 (9)	0 (0)	0 (0)	0 (0)	0 (0)	1 (9)
Case #32	1 (9)	**6 (54)**	3 (27)	0 (0)	1 (9)	0 (0)	0 (0)
Case #33	**11 (100)**	0 (0)	0 (0)	0 (0)	0 (0)	0 (0)	0 (0)
Case #34	**10 (91)**	0 (0)	0 (0)	0 (0)	0 (0)	1 (9)	0 (0)
Case #35	**9 (82)**	1 (9)	0 (0)	0 (0)	0 (0)	1 (9)	0 (0)

Bold indicates diagnosis that was rendered with the highest frequency.

0.69 (combined 0.46), which was indicative of a "moderate" level of inter-observer agreement for the group. Subgroups of "confirmed CCC" [cases diagnosed as such by at least 8 (73%) of the 11 observers, n = 14] and "possible CCC" (cases diagnosed as CCC by ≥ 1 but < 8 observers, n = 13) were compared with regard to a variety of semiquantified morphologic features. By combining selected morphologic features that displayed statistically significant differences between the 2 groups on univariate analyses, the following approximate morphologic profile emerged for the confirmed CCC group: papillae with hyalinized cores in ≥ 33% of the lesion, clear cells in ≥ 33% of the lesion, hyperchromasia in ≥ 33% of the lesion, the absence of nuclear pseudostratification in > 3 cells on the papillae, the absence of nuclear pseudostratification in glands in ≥ 33% of the lesion, the absence of diffuse grade 3 nuclei, the absence of long and slender papillae in $\geq 33\%$ of the lesion, and glands and papillae lined by cuboidal to flat, noncolumnar cells. In a backward stepwise logistic regression analysis, features from the profile that predicted the confirmed CCC group included: (1) absence or minimality of diffuse sheets of grade 3 nuclei [$P = 0.025$; 95% confidence interval (CI), 0.0266–0.363]; (2) absence or minimality of nuclear stratification in glands and papillae ($P = 0.040$; 95% CI, −0.228 to −0.0054); and (3) glands and papillae lined by cuboidal to flat, noncolumnar cells ($P = 0.008$; 95% CI, 0.0911–0.566). The 2 groups displayed significant overlap regarding a wide variety of features, and no single case displayed a full complement of potentially diagnostic features. Morphologic patterns associated with cases with very high levels of interobserver variability (defined as cases with ≥ 4 different diagnoses rendered for them, n = 9) included the near-exclusive or exclusively solid pattern of clear cells (3/9) and glandular/papillary proliferations whose only CCC-like feature was the presence of clear cells (2/9). In conclusion, the diagnosis of endometrial carcinomas with clear cells by gynecologic pathologists is associated with a moderate level of interobserver variability. However, there is a morphologic profile that characterizes cases that gynecologic pathologists more uniformly classify as CCC, and the presence of these features is supportive of a CCC diagnosis in an endometrial carcinoma with clear cells. Cases that display broad and significant qualitative deviations from the aforementioned profile should prompt the consideration of a diagnosis other than CCC (Table 1).

▶ The histologic subtype of carcinoma has major implications regarding the adjuvant treatment and prognosis for patients with endometrial cancer. One of the more problematic areas in gynecologic pathology is how to render a definitive diagnosis in cases of endometrial carcinomas containing clear cells, as these can be seen in multiple different entities and a variety of architectural patterns. This study attempted to determine the degree of interobserver variability in rendering a diagnosis of clear cell carcinoma and to define a set of morphologic features most predictive of this diagnosis. Despite utilizing the extensive experience of a group of 11 specialized gynecologic pathologists (who averaged 10 years of experience), there was only moderate agreement (average kappa = 0.46) between any 2 pathologists over a set of 35 cases. Further, 9 cases received at least 4 separate diagnoses (Table 1). This lack of consistent agreement may account for the uncharacteristically heterogeneous frequency of clear cell carcinoma (1%–7% of endometrial cancers in various studies) and the widely varied prognosis (44.2%–85% 5-year survival for stage I disease and 27%–72% 5-year survival for stage II disease). Analysis of those cases with the highest levels of agreement regarding diagnosis did allow for identification of 8 morphologic features most supportive of a clear cell carcinoma diagnosis, although many of these features are defined as the absence of certain patterns or cell morphologies, a potentially confusing standard to apply in daily practice. Although they do touch briefly on potentially useful ancillary studies such as immunohistochemistry, the authors point out that the main utility of such studies is to exclude other entities in the differential diagnosis rather than to confirm a diagnosis of clear cell carcinoma. The take-away message after reading this article is that endometrial clear cell carcinoma is still a relatively poorly classified entity with surprising heterogeneity in diagnosis, even among experienced gynecologic pathologists, and more standardized definitions are needed to create a widely reproducible scheme for diagnosis.

M. D. Post, MD

Identification of Molecular Pathway Aberrations in Uterine Serous Carcinoma by Genome-wide Analyses
Kuhn E, Wu R-C, Guan B, et al (Johns Hopkins Med Institutions, Baltimore, MD; et al)
J Natl Cancer Inst 104:1503-1513, 2012

Background.—Uterine cancer is the fourth most common malignancy in women, and uterine serous carcinoma is the most aggressive subtype. However, the molecular pathogenesis of uterine serous carcinoma is largely unknown. We analyzed the genomes of uterine serous carcinoma samples to better understand the molecular genetic characteristics of this cancer.

Methods.—Whole-exome sequencing was performed on 10 uterine serous carcinomas and the matched normal blood or tissue samples. Somatically acquired sequence mutations were further verified by Sanger sequencing. The most frequent molecular genetic changes were further validated by Sanger sequencing in 66 additional uterine serous carcinomas and in nine serous endometrial intraepithelial carcinomas (the preinvasive precursor of uterine serous carcinoma) that were isolated by laser capture microdissection. In addition, gene copy number was characterized by single-nucleotide polymorphism (SNP) arrays in 23 uterine serous carcinomas, including 10 that were subjected to whole-exome sequencing.

Results.—We found frequent somatic mutations in *TP53* (81.6%), *PIK3CA* (23.7%), *FBXW7* (19.7%), and *PPP2R1A* (18.4%) among the 76 uterine serous carcinomas examined. All nine serous carcinomas that had an associated serous endometrial intraepithelial carcinoma had concordant *PIK3CA*, *PPP2R1A*, and *TP53* mutation status between uterine serous carcinoma and the concurrent serous endometrial intraepithelial carcinoma component. DNA copy number analysis revealed frequent genomic amplification of the *CCNE1* locus (which encodes cyclin E, a known substrate of FBXW7) and deletion of the *FBXW7* locus. Among 23 uterine serous carcinomas that were subjected to SNP array analysis, seven tumors with *FBXW7* mutations (four tumors with point mutations, three tumors with hemizygous deletions) did not have *CCNE1* amplification, and 13 (57%) tumors had either a molecular genetic alteration in *FBXW7* or *CCNE1* amplification. Nearly half of these uterine serous carcinomas (48%) harbored *PIK3CA* mutation and/or *PIK3CA* amplification.

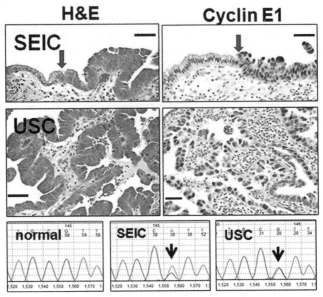

FIGURE 3.—Mutation profiles of the most commonly mutated genes and cyclin E expression in uterine serous carcinoma (USC) and serous endometrial intraepithelial carcinoma (SEIC). **B**) A uterine serous carcinoma with a serous endometrial intraepithelial carcinoma component. Top panel, SEIC; middle panel, USC. The tumor cells in both lesions show highly atypical and enlarged nuclei. The **arrow** indicates the junction between normal-appearing uterine surface epithelium (left) and serous endometrial intraepithelial carcinoma (right). Cyclin E immunoreactivity (**brown**) was detected in both uterine serous carcinoma and serous endometrial intraepithelial carcinoma cells but not in adjacent normal epithelium or stromal cells (scale bar = 100 μm). Bottom panels: Mutational analysis showing an identical somatic mutation of *FBXW7*, from CGT to CAT (**arrows**), leading to the amino acid change R465H in both the serous endometrial intraepithelial carcinoma and the uterine serous carcinoma. For interpretation of the references to color in this figure legend, the reader is referred to web version of this article. (Reprinted from Kuhn E, Wu R-C, Guan B, et al. Identification of molecular pathway aberrations in uterine serous carcinoma by genome-wide analyses. *J Natl Cancer Inst.* 2012;104:1503-1513, by permission of Oxford University Press.)

Conclusion.—Molecular genetic aberrations involving the p53, cyclin E–FBXW7, and PI3K pathways represent major mechanisms in the development of uterine serous carcinoma (Fig 3B).

▶ Historically, ovarian and endometrial tumors have been defined via phenotypic analysis; however, with rapidly advancing molecular technologies, we are now poised to explore a deeper understanding of the molecular events driving carcinogenesis. The authors used a variety of techniques to analyze genetic mutations in 76 uterine serous carcinomas. In concordance with prior studies, they found a high rate of mutation in the *TP53* gene and reinforced the link between positive immunohistochemistry for *p53* and gene mutation status. Interestingly, the other 3 genes found to be mutated frequently in uterine serous carcinoma (*PIK3CA*, *FBXW7*, and *PPP2R1A*) are not mutated at nearly the same rate in ovarian serous carcinoma, suggesting markedly different paths of tumor development in these morphologically similar entities. They also found a putative link between serous carcinogenesis and the Cyclin E-BFXW7 pathway (Fig 3B). Positive staining for

Cyclin E used as part of that analysis may offer another ancillary tool for pathologists who confront morphologically ambiguous tumors, although more work is needed to determine the specificity of this marker for serous (as opposed to endometrioid) carcinogenesis. Lastly, they found the co-occurrence of mutations in paired serous carcinomas and their precursor lesions, endometrial intraepithelial carcinoma. They offer the tantalizing possibility of detecting molecular alterations in endometrial curetting specimens, which may indicate the presence of a clinically occult malignancy. This would obviously have major implications for the screening and counseling of patients in the future. Although seemingly far removed from the daily practice of diagnostic pathology, this article helps to increase our understanding of the molecular genetic events underlying uterine serous carcinogenesis and allows for the future development of tools to detect these lesions earlier, with the ultimate goal of developing more specific and effective treatment for women afflicted by this deadly disease.

M. D. Post, MD

Transitional Cell Carcinoma of the Ovary is Related to High-grade Serous Carcinoma and is Distinct From Malignant Brenner Tumor

Ali RH, Seidman JD, Luk M, et al (Vancouver General Hosp, British Columbia, Canada; Washington Hosp Ctr, DC)
Int J Gynecol Pathol 31:499-506, 2012

Transitional cell tumors of the ovary include benign, borderline (atypically proliferating), and malignant Brenner tumors (BT), as well as transitional cell carcinoma (TCC). Some TCCs could conceivably be examples of malignant BT where the benign component has been overgrown. Our objectives were: (A) compare the immunophenotypes of BT and TCC and (B) examine a large cohort of ovarian carcinomas for cases with the immunophenotype of BT and transitional features but lacking a benign BT component. Seven BTs (3 benign, 3 borderline/atypically proliferating, 1 malignant) and 7 TCCs were stained for WT1, ER, p53, and $p16^{INK4a}$. The BTs were negative for WT1, p53 overexpression, ER (except for weak positivity in 1), and negative or weakly positive for $p16^{INK4a}$. In contrast, the TCCs stained as follows: 4/6 positive for WT1, 5/7 positive for ER, 2/7 strongly positive for $p16^{INK4a}$, and 6/7 showed abnormal p53, an immunophenotype resembling that of high-grade serous carcinoma. A database of 500 cases of ovarian carcinoma was searched and 116 showed an immunoprofile characteristic of BT: WT1 negative, ER negative, $p16^{INK4a}$ negative or weak positive, p53 negative (77 clear cell carcinoma, 14 endometrioid carcinoma, 12 mucinous carcinoma, 8 high-grade serous carcinoma). None of these tumors showed transitional features on review, indicating that if examples of malignant BT where there has been overgrowth of benign BT components exist, they are rare.

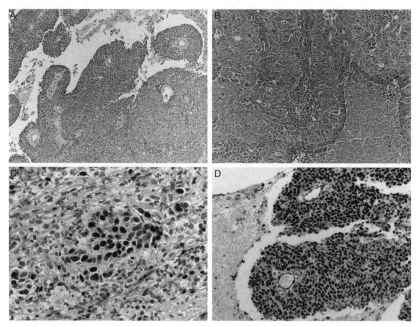

FIGURE 4.—Transitional cell carcinoma of the ovary is composed of multilayered papillae (A). High-grade cytologic features can be seen on higher power (B) as well as foci of necrosis. ER (C) and WT1 (D) immunostains are both positive. (Reprinted from Ali RH, Seidman JD, Luk M, et al. Transitional cell carcinoma of the ovary is related to high-grade serous carcinoma and is distinct from malignant brenner tumor. *Int J Gynecol Pathol.* 2012;31:499-506, with permission from International Society of Gynecological Pathologists.)

Our results suggest that BT and TCC are unrelated, and should not be combined for classification purposes (Fig 4).

▶ The World Health Organization (WHO) Classification of Tumors of the Breast and Female Genital Organs from 2003 is a widely used resource for categorizing ovarian neoplasms and includes a category of "transitional cell tumors" whose malignant end includes both Brenner tumors and non-Brenner transitional cell carcinomas. This grouping is based on morphologic similarities between the 2 tumor types; however, this study and others have amassed substantial evidence that these are, in fact, 2 distinct disease entities with different molecular genetic and immunophenotypic profiles. Increasingly, transitional cell carcinomas of the ovary without a benign Brenner component are being regarded as a variant of serous carcinoma based on *TP53* gene mutations and immunoprofile (WT1, ER, p53 and p16 positive; Fig 4). It has not yet been shown whether there is a significant prognostic difference between these 2 groups; however, precise classification of tumors is helpful for future research studies and potential application of novel therapies. The main limitations of the current study are that they used relatively few tumors for their analysis (14) and that immunostaining was performed on tissue microarray specimens, which, because of their small size, may skew results of patchy stains. Although additional studies exploring the implications of separating out ovarian transitional cell carcinoma from malignant Brenner tumors are needed, our evolving understanding of the disease pathogenesis points toward a revision in the next edition of the WHO.

M. D. Post, MD

Oncofetal protein IMP3: a useful diagnostic biomarker for leiomyosarcoma
Cornejo K, Shi M, Jiang Z (Univ of Massachusetts Med School, Worcester)
Hum Pathol 43:1567-1572, 2012

An accurate diagnosis between leiomyoma and leiomyosarcoma is essential for patient management. IMP3 is a member of the insulin-like growth factor (IGF-II) mRNA binding protein (IMP) family that consist of IMP1, IMP2, and IMP3. IMP3 is an oncofetal protein associated with aggressive and advanced tumors and is specifically expressed in malignant tumors but not found in benign tissues. The aim of this study was to determine the expression and diagnostic value of IMP3 in leiomyoma and leiomyosarcoma. A total of 216 cases (resection, n = 183; biopsy, n = 33) consisting of 82 leiomyosarcomas (uterine, n = 15; soft tissue, n = 67), 62 leiomyomas (uterine, n = 50; soft tissue, n = 12), and 72 uterine-variant leiomyomas (atypical, n = 19 [14%]; cellular, n = 21 [16%]; mitotically active, n = 12 [9%]; myxoid, n = 11 [8%]; vascular, n = 3 [2%]; epithelioid, n = 1 [1%]; benign metastasizing, n = 1 [1%]; and smooth muscle tumors of uncertain malignant potential, n = 4) were examined by immunohistochemistry for IMP3 expression. IMP3 showed strong cytoplasmic staining in 43 (52%) of 82 leiomyosarcomas, regardless of histologic grades. There was no difference in IMP3 expression between uterine and soft tissue leiomyosarcomas. In contrast to malignant tumors, IMP3 expression was not found in any of the typical leiomyomas (0/62 cases). All uterine-variant leiomyomas were negative, except for 3 cases (atypical variant, n = 2; cellular variant, n = 1) for IMP3 staining. In summary, we are the first to describe IMP3 expression in smooth muscle tumors. Our findings indicate that the expression of IMP3 in both uterine and soft tissue leiomyosarcomas can be used as a positive biomarker to increase the level of confidence in establishing a definitive diagnosis of a malignant smooth muscle tumor (Fig 1).

▶ One of the more common specimens received in surgical pathology laboratories is a hysterectomy removed for fibroids. While most cases are straightforward diagnostically solely on the basis of hematoxylin and eosin (H&E) staining, there are a small subset with ambiguous features, raising the concern for leiomyosarcoma. Although many markers currently exist for identifying smooth muscle differentiation, none are regularly used in clinical practice to distinguish benign from malignant tumors because of the significant overlap between these categories or difficulties in accurate stain interpretation. Distinguishing these entities is of vital importance as the subsequent management and patient counseling are dramatically different. In this article, the authors examine 216 cases of benign and

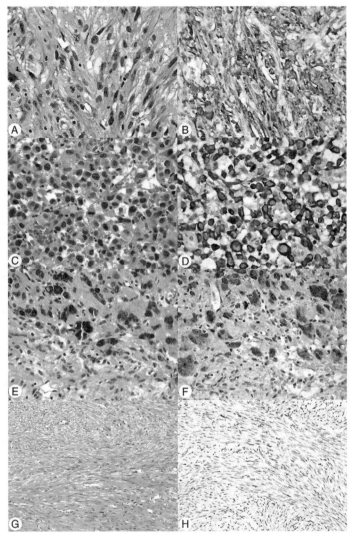

FIGURE 1.—Smooth muscle tumors with hematoxylin and eosin stains (left column, A, C, E, G) and immunohistochemical stains for IMP3 (right column, B, D, F, H). Leiomyosarcomas (spindle [A and B] and epithelioid [C and D]) and a uterine atypical leiomyoma (E and F) showed diffuse, dark-brown, cytoplasmic staining of IMP3. However, no IMP3 expression was detected in typical leiomyoma (G and H). For interpretation of the references to color in this figure legend, the reader is referred to web version of this article. (Reprinted from Cornejo K, Shi M, Jiang Z. Oncofetal protein IMP3: a useful diagnostic biomarker for leiomyosarcoma. *Hum Pathol.* 2012;43:1567-1572, Copyright 2012, with permission from Elsevier.)

malignant smooth muscle tumors from both uterine and extrauterine sites to determine insulin-like growth factor mRNA binding protein (IMP3) staining patterns and the suitability of this antibody as a distinguishing feature between the two. IMP3 has previously been found to be a cancer-specific biomarker associated with more aggressive tumor behavior in such diverse sites as renal cell carcinoma, mesothelioma, and endometrial cancers. It is an oncofetal protein involved in embryogenesis and carcinogenesis, which may play an important role in the pathogenesis of leiomyosarcoma via its modulation of cell proliferation, invasion, and migration. The authors found that 52% of studied leiomyosarcomas expressed IMP3, whereas no typical leiomyomas did, and only 4% of leiomyoma variants did. This offers hope that pathologists can find markers to provide diagnostic aid in histologically challenging or ambiguous cases. Strengths of the study include the relatively large number of cases and the dramatic distinction between benign and malignant entities. The main limitation is that the adoption of immunostains in some cases detracts from classic histologic diagnosis, and it is worth keeping in mind that any ancillary study is just that, to be interpreted in the context of H&E stained slides. With that caveat in mind, looking at Fig 1 of the article, this new immunomarker seems to offer a powerful new tool for use in challenging cases.

M. D. Post, MD

β-Catenin and E-cadherin expression in stage I adult-type granulosa cell tumour of the ovary: correlation with tumour morphology and clinical outcome

Stewart CJR, Doherty D, Guppy R, et al (King Edward Memorial Hosp, Perth, Western Australia, Australia; Univ of Western Australia, Perth, Australia; et al)
Histopathology 2012 [Epub ahead of print]

Aims.—To study E-cadherin and β-catenin expression in stage I adult-type granulosa cell tumours (AGCTs) and correlate the findings with tumour morphology and clinical outcome.

Methods and Results.—The study group comprised 62 FIGO stage I AGCTs, including 48 stage IA and 14 stage IC cases. Fifty patients (80.6%) had negative clinical follow-up over periods from 3.0 to 19.2 years (median 6.4 years), and 12 patients (19.4%) developed metastases at intervals of 3.6–16.2 years (median 8.6 years). β-Catenin and E-cadherin were expressed in 62 (100%) and 53 (85%) primary tumours, respectively, and staining was more consistent and intense in areas showing sex cord-like morphology. In contrast, diffuse tumour areas often showed weak or moderate staining (β-catenin) or were negative (E-cadherin), and there was reduced expression of both proteins in luteinized cells. Reduced β-catenin expression in primary tumours correlated with increased risk of recurrence ($P = 0.002$) and a shorter time interval to recurrence, whereas there was no correlation between E-cadherin staining and the risk of metastases.

Conclusions.—Localized variations in adhesion protein expression may partly explain the diverse morphological patterns exhibited by AGCT, and reduced β-catenin staining in primary tumours may have value as an adverse prognostic factor (Fig 2).

▶ Adult-type granulosa cell tumors are the frequently encountered sex-cord stromal tumors of the ovary, with a propensity for late recurrence and metastasis.

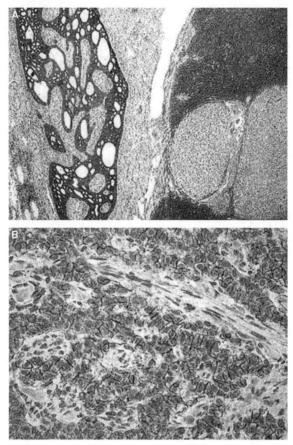

FIGURE 2.—**A,** Tumour cells showing microfollicular (left field) and watered silk (right upper field) patterns are β-catenin-positive, whereas nodular luteinized areas (lower right field) are not stained. **B,** There is strong membranous β-catenin expression in trabecular tumour areas. (Reprinted from Stewart CJR, Doherty D, Guppy R, et al. β-Catenin and E-cadherin expression in stage I adult-type granulosa cell tumour of the ovary: correlation with tumour morphology and clinical outcome. *Histopathology.* 2012 [Epub ahead of print], with permission from Hepatology and John Wiley and Sons, www.interscience.wiley.com.)

It is well known that stage is the most important prognostic factor, but the authors here seek to determine whether there are divisions that can be made within stage I tumors to offer additional clinically relevant information. They undertook to explore the staining patterns of 2 readily available immunohistochemical markers, beta-catenin and E-cadherin, in 62 cases of stage I adult-type granulosa cell tumors and to correlate their findings with clinical outcomes. They found that virtually all tumors expressed beta-catenin and that more diffuse expression was correlated to longer disease-free interval and lower recurrence rates. Interestingly, there was no correlation between primary tumor size and frequency of recurrence, despite tumor size being commonly used as a potential risk factor for more aggressive disease. E-Cadherin staining was found in a majority (85%) of tumors;

however, there were no statistically significant correlations between extent or intensity of staining and clinical outcomes. There were similar staining patterns in primary tumors and metastatic/recurrent disease with E-cadherin, in contrast to beta-catenin, which showed no such correlation. Both markers showed heterogeneous staining, with sex-cord-like areas showing the strongest expression (Fig 2). Given the morphological heterogeneity of these tumors, this finding suggests that to be useful as in clinical practice, multiple sections of a given tumor may need to be examined for beta-catenin expression before drawing any conclusions about possible tumor behavior. The authors only included stage I tumors (at time of primary diagnosis), which is understandable given the aims of this study; however, it would have been interesting to see whether higher-stage tumors at initial surgery followed the same trend.

M. D. Post, MD

Placental Histologic Criteria for Diagnosis of Cord Accident: Sensitivity and Specificity

Ryan WD, Trivedi N, Benirschke K, et al (Univ of California San Diego, La Jolla)
Pediatr Dev Pathol 15:275-280, 2012

"Cord accident" (compromised umbilical blood flow) as a cause of stillbirth is underreported, mainly due to a lack of diagnostic criteria. Based on fetal vascular pathology in the placenta, we have previously established histologic criteria for the diagnosis of cord accident. In the current study, we set out to test the sensitivity and specificity of these criteria by reviewing an independent set of stillbirth cases. Placental slides from 26 cases (in which cord accident was deemed the cause of death) and 62 controls (in which the cause of death was anything other than cord accident) were reviewed. The following histologic changes were noted: (1) dilated fetal vessels, (2) thrombosis in fetal vessels, and (3) avascular or near-avascular chorionic villi. "Minimal" criteria were defined as the presence of dilated and thrombosed fetal vessels, while the additional presence of focal or regional avascular or near-avascular villi satisfied the complete criteria. Of the 62 stillbirth controls with cause of death other than cord accident, 13 (21%) met the minimal criteria (specificity 79%) and only 4 (6%) met the complete criteria for cord accident (specificity 94%). In contrast, of the 26 cases with a cause of death related to cord accident, 16 met the minimal criteria (sensitivity 62%) and 12 met the complete criteria (sensitivity 46%). These histologic criteria identify cases of cord accident as a cause of stillbirth with very high specificity. This study confirms the utility of these criteria for diagnosis of cord accident and further stresses placental examination in evaluation of stillbirths (Fig 1).

▶ Placental examination has repeatedly been shown to play a crucial role in determining the etiology of stillbirth (fetal demise at greater than 20 weeks' gestational age); however, lack of standardization and/or pathologist familiarity with potential causes has limited its usefulness. This article tests the utility of a previously

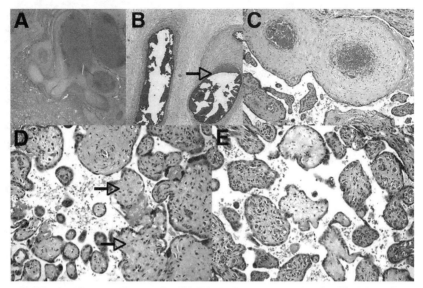

FIGURE 1.—Representative examples of histologic changes associated with stillbirth secondary to cord accident. **A.** Dilated chorionic plate/large stem villous vessels (H&E, original magnification ×20). **B.** Thrombosed chorionic plate vessel (arrow; H&E, original magnification ×40). **C.** Thrombosed stem villous vessel (vessel on the right; H&E, original magnification ×100). **D.** Villi showing villous stromal karyorrhexis (arrows; H&E, original magnification ×200). **E.** Avascular villi (middle of the panel; H&E, original magnification ×200). A color version of this figure is available online. (Reprinted from Ryan WD, Trivedi N, Benirschke K, et al. Placental histologic criteria for diagnosis of cord accident: sensitivity and specificity. *Pediatr Dev Pathol.* 2012;15:275-280, with permission from the Author[s], Pediatric and Developmental Pathology, and Allen Press Publishing Services.)

published set of criteria for diagnosing an umbilical cord accident as the cause of stillbirth.[1] The authors define minimal criteria as the presence of dilated and thrombosed fetal vessels and complete criteria as that plus the presence of fetal thrombotic vasculopathy (as manifested by avascular villi or villous stromal karyorrhexis, Fig 1). A review of 26 cases in which the cause of death had previously been reported as cord accident and 62 cases with a cause of death other than cord accident showed a specificity of 94% when complete criteria were applied. The sensitivity was much lower (62% for minimal criteria and 46% for complete criteria). This is explained by the authors as due to the heterogeneous nature of avascular villi, and they suggest that at least 4 sections of grossly normal placental parenchyma be sampled in cases of otherwise unexplained stillbirth. They acknowledge that the lesions associated with cord accidents do have morphologic overlap with those seen following prolonged in utero retention of a fetal demise, but argue that on balance, applying the criteria for cord accident may allow for a greater proportion of cases to have an assigned cause for the stillbirth, offering explanation to both families and obstetrician colleagues.

M. D. Post, MD

Reference

1. Parast MM, Crum CP, Boyd TK. Placental histologic criteria for umbilical blood flow restriction in unexplained stillbirth. *Hum Pathol.* 2008;39:948-953.

Acute Histologic Chorioamnionitis at Term: Nearly Always Noninfectious
Roberts DJ, Celi AC, Riley LE, et al (Harvard Med School, Boston, MA; et al)
PLoS One 7:e31819, 2012

Background.—The link between histologic acute chorioamnionitis and infection is well established in preterm deliveries, but less well-studied in term pregnancies, where infection is much less common.

Methodology/Principal Findings.—We conducted a secondary analysis among 195 low-risk women with term pregnancies enrolled in a randomized trial. Histologic and microbiologic evaluation of placentas included anaerobic and aerobic cultures (including mycoplasma/ureaplasma species) as well as PCR. Infection was defined as $\geq$1,000 cfu of a single known pathogen or a $\geq$2 log difference in counts for a known pathogen versus other organisms in a mixed culture. Placental membranes were scored and categorized as: no chorioamnionitis, Grade 1 (subchorionitis and patchy acute chorioamnionitis), or Grade 2 (severe, confluent chorioamnionitis). Grade 1 or grade 2 histologic chorioamnionitis was present in 34% of placentas (67/195), but infection was present in only 4% (8/195). Histologic chorioamnionitis was strongly associated with intrapartum fever > 38°C [69% (25/36) fever, 26% (42/159) afebrile, *P* < .0001]. Fever occurred in 18% (n = 36) of women. Most febrile women [92% (33/36)] had received epidural for pain relief, though the association with fever was present with and without epidural. The association remained significant in a logistic regression controlling for potential confounders (OR = 5.8, 95% CI = 2.2,15.0). Histologic chorioamnionitis was also associated with elevated serum levels of interleukin-8 (median = 1.3 pg/mL no histologic chorioamnionitis, 1.5 pg/mL Grade 1, 2.1 pg/mL Grade 2, *P* = 0.05) and interleukin-6 (median levels = 2.2 pg/mL no chorioamnionitis, 5.3 pg/mL Grade 1, 24.5 pg/mL Grade 2, *P* = 0.02) at admission for delivery as well as higher admission WBC counts (mean = 12,000 cells/mm³ no chorioamnionitis, 13,400 cells/mm³ Grade 1, 15,700 cells/mm³ Grade 2, *P* = 0.0005).

Conclusion/Significance.—Our results suggest histologic chorioamnionitis at term most often results from a noninfectious inflammatory process. It was strongly associated with fever, most of which was related to epidural used for pain relief. A more 'activated' maternal immune system at admission was also associated with histologic chorioamnionitis.

▶ Many placentas come to the pathology department with a history of clinical acute chorioamnionitis; however, the correlation between clinical and histologic chorioamnionitis is known to be extremely poor. Dogma has traditionally held that acute chorioamnionitis is exclusively due to intrauterine amniotic fluid infection, despite persistently negative cultures in many cases. This study attempted to further explore the possibility of noninfectious histologic chorioamnionitis in term deliveries. The authors found that of 195 deliveries in a preselected, very-low-risk population, 34% had histologic chorioamnionitis. However, only 4% of these had a demonstrable infectious cause, despite extensive workup for organisms. Rather than infectious agents, histologic chorioamnionitis in this population was associated with intrapartum fever, spontaneous onset of labor, and rupture of membranes for longer than 12 hours. Interestingly, cytokines interleukin-6 and interleukin-8 were higher in maternal serum and umbilical cord blood in those cases with histologic chorioamnionitis. There does seem to be mounting evidence that not all (and indeed, perhaps a minority of cases) of histologic chorioamnionitis cases are due to infection, but rather are related to inflammatory events. Specifically, the authors found that epidural analgesia was strongly associated with both fever and increased inflammatory cytokines. Some limitations of the study are the narrowly selected population that may underrepresent cases of infectious chorioamnionitis, the possibility that despite their best efforts, there were organisms present that could not be cultured, and the lack of examination of a fetal histologic response (previously supposed to be a better indicator of infection). Ultimately the significance of this study lies in beginning to develop means to preemptively identify cases of infection, thereby allowing for the more judicious use of intrapartum antibiotics.

M. D. Post, MD

10 Urinary Bladder and Male Genital Tract

Foamy gland adenocarcinoma of the prostate: incidence, Gleason grade, and early clinical outcome
Hudson J, Cao D, Vollmer R, et al (Washington Univ School of Medicine, St Louis, MO; VA and Duke Univ Med Ctrs, Durham, NC)
Hum Pathol 43:974-979, 2012

Foamy gland carcinoma is a variant of prostatic acinar adenocarcinoma characterized by abundant foamy cytoplasm and often pyknotic nuclei. Limited data exist regarding outcome and the clinicopathologic attributes of this variant. We screened 477 radical prostatectomies for foamy gland carcinoma to determine the incidence, amount, and Gleason grade/score of foamy gland carcinoma within the prostate. Time until prostate-specific antigen biochemical recurrence after radical prostatectomy was compared for both foamy and control/nonfoamy cases. For validation of incidence, Gleason grade, and pathologic stage, a second series of 100 consecutive radical prostatectomies was screened for foamy gland carcinoma. Foamy gland carcinoma was found in 69 (14.5%) of 477 cases. The median Gleason score of the foamy component was 7, which was not significantly different from the Gleason score of the nonfoamy component within those cases or the 408 nonfoamy cases. The most common Gleason score was 7 (44/69). There was no difference between foamy gland and non-foamy gland cases in recurrence rate (23% versus 22%) or the average time to prostate-specific antigen recurrence (130 versus 151 months). In the second series, foamy gland carcinoma was found in 23% of cases and had a median Gleason score of 7; and the most common Gleason score was 7 (11/23). Foamy gland carcinoma exists in a significant subset of prostatic carcinomas. This variant does not appear to harbor a different prognosis compared with usual acinar adenocarcinoma, but diagnostic recognition of foamy gland carcinoma is important because there is a Gleason grade 4 element in the majority of cases (Fig 2, Table 1).

▶ Foamy gland carcinoma is a variant of prostatic acinar adenocarcinoma characterized by abundant foamy cytoplasm and often pyknotic nuclei. Limited data exist regarding outcome and the clinicopathologic attributes of this variant. The authors have screened 477 radical prostatectomies for foamy gland carcinoma to determine the incidence, amount, and Gleason grade/score of foamy gland

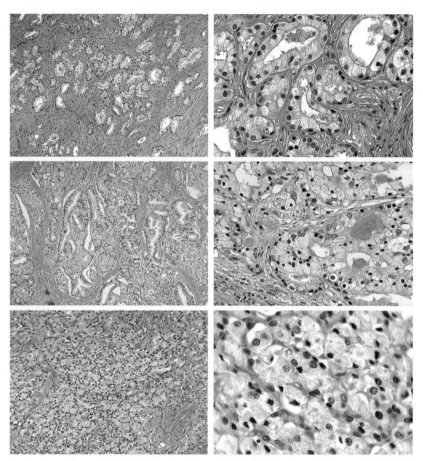

FIGURE 2.—Foamy gland adenocarcinoma: Gleason grade 3 (top), 4 (middle), and 5 (bottom). (Reprinted from Hudson J, Cao D, Vollmer R, et al. Foamy gland adenocarcinoma of the prostate: incidence, Gleason grade, and early clinical outcome. *Hum Pathol.* 2012;43:974-979, Copyright 2012, with permission form Elsevier.)

carcinoma within the prostate. Time until prostate-specific antigen biochemical recurrence after radical prostatectomy was compared for both foamy and control/nonfoamy cases. The World Health Organization classification book states that this variant is best characterized as an intermediate-grade carcinoma. There are limited data on the incidence and the clinicopathologic attributes of foamy gland adenocarcinoma. Little is known of the outcome for patients with this prostate cancer variant. In this study, foamy gland carcinoma was found in 69 (14.5%) of 477 nonconsecutive radical prostatectomy cases. The clinical features and pathologic features of Gleason grade, pathologic stage, and margin status for foamy versus nonfoamy carcinoma cases are studied (Table 1). These carcinomas are also graded (Fig 2). The significance of foamy gland carcinoma

TABLE 1.—Clinical and Pathologic Features of Radical Prostatectomy Cases with Foamy Gland *vs* Nonfoamy Gland Carcinoma: Series 1

Variable	Nonfoamy Cases	Foamy Cases	P Value
n	408	69	
Mean age (range)	61 (37-78)	62 (42-78)	>.1[a]
Mean preoperative PSA (ng/mL)	8.4 (0.7-85)	7.7 (1.5-31)	>.1[a]
Median Gleason score (range)	7 (5-9)	Foamy 7 (6-9)	.4[a]
		Nonfoamy 7 (6-9)	.8[a]
% Stage pT > 2	35	46	.08[b]
% With positive margins	93	83	.03[b]
Mean follow-up time (mo)	46	36	.026[a]
% With recurrence	22	23	>.9[b]

[a]*P* values from Kruskal-Wallis test.
[b]*P* values from χ² tests.

diagnostic recognition is that it can be deceptively benign appearing and it is often of high Gleason grade. For further reading, see reference list.[1,2]

S. A. Chandrakanth, MD, FRCPC

References

1. Zhao J, Epstein JI. High-grade foamy gland prostatic adenocarcinoma on biopsy or transurethral resection: a morphologic study of 55 cases. *Am J Surg Pathol.* 2009;33:583-590.
2. Tran TT, Sengupta E, Yang XJ. Prostatic foamy gland carcinoma with aggressive behavior: clinicopathologic, immunohistochemical, and ultrastructural analysis. *Am J Surg Pathol.* 2001;25:618-623.

Utility of GATA3 Immunohistochemistry in Differentiating Urothelial Carcinoma From Prostate Adenocarcinoma and Squamous Cell Carcinomas of the Uterine Cervix, Anus, and Lung

Chang A, Amin A, Gabrielson E, et al (The Johns Hopkins Hosp, Baltimore, MD)
Am J Surg Pathol 36:1472-1476, 2012

Distinguishing invasive high-grade urothelial carcinoma (UC) from other carcinomas occurring in the genitourinary tract may be difficult. The differential diagnosis includes high-grade prostatic adenocarcinoma, spread from an anal squamous cell carcinoma (SCC), or spread from a uterine cervical SCC. In terms of metastatic UC, the most common problem is differentiating spread of UC to the lung from a primary pulmonary SCC. Immunohistochemical analysis (IHC) for GATA binding protein 3 (GATA3), thrombomodulin (THROMBO), and uroplakin III was performed on a tissue microarray (TMA) containing 35 cases of invasive high-grade UC. GATA3 IHC was also performed on TMAs containing 38 high-grade (Gleason score ≥ 8) prostatic adenocarcinomas, representative tissue sections from 15 invasive anal SCCs, representative tissue sections from 19 invasive cervical SCCs, and TMAs with 12 invasive cervical carcinomas of the cervix

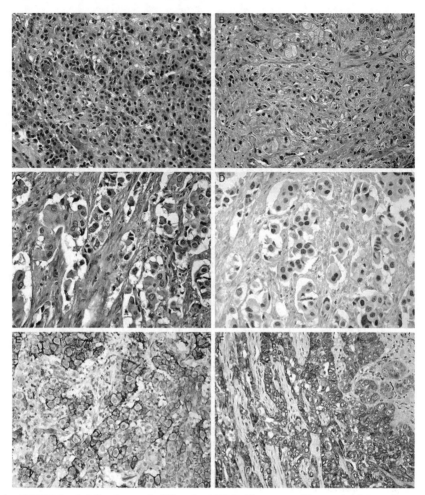

FIGURE 1.—A, Infiltrating poorly differentiated UC. B, Gleason score 10 prostatic adenocarcinoma. C, Invasive poorly differentiated UC. D, GATA3 with both moderate and strong nuclear staining [same case shown in (C)]. E, UC showing diffuse and strong staining with THROMBO. F, UC showing diffuse and strong staining with uroplakin III. (Reprinted from Chang A, Amin A, Gabrielson E, et al. Utility of GATA3 immunohistochemistry in differentiating urothelial carcinoma from prostate adenocarcinoma and squamous cell carcinomas of the uterine cervix, anus, and lung. *Am J Surg Pathol.* 2012;36:1472-1476, with permission from Lippincott Williams & Wilkins.)

[SCC (n = 10), SCC with neuroendocrine features (n = 1), and adenosquamous carcinoma (n = 1)]. In addition, GATA3 IHC was performed on representative tissue sections from 15 pulmonary UC metastases and a TMA with 25 SCCs of the lung and 5 pulmonary non–small cell carcinomas with squamous features. GATA3, THROMBO, and uroplakin III were positive in 28 (80%), 22 (63%), and 21 (60%) cases of high-grade UC, respectively. All cases of GATA3-positive staining were nonfocal; 25 (89%) cases demonstrated moderate to strong staining, and 3 (11%) demonstrated weak

TABLE 1.—Sensitivity of "Urothelial Markers" in High-grade UC

GATA3	28/35 (80%)
Weak	3 (11%)
Moderate-strong	25 (89%)
Thrombomodulin	22/35 (63%)
Uroplakin III	21/35 (60%)

staining. Of the 7 cases that failed to express GATA3, 5 were positive for THROMBO and/or uroplakin III, whereas 2 were negative for all 3 markers. None of the 38 high-grade prostatic adenocarcinomas was positive for GATA3. Weak GATA3 staining was present in occasional basal cells of benign prostate glands, in a few benign atrophic glands, and in urothelial metaplasia. Of the 15 cases of anal SCCs, 2 (7%) cases showed focal weak staining, and 1 (3%) showed focal moderate staining. Weak staining was also rarely observed in the benign anal squamous epithelium. Of the 31 uterine cervical carcinomas, 6 (19%) showed weak GATA3 staining (3 nonfocal and 3 focal), and 2 (6%) demonstrated focal moderate staining. Twelve (80%) of the metastatic UCs to the lung were positive for GATA3, with 11 cases showing diffuse moderate or strong staining and 1 case showing focal moderate staining. None of the pulmonary SCCs or non—small cell carcinomas with squamous features was GATA3 positive. GATA3 IHC is a sensitive marker for UC, and positive staining in UC is typically nonfocal and moderate or strong in intensity. GATA3 is also highly specific in excluding high-grade prostate adenocarcinoma. Although some cervical and anal SCCs can be GATA3 positive, unlike in UC, staining is more commonly focal and weak. GATA3 is also a useful maker when diagnosing metastatic UC to the lung (Fig 1, Table 1).

▶ This is a very useful article highlighting how to distinguish invasive high-grade urothelial carcinoma (UC) from other carcinomas occurring in the genitourinary tract. The differential diagnosis includes high-grade prostatic adenocarcinoma, spread from an anal squamous cell carcinoma (SCC), or spread from a uterine cervical SCC. In terms of metastatic UC, the most common problem is differentiating spread of UC to the lung from a primary pulmonary SCC. GATA-binding protein 3 (GATA3) is a zinc finger transcription factor with a diverse range of biological roles. GATA3 contributes to early T-cell development.

This study evaluates the sensitivity of GATA3 immunohistochemical (IHC) testing for detecting high-grade UC and compares it with the sensitivities of thrombomodulin and uroplakin III. The specificity of GATA3 IHC for high-grade UC and the utility of GATA3 IHC in assessing metastatic UC to the lung are also examined (Table 1). Invasive high-grade UC can be difficult to differentiate from other high-grade carcinomas because the morphology of high-grade UC is not always specific. In most cases, high-grade prostatic adenocarcinoma must be excluded.

This scenario is frequently encountered during transurethral resections of large tumors involving the bladder neck, in which clinically it is virtually impossible to distinguish between a prostate and bladder primary (Fig 1). In conclusion, the authors demonstrate GATA3 IHC is a sensitive marker for UC, and positive staining in UC is typically nonfocal and moderate or strong in intensity. GATA3 is also highly specific in excluding high-grade prostate adenocarcinoma.

Although some cervical and anal SCCs can be GATA3 positive, unlike UC, staining is more commonly focal and weak. GATA3 is also a useful maker when diagnosing metastatic UC to the lung. For additional reading, please see reference list.[1]

S. A. Chandrakanth, MD, FRCPC

Reference

1. Higgins JP, Kaygusuz G, Wang L, et al. Placental S100 (S100P) and GATA3: markers for transitional epithelium and urothelial carcinoma discovered by complementary DNA microarray. *Am J Surg Pathol.* 2007;31:673-680.

Inflammation and preneoplastic lesions in benign prostate as risk factors for prostate cancer

Kryvenko ON, Jankowski M, Chitale DA, et al (Henry Ford Hosp, Detroit, MI; et al)
Mod Pathol 25:1023-1032, 2012

Benign changes ranging from atrophy and inflammation to high-grade prostatic intraepithelial neoplasia (HGPIN) are common findings on prostate core needle biopsies. Although atrophy and inflammation may be precursors of prostate cancer, only HGPIN is currently recommended to be included in surgical pathology reports. To determine whether these benign findings increase prostate cancer risk, we conducted a case–control study nested within a historical cohort of 6692 men with a benign prostate specimen collected between 1990 and 2002. The analytic sample included 574 case–control pairs comprised of cases diagnosed with prostate cancer a minimum of 1 year after cohort entry and controls matched to cases on date and age at cohort entry, race, and type of specimen. The initial benign specimen was reviewed for presence of HGPIN, atrophy (simple, lobular, and partial) and inflammation (glandular and/or stromal). HGPIN significantly increased risk for prostate cancer (odds ratio (OR) = 2.00; 95% confidence interval (CI) = 1.25−3.20). Inflammation within the stromal compartment was associated with decreased risk (OR = 0.66; CI = 0.52−0.84), and diffuse stromal inflammation of severe grade had the strongest inverse association with risk (OR = 0.21; CI = 0.07−0.62). In a model adjusted for prostate-specific antigen (PSA) level at cohort entry and inflammation, simple atrophy was associated with a 33% increased prostate cancer risk that was marginally significant ($P = 0.03$). Clinicians should consider patterns and extent of inflammation when managing high-risk patients with negative biopsy results. Identifying benign inflammatory processes that underlie high PSA levels would help

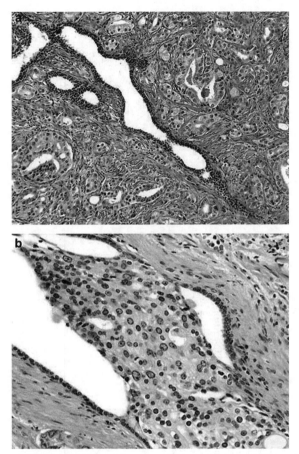

FIGURE 4.—(a) Gland with simple atrophy surrounded by prostate cancer. (b) Intraductal spread of prostate cancer. Note atrophic native epithelium at the periphery of the duct and markedly enlarged and pleomorphic nuclei of intraductal carcinoma. (Reprinted by permission from Macmillan Publishers Ltd: Modern Pathology. Kryvenko ON, Jankowski M, Chitale DA, et al. Inflammation and preneoplastic lesions in benign prostate as risk factors for prostate cancer. *Mod Pathol*. 2012;25:1023-1032, Copyright 2012 by USCAP, Inc.)

to reduce the number of unnecessary repeated prostate biopsies (Fig 4, Tables 4-6).

▶ This is an interesting study that emphasizes the relation of benign prostatic diseases to subsequent development of prostate cancer. Benign changes ranging from atrophy and inflammation to prostatic intraepithelial neoplasia are common findings on prostate needle core biopsies (Fig 4, Table 4). Of these, only high-grade prostatic intraepithelial neoplasia (HGPIN) is routinely recorded on pathologic reports because of its well-known association with prostate cancer. This study confirms previously reported associations of HGPIN with increased risk of subsequent prostate cancer diagnosis. In this nested cohort, the presence of HGPIN was associated with a 2-fold increased risk for prostate cancer. Overall,

TABLE 4.—Multivariable Models Estimating Independent Effects of HGPIN, Atrophy, and Inflammation on Prostate Cancer Risk ($n = 574$ Pairs)

	Initial Model		'Type of Atrophy' Model		'Type of Inflammation' Model	
	OR (95% CI)	P-Value	OR (95% CI)	P-Value	OR (95% CI)	P-Value
PSA (ng/ml)	1.08 (1.05–1.11)	<0.001	1.08 (1.05–1.11)	<0.001	1.08 (1.05–1.11)	<0.001
HGPIN	2.33 (1.41–3.83)	0.001	2.30 (1.39–3.80)	0.001	2.23 (1.36–3.67)	0.002
Presence of atrophy	1.30 (1.02–1.67)	0.04			1.28 (1.00–1.64)	0.05
Simple atrophy			1.33 (1.03–1.70)	0.03		
Post-atrophic hyperplasia			2.03 (0.68–6.04)	0.20		
Partial atrophy			0.92 (0.39–2.15)	0.84		
Presence of inflammation	0.59 (0.46–0.77)	<0.001	0.59 (0.45–0.77)	<0.001		
Stromal inflammation					0.63 (0.49–0.83)	<0.001
Glandular inflammation					1.12 (0.76–1.67)	0.57
Periglandular inflammation					0.93 (0.68–1.27)	0.65

TABLE 5.—Modeling Effect of Extent and Grade of Stromal Inflammation on Prostate Cancer Risk (574 Pairs)[a]

Extent	Grade	OR (95% CI)	P-Value
Focal	Mild	0.68 (0.48−0.95)	0.02
	Moderate	0.56 (0.29−1.08)	0.08
	Severe	0.68 (0.37−1.25)	0.21
Multifocal	Mild	0.75 (0.44−1.27)	0.29
	Moderate	0.48 (0.26−0.89)	0.02
	Severe	0.79 (0.47−1.33)	0.38
Diffuse	Mild[b]	NA	NA
	Moderate	0.38 (0.11−1.36)	0.14
	Severe	0.20 (0.07−0.60)	0.004

[a]Model adjusted for PSA and presence of HGPIN.
[b]There were no individuals in this category.

TABLE 6.—Stratified multivariable model estimating effects of HGPIN, stromal inflammation, and simple atrophy on prostate cancer risk (574 pairs)[a]

	OR (95% CI)	OR (95% CI)
Age[b]	Age <66.2 years (n = 281 pairs)	Age ≥66.2 years (n = 293 pairs)
HGPIN	2.84 (1.32−6.12)	1.89 (0.98−3.64)
Stromal inflammation	0.61 (0.42−0.88)	0.63 (0.44−0.91)
Simple atrophy	1.29 (0.90−1.86)	1.26 (0.89−1.77)
Race	White (n = 345 pairs)	African American (n = 229 pairs)
HGPIN	2.47 (1.28−4.79)	2.09 (0.97−4.52)
Stromal inflammation	0.69 (0.50−0.96)	0.54 (0.36−0.82)
Simple atrophy	1.16 (0.84−1.59)	1.43 (0.96−2.13)
Time to diagnosis[c]	<3.98 years (n = 287 pairs)	≥3.98 years (n = 287 pairs)
HGPIN	5.68 (2.18−13.71)	1.23 (0.65−2.33)
Stromal inflammation	0.72 (0.50−1.03)	0.57 (0.39−0.82)
Simple atrophy	1.14 (0.79−1.64)	1.41 (1.00−1.99)
Date of cohort entry[d]	Before March 1995 (n = 287 pairs)	March 1995 or later (n = 287 pairs)
HGPIN	1.34 (0.66−2.73)	3.62 (1.73−7.56)
Stromal inflammation	0.65 (0.45−0.94)	0.62 (0.43−0.88)
Simple atrophy	1.23 (0.87−1.74)	1.30 (0.90−1.86)
Gleason grade[e]	Non-advanced (n = 410 pairs)	Advanced (n = 155 pairs)
HGPIN	2.31 (1.29−4.15)	2.26 (0.85−6.00)
Stromal inflammation	0.66 (0.49−0.88)	0.57 (0.34−0.94)
Simple atrophy	1.37 (1.02−1.83)	1.15 (0.71−1.87)

[a]All models adjusted for PSA at date of cohort entry.
[b]Stratified on median age = 66.2.
[c]Stratified on median time to diagnosis.
[d]Stratified on median date of entry into the cohort.
[e]Advanced grade = total Gleason 7 (4 + 3) or ≥ 8.

prostate cancer was diagnosed in 65% (56/86) of patients with HGPIN present in their initial benign prostate specimen, the majority being diagnosed within 4 years of follow-up. This study suggests that simple atrophy may modestly increase risk of prostate cancer, whereas presence of stromal inflammation significantly decreases risk (Tables 5 and 6). Moreover, characterizing the type and extent of inflammation may explain the main cause of elevated prostate-specific antigen in patients with negative prostate biopsy results. Such characterization would aid in the clinical treatment of these patients by reducing the number of unnecessary repeated prostate biopsies. For further reading, see reference list.[1,2]

S. A. Chandrakanth, MD, FRCPC

References

1. Netto GJ, Epstein JI. Widespread high-grade prostatic intraepithelial neoplasia on prostatic needle biopsy: a significant likelihood of subsequently diagnosed adenocarcinoma. *Am J Surg Pathol.* 2006;30:1184-1188.
2. Merrimen JL, Jones G, Srigley JR. Is high grade prostatic intraepithelial neoplasia still a risk factor for adenocarcinoma in the era of extended biopsy sampling? *Pathology.* 2010;42:325-329.

Loss of PTEN expression is associated with increased risk of recurrence after prostatectomy for clinically localized prostate cancer
Chaux A, Peskoe SB, Gonzalez-Roibon N, et al (Johns Hopkins Univ School of Medicine, Baltimore, MD; Johns Hopkins Bloomberg School of Public Health, Baltimore, MD)
Mod Pathol 25:1543-1549, 2012

PTEN (phosphatase and tensin homolog on chromosome 10) is one of the most frequently lost tumor suppressor genes in human cancers and it has been described in more than two-thirds of patients with advanced/ aggressive prostate cancer. Previous studies suggest that, in prostate cancer, genomic *PTEN* loss is associated with tumor progression and poor prognosis. Thus, we evaluated whether immunohistochemical PTEN expression in prostate cancer glands was associated with higher risk of recurrence, using a nested case—control study that included 451 men who recurred and 451 men who did not recur with clinically localized prostate cancer treated by radical prostatectomy. Recurrence was defined as biochemical recurrence (serum prostate-specific antigen > 0.2 ng/ml) or clinical recurrence (local recurrence, systemic metastases, or prostate cancer-related death). Cases and controls were matched on pathological T stage, Gleason score, race/ethnicity, and age at surgery. Odds ratios of recurrence and 95% confidence intervals were estimated using conditional logistic regression to account for the matching factors and to adjust for year of surgery, preoperative prostate-specific antigen concentrations, and status of surgical margins. Men who recurred had a higher proportion of PTEN negative expression (16 *vs* 11%, *P* = 0.05) and PTEN loss (40 vs 31%, *P* = 0.02) than controls. Men with markedly decreased PTEN staining had a higher risk of recurrence (odds ratio = 1.67; 95% confidence intervals 1.09, 2.57; *P* = 0.02) when compared with all other men. In summary, in patients with clinically localized prostate cancer treated by prostatectomy, decreased PTEN expression was associated with an increased risk of recurrence, independent of known clinicopathological factors (Fig 1, Tables 1 and 2).

▶ This is one of the recent articles on phosphatase and tensin homolog on chromosome 10 (PTEN) and its relation with prostate cancer. PTEN is one of the most

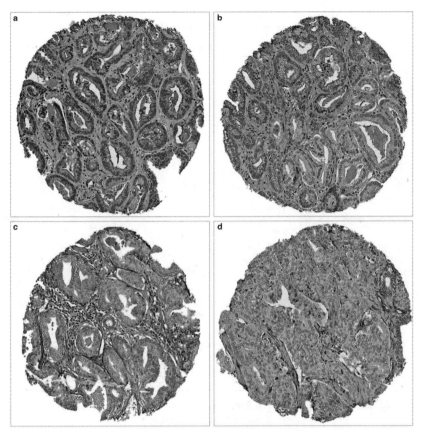

FIGURE 1.—Patterns of PTEN (phosphatase and tensin homolog on chromosome 10) expression in prostate carcinoma. (a) Diffuse cytoplasmic PTEN expression. (b) Reduced PTEN expression, more obvious in the glands at the lower right. (c, d) Markedly decreased to negative PTEN expression in all glands. Note the PTEN positivity in the stromal cells. Tissue microarray spots at (b–d) were classified as 'markedly decreased PTEN expression'. (Reprinted by permission from Macmillan Publishers Ltd: Modern Pathology. Chaux A, Peskoe SB, Gonzalez-Roibon N, et al. Loss of PTEN expression is associated with increased risk of recurrence after prostatectomy for clinically localized prostate cancer. *Mod Pathol.* 2012;25:1543-1549, Copyright 2012, by USCAP, Inc.)

frequently lost tumor suppressor genes in human cancers and has been described in more than two-thirds of patients with advanced/aggressive prostate cancer (Fig 1). Earlier studies suggest that, in prostate cancer, genomic PTEN loss is associated with tumor progression and poor prognosis. PTEN functions as a tumor suppressor protein, negatively controlling the activation of the phosphoinosite 3-kinase pathway. Loss of PTEN leads to accumulation of phosphoinosite 3,4,5-triphosphate, which in turns leads to overactivation of AKT, a key regulator of the mammalian target of rapamycin (mTOR) pathway. Activation of mTOR is associated with increased cell growth and cell proliferation, favoring the survival of cells with dysregulation of this pathway.

This is one of the largest studies to date evaluating PTEN in association with recurrence in patients with prostate cancer (Table 1). Decreased or loss of

TABLE 1.—Characteristics of Recurrence Cases and Controls

	Cases	Controls	P-Value
Age at surgery, years			
Mean (s.d.)	58.7 (6.1)	58.9 (5.8)	Matched
Race, %			
Caucasian	85	88	Matched
Pre-operative serum PSA, ng/ml			
Mean (s.d.)	12.3 (10.4)	11.2 (8.5)	0.21
Median (IQR)	9.1 (8.6)	8.7 (7.2)	0.22
Follow-up time, years			
Mean (s.d.)	2.5 (1.9)	5.9 (2.4)	< 0.001
Median (IQR)	2 (2)	6 (4)	< 0.001
Gleason score, %			Matched
≤ 6	15	15	
7	61	63	
≥ 8	24	22	
Pathological stage, %			Matched
T2	13	13	
T3a	51	51	
T3b or N1	36	36	
PTEN mean H-Score			
Mean (s.d.)	105.5 (93.6)	112.4 (85.3)	0.19
Median (IQR)	100 (175.8)	102.5 (166)	0.08
PTEN expression, %			
Mean H-score = 0	16	11	0.05
All TMA spots markedly decreased[a]	40	31	0.02

Abbreviations: IQR, interquartile range; TMA, tissue microarray.
[a]Limited to matched pairs with three to six TMA spots evaluated per patient (N = 714).

TABLE 2.—PTEN Expression and Risk of Recurrence After Prostatectomy for Clinically Localized Prostate Cancer

PTEN Expression	Biochemical or Clinical Recurrence Odds Ratio[a]	P-Value	Biochemical Recurrence First Odds Ratio[a]	P-Value	Clinical Recurrence First Odds Ratio[a]	P-Value
	N = 902 (452 pairs)		N = 574 (287 pairs)		N = 328 (164 pairs)	
Mean H-score = 0	1.41 (0.81, 2.45)	0.22	1.34 (0.63, 2.85)	0.44	2.52 (1.07, 5.95)	0.03
Mean H-score < 10	2.20 (1.33, 3.63)	0.002	2.09 (1.10, 3.96)	0.02	1.50 (0.65, 3.47)	0.34
Any spot markedly decreased[b]	1.32 (0.90, 1.94)	0.15	1.26 (0.76, 2.09)	0.37	1.36 (0.74, 2.50)	0.32
	N = 714 (357 pairs)		N = 462 (231 pairs)		N = 252 (126 pairs)	
All spots markedly decreased[c]	1.67 (1.09, 2.57)	0.02	1.33 (0.78, 2.26)	0.30	2.19 (0.98, 4.91)	0.06

[a]Adjusted for year of surgery, preoperative serum PSA concentration, surgical margin status, and the residual difference in pathological stage between the cases and controls. Values in parenthesis correspond to 95% confidence intervals.
[b]Irrespective of the number of TMA spots evaluated per patient.
[c]Limited to matched pairs with 3 to 6 spots evaluated per patient. The number of matched pairs is included in parenthesis.

PTEN expression was associated with higher risk of recurrence, independent of established clinicopathological prognostic factors. The current study provides further support for the role of PTEN expression as a predictor of biochemical recurrence in patients with prostate cancer. However, in other studies, PTEN expression was not a predictor of biochemical recurrence when evaluated alone, but it was when associated with other biomarkers. This study is consistent with prior studies on genomic loss of PTEN that showed that a decrease or loss of PTEN immunohistochemical expression was associated with higher risk of recurrence in men with clinically localized prostate cancer (Table 2) who were treated by radical prostatectomy, independent of established clinicopathological prognostic factors. For further reading, see reference list.[1,2]

S. A. Chandrakanth, MD, FRCPC

References

1. Halvorsen OJ, Haukaas SA, Akslen LA. Combined loss of PTEN and p27 expression is associated with tumor cell proliferation by Ki-67 and increased risk of recurrent disease in localized prostate cancer. *Clin Cancer Res.* 2003;9:1474-1479.
2. Dreher T, Zentgraf H, Abel U, et al. Reduction of PTEN and p27kip1 expression correlates with tumor grade in prostate cancer. Analysis in radical prostatectomy specimens and needle biopsies. *Virchows Arch.* 2004;444:509-517.

A Close Surgical Margin After Radical Prostatectomy is an Independent Predictor Of Recurrence

Lu J, Wirth GJ, Wu S, et al (Harvard Med School, Boston, MA)
J Urol 188:91-97, 2012

Purpose.—The term close surgical margin refers to a tumor extending to the inked margin of the specimen without reaching it. Current guidelines state that a close surgical margin should simply be reported as negative. However, this recommendation remains controversial and relies on limited evidence. We evaluated the impact of close surgical margins on the long-term risk of biochemical recurrence after radical prostatectomy.

Materials and Methods.—We identified 1,195 consecutive patients who underwent radical prostatectomy and lymphadenectomy for localized prostate cancer at our institution from 1993 to 1999. In 894 of these patients associations between margin status and location, Gleason score, pathological stage, preoperative prostate specific antigen, prostate weight and age with the risk of biochemical recurrence were examined.

Results.—Of these 894 patients 644 (72%) had negative margins and of these patients 100 (15.5%) had close surgical margins. In the group with prostate specific antigen failure, median time to recurrence was 3.5 years. In the group without recurrence median followup was 9.9 years. Cumulative recurrence-free survival differed significantly among positive, negative and close surgical margins ($p < 0.001$). On multivariate analysis a close surgical margin constituted a significant, independent predictor of recurrence (HR 2.1, 95% CI 1.04—4.33). Gleason score and positive margins were the strongest prognostic factors.

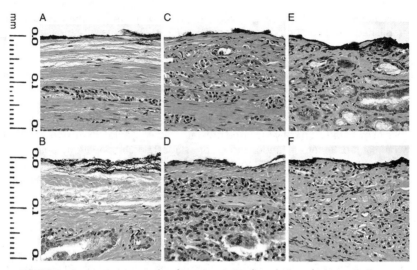

FIGURE 1.—Representative examples of negative (A—B), close (C—D) and positive (E—F) prostatectomy margins. H&E, reduced from ×400. (Reprinted from Lu J, Wirth GJ, Wu S, et al. A close surgical margin after radical prostatectomy is an independent predictor of recurrence. *J Urol.* 2012;188:91-97, Copyright 2012, with permission from the American Urological Association.)

TABLE 1.—Clinicopathological Characteristics

	Overall	NSM	CSM	PSM	P Value
No. pts (%)	894	544 (60.9)	100 (11.1)	250 (28.0)	
Median pt age (IQR)	62 (57—66)	62 (56—66)	62 (57—66)	62 (57—66)	0.782
Median ng/ml PSA (IQR)	6.0 (4.5—8.6)	5.9 (4.5—8.0)	6.1 (4.6—9.5)	6.2 (4.5—9.3)	0.048
No. Gleason score (%):					<0.001
6 or Less	420 (47.0)	293 (53.9)	47 (47)	80 (32.0)	
7	376 (42.0)	211 (38.8)	38 (38)	127 (50.8)	
8 or Greater	98 (11.0)	40 (7.3)	15 (15)	43 (17.2)	
No. stage (%):					<0.001
pT2	703 (78.6)	468 (66.6)	74 (10.5)	161 (22.9)	
pT3	191 (21.4)	76 (39.8)	26 (13.6)	89 (46.6)	
Median gm prostate wt (IQR)	43 (34—55)	44 (34—58)	44 (35—52)	40.2 (33.5—50)	0.014
No. margin location (%):					<0.001
Apex			17 (17)	60 (24)	
Peripheral			81 (81)	128 (51)	
Bladder neck			1 (1)	10 (4)	
Multiple			1 (1)	52 (21)	
Median yrs follow-up (IQR)	9.9 (6.1—11.3)	10.0 (6.5—11.3)	10.2 (4.5—12.4)	9.6 (6.0—11.0)	0.355
No. recurrence (%)	277 (31)	114 (21.0)	39 (39.0)	124 (49.6)	<0.001
Median yrs to recurrence (IQR)	3.5 (1.8—6.2)	3.7 (2.0—6.4)	5.5 (2.5—8.4)	3.1 (1.4—5.1)	0.007

Conclusions.—In this cohort close surgical margins were independently associated with a twofold risk of postoperative biochemical recurrence. Further evaluation of the clinical significance of close surgical margins is

TABLE 2.—Association of Margin Status and Other Clinical and Pathological Factors with BCR

	HR	P Value	95% CI
Univariate analyses			
PSA	1.06	0.000	1.04—1.08
Stage:			
pT2	1.00	0.000	
pT3	2.52	0.000	1.97—3.23
Gleason score:			
6 or Less	1.00		
7	2.46	0.000	1.84—3.30
8	5.62	0.000	3.34—9.46
9 or Greater	11.6	0.000	8.18—16.47
Margin:			
Neg	1.00		
Close	1.93	0.000	1.34—2.78
Pos	2.97	0.000	2.30—3.83
Yr of surgery	0.88	0.000	0.82—0.94
Age	1.02	0.053	1.00—1.03
Prostate wt	0.99	0.010	0.98—1.00
Nerve sparing*	0.89	0.342	0.70—1.13
Multivariate analysis: neg, close + pos margins[†,‡]			
PSA	1.05	0.000	1.02—1.07
Stage:			
pT2	1.00		
pT3	1.34	0.079	0.97—1.86
Gleason score:			
6 or Less	1.00		
7	2.71	0.000	1.73—4.21
8	3.64	0.011	1.35—9.84
9 or Greater	29.54	0.000	16.59—52.61
Margin:			
Neg	1.00		
Close	2.12	0.039	1.04—4.33
Pos	3.52	0.000	1.97—6.29
Yr of surgery	0.89	0.007	0.82—0.97
Multivariate analysis: neg + pos margins[†,§]			
PSA	1.04	0.000	1.02—1.07
Stage:			
pT2	1.00		
pT3	1.40	0.037	1.02—1.93
Gleason score:			
6 or Less	1.00		
7	2.47	0.000	1.70—3.60
8	4.01	0.001	1.78—9.02
9 or Greater	13.26	0.000	8.00—22.00
Margin:			
Neg	1.00		
Pos	2.98	0.000	1.75—5.05
Yr of surgery	0.90	0.005	0.83—0.97

*Also nonsignificant when analyzed as 3 groups (none, unilateral, bilateral).
[†]Bootstrap corrected, multivariate Cox regression models fit with PSA, tumor stage, Gleason score, margin status and year of surgery.
[‡]Close margins treated as an independent group.
[§]Close margins considered negative.

indicated as they might be an indicator of local recurrence and of relevance when considering salvage therapy (Fig 1, Tables 1 and 2).

▶ This is an informative article on surgical margins in prostatectomy.

The term "close surgical margin" refers to a tumor extending to the inked margin of the specimen without reaching it. Current guidelines state that a close surgical margin should simply be reported as negative; however, this recommendation remains controversial and relies on limited evidence. The current study evaluates the effect of close surgical margins on the long-term risk of biochemical recurrence after radical prostatectomy. This includes one of the largest series of cases. The authors used the following data in their study. Surgical margins were classified as negative, close, or positive. By consensus, close surgical margins were reported when the tumor approached the margin by less than 0.1 mm, which corresponds to a few layers of fibroblasts, without being in contact with the ink (Fig 1). When the layer of benign tissue between the inked margin and the tumor was larger (> 0.1 mm), the margins were considered negative. Finally, when tumor cells were in direct contact with ink, the margin was considered positive. Margin status and prostate weight were retrieved from the original pathology reports. Gleason scores and tumor stages were updated according to the International Society of Urological Pathology 10 and the American Joint Committee on Cancer (TNM classification, 7th edition), respectively. This study also demonstrates the association of margin status and other clinical and pathological factors with BCR (Tables 1 and 2).

The current study is that it includes a large cohort of patients with a long follow-up, that the patients were treated in the prostate-specific antigen era, and that an internally validated Cox regression was performed. However, it is subject to limitations inherent to the retrospective design. For further reading, see the reference list.[1,2]

S. A. Chandrakanth, MD, FRCPC

References

1. Swanson GP, Lerner SP. Positive margins after radical prostatectomy: implications for failure and role of adjuvant treatment. *Urol Oncol.* July 18, 2011. Epub ahead of print.
2. Boorjian SA, Karnes RJ, Crispen PL, et al. The impact of positive surgical margins on mortality following radical prostatectomy during the prostate specific antigen era. *J Urol.* 2010;183:1003-1009.

Urethral caruncle: clinicopathologic features of 41 cases
Conces MR, Williamson SR, Montironi R, et al (Indiana Univ School of Medicine, Indianapolis; Polytechnic Univ of the Marche Region (Ancona), Italy; et al)
Hum Pathol 43:1400-1404, 2012

Urethral caruncle is a benign polypoid mass of the urethral meatus in primarily postmenopausal women. Although a conclusive association with malignancy, urologic disorder, or systemic disease has not been established, often the lesion carries a challenging clinical differential diagnosis that

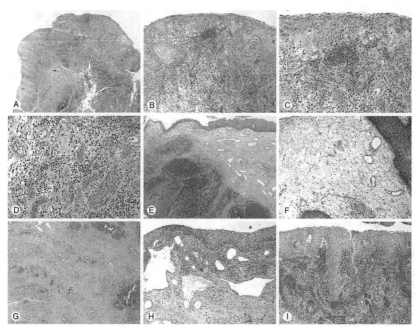

FIGURE 1.—Urethral caruncle. A, Low magnification, demonstrating a polypoid lesion lined by hyperplastic squamous epithelium with stromal inflammatory infiltrates and dilated blood vessels (40×). B and C, Intermediate and high magnification, showing lymphoplasmacytic infiltrates with intermingled acute inflammatory cells and extravasation of erythrocytes (B, 100×; C, 200×). D, Plasma cells are abundant, with occasional Mott cells (200×). E, Another case, showing hyperplastic urothelium overlying stromal pools of blood with organizing thrombus and dilated vessels (40×). F, A case with prominent stromal edema and scattered inflammatory cells (100×). G, Another case, showing a more sclerotic stroma with invaginations of urothelium, containing central cystic/glandular lumens within urothelial nests (40×). H, Subepithelial localization of the inflammatory cell infiltrate in another case (100×). I, Prominent extravasation of erythrocytes and stromal mononuclear cell infiltrates (100×). (Reprinted from Conces MR, Williamson SR, Montironi R, et al. Urethral caruncle: clinicopathologic features of 41 cases. *Hum Pathol.* 2012;43:1400-1404, Copyright 2012, with permission from Elsevier.)

includes malignancy. Conversely, unexpected malignancy is identified in some cases resembling caruncle clinically. We examined clinical and histopathologic characteristics in 41 patients. Medical records were assessed for presentation, clinical diagnosis, associated urothelial carcinoma, radiation treatment, tobacco use, immunologic/urologic disorder, and treatment strategy/outcome. Average patient age was 68 years (range, 28-87 years). Presenting symptoms were pain (37%), hematuria (27%), and dysuria (20%), in contrast to asymptomatic (32%). Clinical diagnosis favored malignancy in 10% of cases. Concurrent or subsequent urothelial carcinoma was present for 5 patients (12%), although none developed urethral carcinoma. Histologic features included mixed hyperplastic urothelial and squamous lining, overlying a variably fibrotic, edematous, inflamed, and vascular stroma. Invaginations of urothelium extending into the stroma were common (68%), showing rounded nests with cystic or glandular luminal spaces, similar to urethritis cystica/glandularis, without intestinal metaplasia. Two lesions included an organizing thrombus, 1 with intravascular papillary

TABLE 1.—Summary of Clinical Findings in 41 Cases of Urethral Caruncles

Total number of cases	41
Age (y), mean	68
Location at urethral meatus	
Posterior	18 (44%)
Anterior	6 (15%)
Distal urethra, not specified	17 (41%)
Symptoms	
Pain	15 (37%)
Hematuria	11 (27%)
Dysuria	8 (20%)
Asymptomatic	13 (32%)
Clinical diagnosis	
Urethral caruncle	18 (44%)
Urethral polyp	7 (17%)
Urethral prolapse	6 (15%)
Periurethral gland abscess	5 (12%)
Urethral carcinoma	3 (7%)
Diagnosis of urothelial carcinoma[a]	5 (12%)
Prior exposure to radiation	4 (10%)
Positive history of tobacco use	15 (37%)
Autoimmune disease	2 (5%)

[a]Urothelial carcinoma was present concurrently or subsequent to the diagnosis of the urethral caruncle and was not present in the urethra.

endothelial hyperplasia. Twenty patients were treated with topical medications without resolution. Three lesions recurred (7%) after excision. A subset of patients had history of smoking or previous pelvic irradiation. Urethral caruncle is an uncommon lesion that may clinically mimic benign and malignant conditions. Awareness of the spectrum of clinical and histologic differential diagnoses is important in dealing with this unusual disease (Fig 1, Table 1).

▶ This article deals with the urethral caruncle, which is a benign polypoid mass of the urethral meatus primarily in postmenopausal women. Although a conclusive association with malignancy, urologic disorder, or systemic disease has not been established, often the lesion carries a challenging clinical differential diagnosis that includes malignancy. Conversely, unexpected malignancy is identified in some cases resembling caruncle clinically. The authors have examined clinico-histological features of this lesion (Fig 1, Table 1). This article represents 1 of the largest series of urethral carbuncle. This article also highlights the differential diagnosis of urethral or periurethral masses along with clinicopathological features. For additional reading, please see reference list.[1]

S. A. Chandrakanth, MD, FRCPC

Reference

1. Palmer JK, Emmett JL, McDonald JR. Urethral caruncle. *Surg Gynecol Obstet.* 1948;87:611-620.

Invasive Low-Grade Papillary Urothelial Carcinoma: A Clinicopathologic Analysis of 41 Cases

Toll AD, Epstein JI (The Johns Hopkins Hosp, Baltimore, MD)
Am J Surg Pathol 36:1081-1086, 2012

Typically in invasive papillary urothelial carcinoma both the overlying papillary and the invasive components are high grade. We describe a series of patients with invasive low-grade papillary urothelial carcinoma (LPUC) in which both the noninvasive and invasive components are low grade. A retrospective search from The Johns Hopkins Surgical Pathology

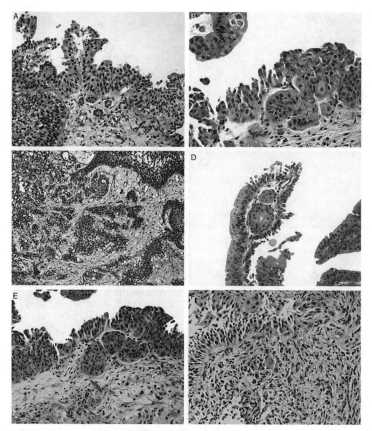

FIGURE 1.—A, Invasive LPUC with surface low-grade papillary carcinoma and underlying small nests with retraction artifact invading the superficial lamina propria. Rounded nest of UC invading the papillary stalk. B, Microinvasive low-grade UC. Note the low-grade papillary carcinoma component (upper left). C, Invasive low-grade UC with myxoid stroma (left) infiltrating the base of a papillary lesion (upper right). D, Small nests of invasive carcinoma within the stalk of the papillary frond of low-grade carcinoma. E, Small rounded nests of invasive carcinoma with moderate atypia and retraction artifact in the superficial lamina propria. F, Single cell invasion at the base of an LPUC. Note the retraction artifact and the stromal inflammatory reaction associated with invasive tumor. (Reprinted from Toll AD, Epstein JI. Invasive low-grade papillary urothelial carcinoma: a clinicopathologic analysis of 41 cases. *Am J Surg Pathol.* 2012;36:1081-1086, with permission from Lippincott Williams & Wilkins.)

TABLE 1.—Invasive Carcinoma

Architecture	
Nested	32/41 (78%)
Small, smooth contours	26/32
Small, irregular contours	5/32
Large, irregular contours	1/32
Non-nested	8/41 (18%)
Small nests and single cells	5/8
Small nests, cords, and sheets	2/8
Single cells	1/8
Microinvasive (< 1 HPF)	18/41 (44%)
Invasion into stalk	8/41 (20%)
Invasion extending from base	33/41 (80%)
Concurrent lesions	11/41 (27%)
Noninvasive LPUC	9/11
Invasive LPUC	1/11
Urothelial dysplasia	1/11
Cytology	
Moderate atypia	38/41 (93%)
Mild atypia	3/41 (7%)
Rare mitoses	8/41 (20%)
No mitoses	33/41 (80%)
Prominent nucleoli	8/41 (20%)
Focal nucleoli	14/41 (34%)
No nucleoli	19/41 (46%)
Paradoxical differentiation	7/41 (17%)

TABLE 3.—Recurrent Tumors

Patient	Age	Sex	Recurrence [Time Interval (mo)]
1	76	Male	Noninvasive bladder HGUC (50)
2	65	Female	T1 bladder HGUC (10)
3	73	Male	T1 bladder HGUC (96)
4	74	Female	T3N2 bladder HGUC (19)
5	60	Male	T2N0 bladder HGUC (9)
6	47	Male	T3N1 bladder HGUC (2)
7	61	Male	T1 bladder LPUC (6), noninvasive ureter LPUC (11)
8	71	Female	Noninvasive ureter LPUC (3)
9	78	Male	Noninvasive bladder LPUC (16 and 23)
10	64	Male	Noninvasive bladder LPUC (59 and 73)

HGUC indicates high-grade UC.

Database and consult cases from one of the author's files from 1998 to 2011 found 54 cases of invasive LPUC, excluding the more common, unique, and already well-characterized nested variant of urothelial carcinoma. Slides were available for 41 cases and formed the basis of the current study. The mean patient age was 68.4 years, with a male predominance. The specimens consisted of 37 bladder biopsies, 1 renal pelvis biopsy, 1 cystoprostatectomy specimen, 1 nephrectomy specimen, and 1 nephroureterectomy specimen. In all cases, invasion was limited to the superficial lamina propria above the muscularis mucosae. None of the histologic features correlated with tumor recurrence. Follow-up information was available for 73% of cases, with an average time interval of 49 months. Recurrent tumor was identified in 10/29 (34%) cases; however, 34% of cases without recurrence had limited follow-up (< 24 mo). Three patients showed progression in tumor grade, and 3 additional patients progressed in both grade and stage (60% stage/grade progression). Four patients developed recurrence with ureteral noninvasive LPUC (2 in the bladder and 2 in the ureter). All are alive without disease. As this lesion is being increasingly recognized, larger studies are needed to determine whether invasion arising in LPUC is a significant risk factor for future disease (Fig 1, Tables 1 and 3).

▶ Usually in invasive papillary urothelial carcinoma, both the overlying papillary and the invasive components are high grade. Here the authors describe a series of patients with invasive low-grade papillary urothelial carcinoma (LPUC) in which both the noninvasive and invasive components are low grade (Fig 1). Although rarely fatal, noninvasive LPUC recurs commonly, and in a smaller percentage of cases it progresses to higher grade/stage. Prior work on noninvasive LPUC found recurrence in approximately 35% to 50% of cases and grade progression in 18% of cases.

The results of this study on invasive LPUC suggest a rate of recurrence and progression (both grade and stage) (Table 3) at least similar to that of previous work examining noninvasive LPUC. This study also has limitations, which included the retrospective nature of the study, a lack of follow-up on all patients, and a lack of uniform follow-up and treatment. Overall, this is a good study. For further reading, see reference list.[1]

S. A. Chandrakanth, MD, FRCPC

Reference

1. Amin MB, Gomez JA, Young RH. Urothelial transitional cell carcinoma with endophytic growth patterns: a discussion of patterns of invasion and problems associated with assessment of invasion in 18 cases. *Am J Surg Pathol.* 1997;21:1057-1068.

Frozen section assessment in testicular and paratesticular lesions suspicious for malignancy: its role in preventing unnecessary orchiectomy
Subik MK, Gordetsky J, Yao JL, et al (Univ of Rochester Med Ctr, NY)
Hum Pathol 43:1514-1519, 2012

To investigate the role of frozen section assessment in sparing unnecessary orchiectomy for suspected lesions, we retrospectively reviewed intraoperative testicular and paratesticular frozen section assessments performed at our institution between the years 1993 and 2010. Frozen section assessments were performed on 45 testicular lesions (age, 5-60 [mean, 32.2] years; lesion size, 0.5-9.7 [mean, 2.1] cm) and 20 paratesticular lesions (age, 26-76 [mean, 43.5] years; lesion size, 0.4-11.0 [mean, 2.8] cm) before the decision to complete radical orchiectomy. Benign/malignant frozen section assessment diagnoses were reported in 26/19 testicular cases and 17/3 paratesticular

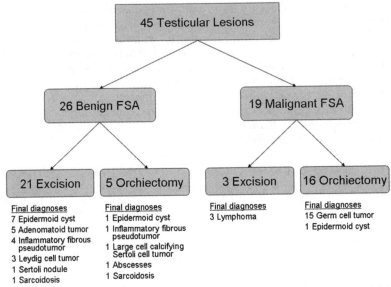

FIGURE 1.—Flow diagram for FSAs in 45 patients with testicular lesions. (Reprinted from Subik MK, Gordetsky J, Yao JL, et al. Frozen section assessment in testicular and paratesticular lesions suspicious for malignancy: its role in preventing unnecessary orchiectomy. *Hum Pathol*. 2012;43:1514-1519, Copyright 2012, with permission from Elsevier.)

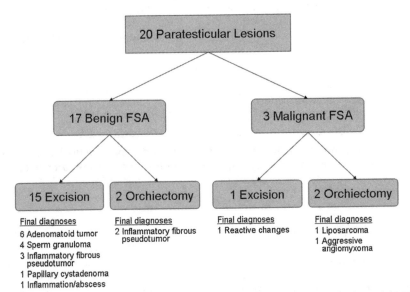

FIGURE 2.—Flow diagram for FSAs in 20 patients with paratesticular lesions. (Reprinted from Subik MK, Gordetsky J, Yao JL, et al. Frozen section assessment in testicular and paratesticular lesions suspicious for malignancy: its role in preventing unnecessary orchiectomy. *Hum Pathol*. 2012;43:1514-1519, Copyright 2012, with permission from Elsevier.)

TABLE 1.—Summary of the Patients Undergoing Potentially Unnecessary Orchiectomy

Age (y)	Lesion (Size)	Frozen Section Diagnosis	Permanent Diagnosis	Reason for Orchiectomy
16	T (1.8 cm)	Suspicious for epidermoid cyst	Epidermoid cyst	Possibility of teratoma
18	T (1.1 cm)	Most consistent with large cell calcifying Sertoli cell tumor	Large cell calcifying Sertoli cell tumor	Clinical suspicion for malignancy
37	T (NA)	Fibrosis, chronic inflammation	Inflammatory fibrous pseudotumor	Questionable testicular viability + severe chronic pain
47	T (NA)	Abscesses	Abscesses	Unknown
28	T (NA)	Fibrous tissue	Sarcoidosis	Clinical suspicion for malignancy
19	T (1.1 cm)	Consistent with mature teratoma	Epidermoid cyst	Frozen section diagnosis of teratoma
50	P (3.6 cm)	Dense fibrosis	Inflammatory fibrous pseudotumor	Questionable testicular function
69	P (2.0 cm)	Dense fibrosis, lymphocytic proliferation	Inflammatory fibrous pseudotumor	Possibility of lymphoproliferative malignancy

Abbreviations: T, testicular lesion; P, paratesticular lesion; NA, not available.

cases, respectively. Of the 26 benign testicular frozen section assessments, 5 cases resulted in orchiectomy, where permanent diagnoses included epidermoid cyst, large cell calcifying Sertoli cell tumor, fibrous pseudotumor, abscesses, and sarcoidosis, caused by a concern for potential malignancy or questionable viability of the testicles. Of the 19 malignant testicular frozen section assessments, orchiectomy was performed in 16 cases with germ cell tumor, but not in the remaining 3 cases with lymphoma. Of the 17 benign paratesticular frozen section assessments, 2 cases, both fibrous pseudotumors, resulted in orchiectomy. There were statistically significant differences in the size of the testicular ($P < .001$) or paratesticular ($P < .001$) lesions between benign and malignant frozen section assessments. Thus, in 36 (83.7%) of 43 cases with benign frozen section assessments, in addition to all 3 cases of lymphoma, orchiectomy was successfully avoided. These results suggest that frozen section assessment is useful for permitting testicular preservation, especially in men with small, nonpalpable, incidentally found masses as well as other benign lesions where a clinical diagnosis of malignancy is in doubt (Figs 1 and 2, Table 1).

▶ This is a good article highlighting the role of frozen section diagnosis of testicular and paratesticular lesions. It also spares the radical surgery for benign lesions, as the authors noted (Figs 1 and 2, Table 1). This study cited several cases in which radical surgery was done for benign diseases for which surgery could have been avoided if frozen section was carried out. The authors also highlight the usefulness of frozen section assessment particularly in assessing small, non-palpable, incidentally found masses in which there is a much higher likelihood of a benign diagnosis as well as other lesions in which a clinical diagnosis is in doubtful. For further reading, see reference list.[1]

S. A. Chandrakanth, MD, FRCPC

Reference

1. Elert A, Olbert P, Hegele A, Barth P, Hofmann R, Heidenreich A. Accuracy of frozen section examination of testicular tumors of uncertain origin. *Eur Urol.* 2002;41:290-293.

Distribution and characterization of subtypes of penile intraepithelial neoplasia and their association with invasive carcinomas: a pathological study of 139 lesions in 121 patients
Chaux A, Velazquez EF, Amin A, et al (Instituto de Patología e Investigación, Asunción, Paraguay; Caris Life Sciences, Newton, MA; Johns Hopkins Univ School of Medicine, Baltimore, MD; et al)
Hum Pathol 43:1020-1027, 2012

We are presenting the morphological features of 121 cases of atypical penile intraepithelial lesions. The term *penile intraepithelial neoplasia* (PeIN) was used to encompass all of them, and lesions were classified into

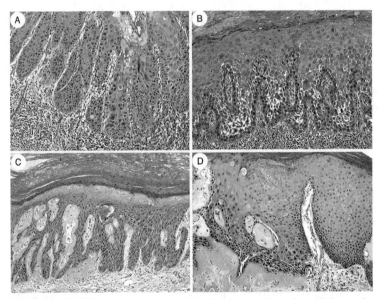

FIGURE 1.—PeIN, differentiated type. A, Atypia is observed throughout the epithelium and is more prominent at the bottom layers; areas of microinvasion cannot be ruled out (right field). B, Differentiated PeIN with acantholysis at the parabasal layers. C, Differentiated PeIN with prominent parakeratosis and lichen sclerosus. D, Squamous hyperplasia (right field) merging with differentiated PeIN (left field); note the association of differentiated PeIN with lichen sclerosus. (Reprinted from Chaux A, Velazquez EF, Amin A, et al. Distribution and characterization of subtypes of penile intraepithelial neoplasia and their association with invasive carcinomas: a pathological study of 139 lesions in 121 patients. *Hum Pathol.* 2012;43:1020-1027, Copyright 2012, with permission from Elsevier.)

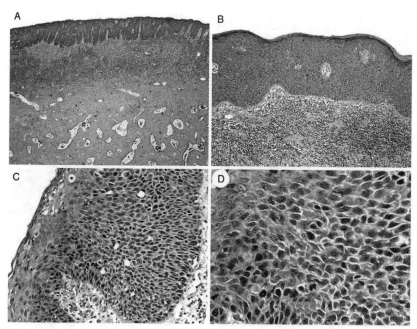

FIGURE 2.—PeIN, basaloid subtype. A, Low-power view of a basaloid PeIN showing a flat, hyperkeratotic surface, irregular rete ridges, and underlying chronic inflammation. B, Basaloid PeIN with the epithelium replaced by a monotonous population of cells with scant cytoplasm, giving an amphophilic/basophilic appearance to the lesion; note the slight hypergranulosis/hyperkeratosis and the chronic inflammatory response in the stroma. C, Basaloid PeIN with occasional koilocytic-like clear cells in the upper layers of the epithelium; however, surface is flat, allowing the distinction between this subtype and warty-basaloid PeIN. D, High-power view of a basaloid PeIN showing the cytologic features of the lesion: tumor cells with scant, basophilic cytoplasm, evident atypia, and high mitotic rate. (Reprinted from Chaux A, Velazquez EF, Amin A, et al. Distribution and characterization of subtypes of penile intraepithelial neoplasia and their association with invasive carcinomas: a pathological study of 139 lesions in 121 patients. *Hum Pathol.* 2012;43:1020-1027, Copyright 2012, with permission from Elsevier.)

2 major groups, differentiated and undifferentiated. The latter was further divided in warty, basaloid, and warty-basaloid subtypes. Ninety-five cases were associated with invasive squamous cell carcinomas. Differentiated lesions predominated (68%), followed by warty-basaloid (14%), basaloid (11%), and warty (7%) subtypes. Multifocality was found in 15% of the cases. Differentiated lesions were preferentially located in foreskin, whereas warty and/or basaloid subtypes were more prevalent in the glans. The former lesions were preferentially seen in association with keratinizing variants of squamous carcinoma, whereas the latter subtypes were found mostly in conjunction with invasive warty, basaloid, and warty-basaloid carcinomas. Lichen sclerosus was present in 51% of cases of differentiated lesions and absent in warty and/or basaloid subtypes. In summary, PeIN can be classified into 4 distinctive morphological subtypes. The proper pathological characterization of these lesions may provide important clues to

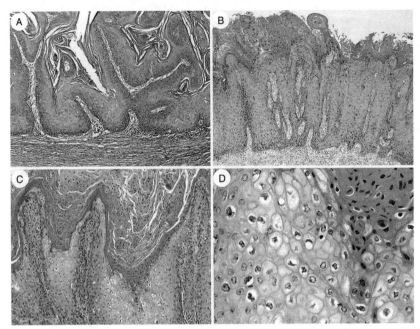

FIGURE 3.—PeIN, warty subtype. A, Warty PeIN with papillomatosis, conspicuous fibrovascular cores and parakeratosis. B and C, Warty PeIN showing prominent parakeratosis and a spiky surface; note also the presence of koilocytes in the upper layers of the epithelium. D, Warty PeIN at medium-power view with abundant koilocytes and atypical parakeratosis. (Reprinted from Chaux A, Velazquez EF, Amin A, et al. Distribution and characterization of subtypes of penile intraepithelial neoplasia and their association with invasive carcinomas: a pathological study of 139 lesions in 121 patients. *Hum Pathol.* 2012;43:1020-1027, Copyright 2012, with permission from Elsevier.)

the understanding of the pathogenesis and natural history of penile cancer (Figs 1-4, Table 2).

▶ This is a very interesting article regarding penile neoplasia. The authors have classified penile neoplasia into 2 major groups, differentiated and undifferentiated. The latter was further divided into warty (Fig 3), basaloid (Fig 2), and warty-basaloid (Fig 4) subtypes. Among 121 cases, 95 were associated with invasive squamous cell carcinomas. Differentiated lesions predominated (68%), followed by warty-basaloid (14%), basaloid (11%), and warty (7%) subtypes. Multifocality was found in 15% of the cases. Differentiated lesions were preferentially located in foreskin (Table 2), whereas warty and/or basaloid subtypes were more prevalent in the glans. The former lesions were preferentially seen in association with keratinizing variants of squamous carcinoma, whereas the latter subtypes were found mostly in conjunction with invasive warty, basaloid, and warty-basaloid carcinomas. Lichen sclerosus was present in 51% of cases of differentiated lesions and absent in warty and/or basaloid subtypes. In summary, penile intraepithelial neoplasia can be classified into 4 distinctive morphological subtypes. The proper pathological characterization of these lesions may provide

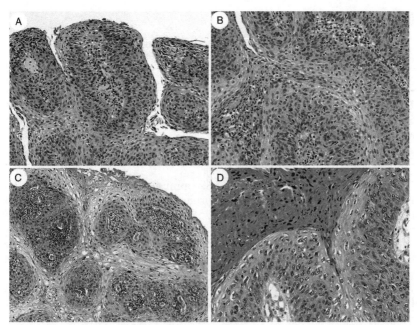

FIGURE 4.—PeIN, warty-basaloid subtype. A, Warty-basaloid PeIN showing a papillomatous surface with evident fibrovascular cores. B and C, Papillae in warty PeIN are lined by basaloid-type cells in the bottom layers and clear, koilocytic-type cells in the surface; note also the conspicuous fibrovascular cores and the parakeratosis at the surface. D, Warty-basaloid PeIN exhibiting prominent parakeratosis; note the fibrovascular cores and the presence of atypical cells in the parakeratotic layer. (Reprinted from Chaux A, Velazquez EF, Amin A, et al. Distribution and characterization of subtypes of penile intraepithelial neoplasia and their association with invasive carcinomas: a pathological study of 139 lesions in 121 patients. *Hum Pathol.* 2012;43:1020-1027, Copyright 2012, with permission from Elsevier.)

TABLE 2.—Subtypes of PeIN by Anatomical Site and Association with Invasive Squamous Cell Carcinoma

	No. Cases (%)[a]	
	Glans	Foreskin
PeIN alone (n = 24)		
Differentiated PeIN	1 (17)	14 (78)
PeIN with warty and/or basaloid features	5 (83)	4 (22)
PeIN plus SCC (n = 44)		
Differentiated PeIN	16 (57)	9 (56)
PeIN with warty and/or basaloid features	12 (43)	7 (44)

[a]Cases with only 1 anatomical compartment involved (n = 68).

important clues to the understanding of the pathogenesis and natural history of penile cancers (Fig 1). For further reading, see reference list.[1]

S. A. Chandrakanth, MD, FRCPC

Reference

1. Cubilla AL, Meijer CJ, Young RH. Morphological features of epithelial abnormalities and precancerous lesions of the penis. *Scand J Urol Nephrol Suppl.* 2000; (205):215-219.

The prognostic value of Ki-67 expression in penile squamous cell carcinoma
Stankiewicz E, Ng M, Cuzick J, et al (Barts Cancer Inst, London, UK; Queen Mary Univ of London, UK; et al)
J Clin Pathol 65:534-537, 2012

Aims.—To determine whether Ki-67 immunoexpression in penile squamous cell carcinoma (PSCC) has a prognostic value and correlates with lymph node metastasis, human papillomavirus (HPV) infection and patient survival.

Methods.—148 formalin-fixed paraffin-embedded PSCC samples were tissue-microarrayed, including 97 usual-type SCCs, 17 basaloid, 15 pure verrucous carcinomas, 2 warty and 17 mixed-type tumours. All samples were immunostained for Ki-67 protein. HPV DNA was detected with INNO-LiPA assay. Follow-up data were available for 134 patients.

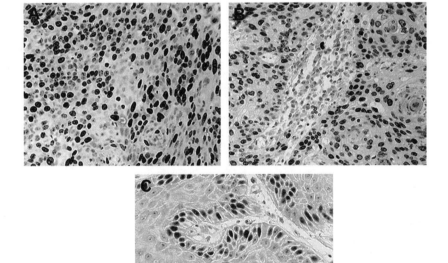

FIGURE 1.—Pattern of Ki-67-positive immunoexpression in subtypes of penile squamous cell carcinoma (PSCC). (A) Basaloid PSCC. (B) Usual type PSCC. (C) Verrucous PSCC. Magnification ×200. (Reprinted from Stankiewicz E, Ng M, Cuzick J, et al. The prognostic value of Ki-67 expression in penile squamous cell carcinoma. *J Clin Pathol.* 2012;65:534-537, with permission from the BMJ Publishing Group Ltd.)

TABLE 1.—Ki-67 Immunoexpression in Different Subtypes of Penile Squamous Cell Carcinoma (PSCC)

PSCC Type	Ki-67 Positive (%)	Mean	Median
All PSCC	57/148 (38.5)	42.2	40
Usual type	38/97 (39.2)	43.6	40
Basaloid	16/17 (94.1)	74.7	70
Verrucous	0/15 (0)	19.3	20

Cut-off >40%.

TABLE 2.—Correlation of Ki-67 immunoexpression with high-risk human papillomavirus (HPV) infection (p<0.0001)

	High-risk HPV Positive	High-risk HPV Negative	Total
Ki-67 positive	31	8	39
Ki-67 negative	20	42	62
Total	51	50	101

Results.—Ki-67 was strongly expressed in 57/148 (38.5%) of PSCCs. Different cancer subtypes showed significant difference in Ki-67 expression ($p < 0.0001$) with highest positivity in basaloid, 16/17 (94%), followed by usual type, 38/97 (39%) and lack of Ki-67 positive cases within verrucous tumours, 0/15. Ki-67 positively correlated with high-risk HPV ($p < 0.0001$) and showed good specificity (84%) but low sensitivity (61%) for high-risk HPV detection. Ki-67 protein strongly positively correlated with tumour grade ($p < 0.0001$) but not with stage ($p = 0.2193$), or lymph node status ($p = 0.7366$). Ki-67 showed no prognostic value for cancer-specific survival (HR = 1.00, 95%, CI 0.99 to 1.02, $p = 0.54$) or overall survival (HR = 1.00, 95%, CI 0.99 to 1.02, $p = 0.45$). High tumour stage, lymph node metastasis, high tumour grade and age at diagnosis were all independent prognostic factors for cancer-specific survival and overall survival.

Conclusions.—Ki-67 is only a moderate surrogate marker for HPV infection in PSCC. It does not show prognostic value for cancer-specific survival and overall survival in PSCC (Fig 1, Tables 1 and 2).

▶ This is an interesting study to determine whether Ki-67 immunoexpression in penile squamous cell carcinoma (PSCC) has a prognostic value and correlates with lymph node metastasis, human papillomavirus (HPV) infection, and patient survival. The authors found that Ki-67 is only a moderate surrogate marker for HPV infection in PSCC. It does not show prognostic value for cancer-specific survival and overall survival in PSCC. The most important prognostic factor in PSCC is lymph node metastasis (LNM). The best treatment option for nodal metastasis is regional lymphadenectomy.

Several studies investigated the risk factors for nodal metastases with the most important being tumor grade and lymphovascular invasion. Further, they found a pattern of Ki-67 immunoexpression in subtypes of PSCC, basaloid PSCC, usual-type PSCC, and verrucous PSCC (Fig 1, Table 1). They also studied the correlation of Ki-67 immunoexpression with high-risk HPV infection (Table 2). This article concludes that high Ki-67 immunoexpression could be an indicator, but not a definitive predictor, of high-risk HPV infection in PSCC.

However, it does not correlate with LNM or show prognostic value for cancer-specific survival and overall survival in PSCC. Further studies on a larger cohort of LNM-positive PSCCs are needed to confirm prognostic usefulness of Ki-67. For additional reading, see reference list.[1-3]

S. A. Chandrakanth, MD, FRCPC

References

1. Narayana AS, Olney LE, Loening SA, Weimar GW, Culp DA. Carcinoma of the penis: analysis of 219 cases. *Cancer.* 1982;49:2185-2191.
2. Stankiewicz E, Kudahetti SC, Prowse DM, et al. HPV infection and immunochemical detection of cell-cycle markers in verrucous carcinoma of the penis. *Mod Pathol.* 2009;22:1160-1168.
3. Graafland NM, Lam W, Leijte JA, et al. Prognostic factors for occult inguinal lymph node involvement in penile carcinoma and assessment of the high-risk EAU subgroup: a two-institution analysis of 342 clinically node-negative patients. *Eur Urol.* 2010;58:742-747.

Frozen section assessment in testicular and paratesticular lesions suspicious for malignancy: its role in preventing unnecessary orchiectomy
Subik MK, Gordetsky J, Yao JL, et al (Univ of Rochester Med Ctr, NY)
Hum Pathol 43:1514-1519, 2012

To investigate the role of frozen section assessment in sparing unnecessary orchiectomy for suspected lesions, we retrospectively reviewed intraoperative testicular and paratesticular frozen section assessments performed at our institution between the years 1993 and 2010. Frozen section assessments were performed on 45 testicular lesions (age, 5-60 [mean, 32.2] years; lesion size, 0.5-9.7 [mean, 2.1] cm) and 20 paratesticular lesions (age, 26-76 [mean, 43.5] years; lesion size, 0.4-11.0 [mean, 2.8] cm) before the decision to complete radical orchiectomy. Benign/malignant frozen section assessment diagnoses were reported in 26/19 testicular cases and 17/3 paratesticular cases, respectively. Of the 26 benign testicular frozen section assessments, 5 cases resulted in orchiectomy, where permanent diagnoses included epidermoid cyst, large cell calcifying Sertoli cell tumor, fibrous pseudotumor, abscesses, and sarcoidosis, caused by a concern for potential malignancy or questionable viability of the testicles. Of the 19 malignant testicular frozen section assessments, orchiectomy was performed in 16 cases with germ cell tumor, but not in the remaining 3 cases with lymphoma. Of the 17 benign paratesticular frozen section assessments, 2 cases, both fibrous pseudotumors, resulted in orchiectomy. There were statistically significant differences in the size of the testicular ($P < .001$) or paratesticular ($P < .001$) lesions between benign and malignant frozen section assessments. Thus, in 36 (83.7%) of 43 cases with benign frozen section assessments, in addition to all 3 cases of lymphoma, orchiectomy was successfully avoided. These results suggest that frozen section assessment is useful for permitting testicular preservation, especially in men with small, nonpalpable, incidentally found masses as well as other benign lesions where a clinical diagnosis of malignancy is in doubt.

▶ Subik et al show the value of pathology communication in improving the quality of patient care through providing immediate information to guide surgical practice in testicular and paratesticular lesions. Fine-needle aspiration services also have been shown to be useful in preventing surgery for cases of malignant lymphoma of the testis. In some of these patients, the lesions are quite large and mimic a nonlymphomatous malignancy. With either an intra-operative consultation of a fine-needle aspiration, clinicians are provided with information that prevents unnecessary surgery. The data indicate that especially for small, nonpalpable lesions of the testes, tissue sampling prior to excision is the management of choice. For additional reading, please see reference list.[1,2]

S. S. Raab, MD

References

1. Steiner H, Höltl L, Maneschg C, et al. Frozen section analysis-guided organ-sparing approach in testicular tumors: technique, feasibility, and long-term results. *Urology.* 2003;62:508-513.
2. Leroy X, Rigot JM, Aubert S, Ballereau C, Gosselin B. Value of frozen section examination for the management of nonpalpable incidental testicular tumors. *Eur Urol.* 2003;44:458-460.

11 Kidney

Banff 2011 Meeting Report: New Concepts in Antibody-Mediated Rejection
Mengel M, as the Banff meeting report writing committee (Univ of Alberta, Edmonton, Canada; Cedars-Sinai Med Ctr, Los Angeles, CA; et al)
Am J Transplant 12:563-570, 2012

The 11th Banff meeting was held in Paris, France, from June 5 to 10, 2011, with a focus on refining diagnostic criteria for antibody-mediated rejection (ABMR). The major outcome was the acknowledgment of C4d-negative ABMR in kidney transplants. Diagnostic criteria for ABMR have also been revisited in other types of transplants. It was recognized that ABMR is associated with heterogeneous phenotypes even within the same type of transplant. This highlights the necessity of further refining the respective diagnostic criteria, and is of particular significance for the design of randomized clinical trials. A reliable phenotyping will allow for definition of robust end-points. To address this unmet need and to allow for an evidence-based refinement of the Banff classification, Banff Working Groups presented multicenter data regarding the reproducibility of features relevant to the diagnosis of ABMR. However, the consensus was that more data are necessary and further Banff Working Group activities were initiated. A new Banff working group was created to define diagnostic criteria for ABMR in kidneys independent of C4d. Results are expected to be presented at the 12th Banff meeting to be held in 2013 in Brazil. No change to the Banff classification occurred in 2011.

▶ Several topics were covered at the 2011 Banff Conference on Allograft Pathology that are worth brief discussion. Much of the focus was on antibody-mediated rejection (ABMR), and one of the major outcomes was the recognition of the ABMR in the absence of C4d deposition in peritubular capillaries, a current requirement for a diagnosis of ABMR in the Banff 2011 update. Despite the formal recognition of this entity, it was felt further data and study were required to develop diagnostic criteria for ABMR in the absence of C4d deposition. Some data were presented that showed an immunophenotype difference in the intimal arteritis (v lesions) seen in cases of cellular-mediated rejection and cases of ABMR. V lesions have universally been associated with cell-mediated rejection, but it seems they may be seen in ABMR as well. It was also recognized that the term *chronic antibody-mediated rejection* refers to the histologic changes, including double contour formation and multilayering in the peritubular capillaries, rather than the time course since transplant. Finally, it was discussed how complement inhibition alone does not prevent the development of chronic

ABMR rejection changes, suggesting that complement activation is not the whole story in ABMR. We can expect changes to the renal Banff classification after the 2013 meeting.

M. L. Smith, MD

The Pathology and Clinical Features of Early Recurrent Membranous Glomerulonephritis
Rodriguez EF, Cosio FG, Nasr SH, et al (Mayo Clinic, Rochester, MN)
Am J Transplant 12:1029-1038, 2012

We assessed the earliest manifestations of recurrent membranous glomerulonephritis (MGN) in renal allografts. Clinical, laboratory and pathologic data were reviewed in 21 patients at the initial biopsy within 4 months post-transplant with evidence of MGN and on follow-up biopsies, compared to a biopsy control group of eight transplants without recurrent MGN. The mean time of first biopsy with pathologic changes was 2.7 months. In each earliest biopsy, immunofluorescence (IF) showed granular glomerular basement membrane (GBM) staining for C4d, IgG, kappa and lambda. IF for C3 was negative or showed trace staining in 16/21. On each MGN biopsy positive by IF, 14/19 showed absence of deposits or rare tiny subepithelial deposits by electron microscopy (EM). At the earliest biopsy, the mean proteinuria was 1.1 g/day; 16 patients had <1 g/day proteinuria. Follow-up was available in all patients (mean 35 months posttransplant). A total of 13 patients developed >1 g/day proteinuria; 12 were treated with: rituximab (n = 8), ACEI and increased prednisone dose (n = 2), ACEI or ARB only (n = 2). All patients showed reduction in proteinuria after treatment. A total of 11/16 patients showed progression of disease by EM on follow-up biopsy. Recognition of early allograft biopsy features aids in diagnosis of recurrent MGN before patients develop significant proteinuria.

▶ This retrospective case control study attempts to define the early light microscopic, immunofluorescence, and electron microscopy findings in recurrent membranous nephropathy (MGN). The earliest finding is that of granular glomerular basement staining by immunofluorescence for immunoglobulins such as IgG, kappa, lambda, and C4d. In renal allograft specimens, many centers only perform immunofluorescence for C4d primarily for the evaluation of peritubular reactivity and evidence of antibody-mediated rejection. The findings in this study support a critical and detailed evaluation of the glomeruli by C4d immunofluorescence to evaluate for early recurrent and/or de novo MGN. The lack of significant C3 staining is interesting and suggests the possibility of a component of immune modulation in the recipient immune system. It should be noted that other immune complex—mediated glomerulopathies will also be positive for C4d and thus, the presence of granular C4d reactivity should trigger a full immunofluorescence panel. Finally, many centers have transitioned to the slightly less sensitive method of C4d by immunohistochemistry. It remains to be seen if cases of early recurrent MGN can be identified by immunohistochemistry for C4d.

M. L. Smith, MD

Predictors of Response to Targeted Therapy in Renal Cell Carcinoma

Eisengart LJ, MacVicar GR, Yang XJ (Northwestern Univ Feinberg School of Medicine, Chicago, IL; the Robert H. Lurie Comprehensive Cancer Ctr of Northwestern Univ, Chicago, IL)
Arch Pathol Lab Med 136:490-495, 2012

Context.—The prognosis for patients with metastatic renal cell carcinoma is poor, with an average 5-year survival of approximately 10%. Use of traditional cytokine therapy, specifically high-dose interleukin 2, is limited by significant toxicity. Better understanding of the molecular pathogenesis of renal cell carcinoma has led to the development of targeted therapies to inhibit specific cellular pathways leading to tumorigenesis. These drugs provide improved survival with a more favorable toxicity profile. There is ongoing investigation of markers that predict response of an individual patient to different targeted therapies.

Objective.—To explain the molecular basis for vascular endothelial growth factor inhibitor (antiangiogenic) and mammalian target of rapamycin inhibitor therapies for renal cell carcinoma, summarize the clinical trials demonstrating the effectiveness of these drugs, and describe the biomarkers shown to correlate with outcome in patients treated with targeted therapy.

Data Sources.—All included sources are from peer-reviewed journals in PubMed (US National Library of Medicine).

Conclusion.—Emerging evidence shows promise that biomarkers will be useful for predicting an individual patient's response to targeted therapy, leading to a more personalized approach to treating renal cell carcinoma.

▶ It is an exciting time to be involved in the study of neoplasms with the promise of targeted therapies slowly coming to fruition. Renal cell neoplasms are no exception to the increasing availability of different therapeutic approaches. This articles reviews some of the newer targeted therapies such as sunitinib, sorafenib, and bevacizumab aimed at the vascular endothelial growth factor pathway and temsirolimus and everolimus aimed at the mammalian target of rapamycin pathway. It becomes evident that basic pathology elements such as tumor type, grade, and other histologic elements, including degree of clear cell change, presence of sarcomatoid features, immunohistochemical expression, and rhabdoid morphology, still have discriminating power in multivariate analysis in the prediction of response to certain targeted therapies. Therefore, the pathologist is still very situated in the cross-hairs of the molecular revolution in cancer treatment. As such, the specialty must continue to work with and adopt emerging technologies, such as gene expression profiling, that may assist in more robust classification of renal neoplasms.

M. L. Smith, MD

Persistent or New Onset Microscopic Hematuria in Patients with Small Vessel Vasculitis in Remission: Findings on Renal Biopsy

Geetha D, Seo P, Ellis C, et al (Johns Hopkins Univ School of Medicine, Baltimore, MD)
J Rheumatol 39:1413-1417, 2012

Objective.—Hematuria is considered a sign of active renal disease in patients with small-vessel vasculitis. In patients who are in apparent clinical remission, presence of persistent or new-onset microscopic hematuria may reflect active vasculitis, damage, or other glomerular pathology.

Methods.—We identified 74 patients from the Johns Hopkins Renal Pathology database between 1995 and 2009 with the diagnosis of pauciimmune glomerulonephritis (GN). Among them we identified 9 who were in clinical remission and underwent a renal biopsy for evaluation of persistent or new-onset hematuria.

Results.—Nine patients with small-vessel vasculitis, 8 antineutrophil cytoplasmic antibody (ANCA)-positive and 1 ANCA-negative, underwent a renal biopsy at variable time periods after remission of vasculitis (6 to 164 months) for persistent microscopic hematuria (n = 6) or new-onset microscopic hematuria (n = 3). All patients were in apparent clinical remission at the time of renal biopsy. Of the 3 patients presenting with new-onset hematuria, 2 had crescentic IgA nephropathy and 1 had healed crescentic pauciimmune GN. Of the 6 patients with persistent hematuria, 2 had arteriosclerosis, 2 had focal segmental glomerulosclerosis, and 2 had global and segmental glomerulosclerosis and healed crescentic GN, and none had active vasculitis.

Conclusion.—Microscopic hematuria in patients with renal vasculitis otherwise in remission could represent chronic glomerular injury from prior episode of vasculitis or may represent new glomerular pathology. Renal biopsy should be considered in these patients to guide therapy.

▶ This is a retrospective, single-institution study that seeks to investigate the renal biopsy findings in patients with antineutrophil cytoplasmic antibody–associated vasculitis in remission. The primary controversy is whether isolated hematuria can be used as a marker of vasculitis activity in this group of patients and thus support increased immunosuppression,[1,2] stabilization or improvement of the serum creatinine, and resolution of hematuria-defined clinical remission. Major drawbacks to this study include the limited sample size and the sampling limitations inherent in a needle core biopsy study with negative (lack of findings of disease activity) results. Although the biopsies were all deemed "adequate," the number of glomeruli seen in each case was only given for the cases that showed disease activity. It must be remembered that screening for hematuria essentially evaluates all functioning nephrons for evidence of bleeding, whereas a biopsy only evaluates those examined microscopically. Further study with more patients in this clinical scenario is required to make a definitive judgment on the clinical importance of isolated hematuria in this patient population.

M. L. Smith, MD

References

1. Hauer HA, Bajema IM, Hagen EC, et al. Long-term renal injury in ANCA-associated vasculitis: an analysis of 31 patients with follow-up biopsies. *Nephrol Dial Transplant.* 2002;17:587-596.
2. Magrey MN, Villa-Forte A, Koening CL, Myles JL, Hoffman GS. Persistent hematuria after induction of remission in Wegener granulomatosis: a therapeutic dilemma. *Medicine.* 2009;88:315-321.

Immunotactoid glomerulopathy: clinicopathologic and proteomic study
Nasr SH, Fidler ME, Cornell LD, et al (Mayo Clinic, Rochester, MN; et al)
Nephrol Dial Transplant 27:4137-4146, 2012

Background.—Immunotactoid glomerulopathy (ITG) is a rare glomerular disease. Here, we report the largest clinicopathologic series of ITG and define its proteomic profile.

Methods.—The characteristics of 16 ITG patients who were identified from our pathology archives are provided between 1993 and 2011. We also performed laser microdissection and mass spectrometry (LMD/MS) in three cases.

Results.—Presentation included proteinuria (100%), nephrotic syndrome (69%), renal insufficiency (50%) and microhematuria (80%). Hypocomplementemia was present in 46% and a serum M-spike in 63%. Hematologic malignancy was present in 38%, including chronic lymphocytic leukemia in 19%, lymphoplasmacytic lymphoma in 13% and myeloma in 13%. The pattern of glomerular injury was membranoproliferative (56%), membranous (31%) or proliferative (13%) glomerulonephritis. The microtubular deposits were immunoglobulin light chain restricted in 69% and had a mean diameter of 31 nm (range 17–52). During an average of 48 months of follow-up for 12 patients, 50% had remission, 33% had persistent renal dysfunction and 17% progressed to end-stage renal disease. Proteomic analysis by LMD/MS revealed the presence of immunoglobulins, monotypic light chains, complement factors of the classical and terminal pathway and small amount of serum amyloid P-component.

Conclusions.—Hematologic malignancy, particularly lymphoma, is not uncommon in ITG. ITG appears to have a better prognosis than other paraprotein-related renal lesions, with a half of patients expected to recover kidney function with immunosuppressive therapy or chemotherapy. The proteomic profile of ITG is consistent with deposition of monotypic immunoglobulins and activation of the classical and terminal pathway of complement (Fig 5).

▶ This is the first study to report the mass spectrometry findings in cases of immunotactoid glomerulopathy (ITG), although it would have been more complete if mass spectrometry (MS) was performed on all samples. MS is becoming the gold standard for the identification of organized deposits in glomeruli and is widely used for amyloid typing. Not surprisingly, based on the immunofluorescence

Probability Legend:
- over 95%
- 80% to 94%
- 50% to 79%
- 20% to 49%
- 0% to 19%

CASES

	#	Identified Proteins	UNIPROT ID	Molecular Weight	#4	#8	#15
A	1	Ig gamma-1 chain C region	IGHG1_HUMAN	36 kDa	72	62	7
	2	Ig lambda-1 chain C regions	LAC1_HUMAN	11 kDa	18	23	2
	3	Ig alpha-1 chain C region	IGHA1_HUMAN	38 kDa			10
	4	Ig kappa chain C region	IGKC_HUMAN	12 kDa			9
	5	Ig gamma-3 chain C region	IGHG3_HUMAN	41 kDa	2	1	2
	6	Ig mu chain C region	IGHM_HUMAN	49 kDa			8
	7	Ig gamma-4 chain C region	IGHG4_HUMAN	36 kDa	4		
	8	Ig kappa chain V-III region SIE	KV302_HUMAN	12 kDa			4
	9	Ig heavy chain V-I region ND	HV104_HUMAN	16 kDa	1		
	10	Ig heavy chain V-I region HG3	HV102_HUMAN	13 kDa			2
	11	Ig heavy chain V-III region CAM	HV307_HUMAN	14 kDa			2
	12	Ig lambda-2 chain C regions	LAC2_HUMAN	11 kDa			2
	13	Ig lambda chain V-III region LOI	LV302_HUMAN	12 kDa			2
	14	Ig heavy chain V-III region KOL	HV311_HUMAN	14 kDa			1
B	1	Complement C1q subcomponent subunit A	C1QA_HUMAN	26 kDa	2		
	2	Complement C1q subcomponent subunit B	C1QB_HUMAN	27 kDa	3		
	3	Complement C1q subcomponent subunit C	C1QC_HUMAN	26 kDa	9	1	
	4	Complement C3	CO3_HUMAN	187 kDa	8	46	13
	5	Complement C4-A	CO4A_HUMAN	193 kDa	8	5	7
	6	Complement C5	CO5_HUMAN	188 kDa		10	2
	7	Complement component C6	CO6_HUMAN	105 kDa		7	
	8	Complement component C7	CO7_HUMAN	94 kDa		9	
	9	Complement component C8 alpha chain	CO8A_HUMAN	65 kDa		9	2
	10	Complement component C8 beta chain	CO8B_HUMAN	67 kDa		4	2
	11	Complement component C9	CO9_HUMAN	63 kDa		29	11
	12	Complement factor H	CFAH_HUMAN	139 kDa		4	8
	13	Complement factor H-related protein 1	FHR1_HUMAN	38 kDa	1	6	6
	14	Complement factor H-related protein 2	FHR2_HUMAN	31 kDa		2	
	15	Complement factor H-related protein 5	FHR5_HUMAN	64 kDa		2	
C	1	Apolipoprotein E	APOE_HUMAN	36 kDa	4	13	3
	2	Clusterin	CLUS_HUMAN	52 kDa		14	3
	3	Serum amyloid P-component	SAMP_HUMAN	25 kDa	4	5	8

FIGURE 5.—Mass spectrometry-based proteomic analysis of glomeruli in ITG. Immunoglobulin (A), complement-related (B), and amyloid-related (C) proteins identified in three cases (4, 8 and 15) are shown. The numbers reflect the number of peptide spectra identified for each protein. The probability score reflects predicted accuracy of protein identification. (Reprinted from Nasr SH, Fidler ME, Cornell LD, et al. Immunotactoid glomerulopathy: clinicopathologic and proteomic study. *Nephrol Dial Transplant.* 2012;27:4137-4146, by permission of Oxford University Press.)

finding in cases of ITG and association with hematologic diseases, MS confirmed the presence of immunoglobulin and complement-associated peptide spectra. What was surprising was the finding of amyloid-associated peptide spectra in all 3 cases analyzed (Fig 5C). Although there were lower values than those seen in amyloid, further MS-based studies are required to understand their significance, if any. The spectrum of glomerular light microscopic abnormalities suggests ITG, despite its rare frequency, should be included in the differential diagnosis of a variety of light microscopic situations, especially in the setting of a lymphoma clinical history. Finally, the outcome was better in this patient group when compared with fibrillary glomerulonephritis (FG). Debate continues as to whether ITG and FG represent a spectrum of the same disease or are distinct entities. Further studies similar to this one will be required.

M. L. Smith, MD

Association of Noninvasively Measured Renal Protein Biomarkers With Histologic Features of Lupus Nephritis

Brunner HI, Bennett MR, Mina R, et al (Cincinnati Children's Hosp Med Ctr and Univ of Cincinnati College of Medicine, OH; et al)
Arthritis Rheum 64:2687-2697, 2012

Objective.—To investigate the relationship of urinary biomarkers and established measures of renal function to histologic findings in lupus nephritis (LN), and to test whether certain combinations of the abovementioned laboratory measures are diagnostic for specific histologic features of LN.

Methods.—Urine samples from 76 patients were collected within 2 months of kidney biopsy and assayed for the urinary biomarkers lipocalin-like prostaglandin D synthase (L-PGDS), α_1-acid glycoprotein (AAG), transferrin (TF), ceruloplasmin (CP), neutrophil gelatinase–associated lipocalin (NGAL), and monocyte chemotactic protein 1

Histological features \ Biomarkers‡	NGAL	MCP1	CP	AAG	TF	L-PGDS	C3	C4	P/C-ratio	GFR	Serum creatinine
Mesangial proliferation		•	•	•	•						
Capillary proliferation		•	•		•						
Cellular crescents	•			•	•				•		
Fibrinoid necrosis			•								
Wire-loops										•	
BAI Score		•	•	•	•				•		
Fibrosis											•
Tubular atrophy					•						
BCI Score										•	•
Epimembranous deposits											
Class 5 lupus nephritis										•	

FIGURE 3.—Summary of significant changes in marker levels in relation to the presence versus absence of histologic features of lupus nephritis (LN). Blue dots represent changes seen in urine samples that were collected within 2 months of the kidney biopsy (n = 76); green dots represent additional significant differences observed in the analysis that included only urine samples collected prior to the kidney biopsy (n = 38). The novel urine biomarkers are differentially excreted in the presence of histologic features of LN activity but not in the presence of membranous changes or features of LN chronicity. The P:C ratio, GFR, and serum creatinine level do not allow for differentiation between active, chronic, or membranous changes of LN. Complement levels do not distinguish between any histologic features. BAI = biopsy activity index; BCI = biopsy chronicity index (see Fig 1 for other definitions). For interpretation of the references to color in this figure legend, the reader is referred to web version of this article. (Reprinted from Brunner HI, Bennett MR, Mina R, et al. Association of noninvasively measured renal protein biomarkers with histologic features of lupus nephritis. *Arthritis Rheum.* 2012;64:2687-2697, with permission from Arthritis & Rheumatism and John Wiley and Sons, www.interscience.wiley.com.)

TABLE 3.—Combinations of Markers Predicting Key Biopsy Features in LN*

Model Outcome Variable	Predictor Variables	Area Under the ROC Curve (95% CI)[†]	Sensitivity, %[‡]	Specificity, %
Biopsy activity index score ≥7	MCP-1, CP, AAG, P:C ratio	0.85 (0.69–1.0)	72	66
Biopsy chronicity index score ≥4	NGAL, GFR, MCP-1	0.83 (0.67–0.93)	73	67
Membranous LN (class V)	MCP-1, GFR, AAG, TF, C4	0.75 (0.62–0.86)	75	48

*LN = lupus nephritis; 95% CI = 95% confidence interval; MCP-1 = monocyte chemotactic protein 1; CP = ceruloplasmin; AAG = α_1-acid glycoprotein; P:C = protein-to-creatinine; NGAL = neutrophil gelatinase–associated lipocalin; GFR = glomerular filtration rate; TF = transferrin.
[†]The area under the receiver operating characteristic (ROC) curve ranges from 0 to 1.
[‡]Clinically relevant point on ROC, with sensitivity of ≥ 70%.

(MCP-1). Using nonparametric analyses, levels of urinary biomarkers and established markers of renal function were compared with histologic features seen in LN, i.e., mesangial expansion, capillary proliferation, crescent formation, necrosis, wire loops, fibrosis, tubular atrophy, and epimembranous deposits. The area under the receiver operating characteristic curve (AUC) was calculated to predict LN activity, chronicity, or membranous LN.

Results.—There was a differential increase in levels of urinary biomarkers that formed a pattern reflective of specific histologic features seen in active LN. The combination of MCP-1, AAG, and CP levels plus protein: creatinine ratio was excellent in predicting LN activity (AUC 0.85). NGAL together with creatinine clearance plus MCP-1 was an excellent diagnostic test for LN chronicity (AUC 0.83), and the combination of MCP-1, AAG, TF, and creatinine clearance plus C4 was a good diagnostic test for membranous LN (AUC 0.75).

Conclusion.—Specific urinary biomarkers are associated with specific tissue changes observed in conjunction with LN activity and chronicity. Especially in combination with select established markers of renal function, urinary biomarkers are well-suited for use in noninvasive measurement of LN activity, LN chronicity, and the presence of membranous LN (Fig 3, Table 3).

▶ Renal biopsy is costly to the health system, is an uncomfortable procedure to undergo, and is associated with a major complication rate of about 1%. Because of these limitations, the clinical decision for biopsy is cautiously made. Currently, renal biopsy is the primary factor in making treatment decisions in lupus nephritis. One limitation of biopsy is the inability to follow the resolution or progression of disease over time without the increased risk of subsequent biopsies. From a clinical perspective, noninvasive means of detecting renal pathology and following it over time would be a vast improvement. These data suggest that a series of different urine-based proteins in patients with lupus nephritis has the ability to predict renal pathology. How the various biomarkers correlate with histologic findings is given in Fig 3. Panels of biomarkers were developed to predict very specific histologic outcomes (activity index score ≥7, chronicity index score of ≥4, and membranous lupus nephritis). Although the areas under the curve are decent, sensitivity and specificity were limited (Table 3). There is still much work to be done on this topic. It is likely many other biomarkers will be needed for better discrimination. Furthermore, prospective trials on biomarker usefulness on disease monitoring and treatment response are needed. For now, renal biopsy will remain the gold standard.

M. L. Smith, MD

Membranoproliferative glomerulonephritis and C3 glomerulopathy: resolving the confusion

Sethi S, Nester CM, Smith RJH (Mayo Clinic, Rochester, MN; Carver College of Medicine, Iowa City, IA)
Kidney Int 81:434-441, 2012

Membranoproliferative glomerulonephritis (MPGN) denotes a general pattern of glomerular injury that is easily recognized by light microscopy. With additional studies, MPGN subgrouping is possible. For example, electron microscopy resolves differences in electron-dense deposition that are classically referred to as MPGN type I (MPGN I), MPGN II, and MPGN III, while immunofluorescence typically detects immunoglobulins in MPGN I and MPGN III but not in MPGN II. All three MPGN types stain positive for complement component 3 (C3). Subgrouping has led to unnecessary confusion, primarily because immunoglobulin-negative MPGN I and MPGN III are more common than once recognized. Together with MPGN II, which is now called dense deposit disease, immunoglobulin-negative, C3-positive glomerular diseases fall under the umbrella of C3 glomerulopathies (C3G). The evaluation of immunoglobulin-positive MPGN should focus on identifying the underlying trigger driving the chronic antigenemia or circulating immune complexes in order to begin disease-specific treatment. The evaluation of C3G, in contrast, should focus on the complement cascade, as dysregulation of the alternative pathway and terminal complement cascade underlies pathogenesis. Although there are no disease-specific treatments currently available for C3G, a better understanding of their pathogenesis would set the stage for the possible use of anti-complement drugs (Fig 1, Table 1).

▶ Although this retrospective review is primarily based on expert opinion, it is useful for the practicing pathologist in the understanding of C3 glomerulopathy (C3G) and its relationship to membranoproliferative glomerulonephritis (MPGN). Fig 1 shows how the traditional classification of MPGN, based primarily on the distribution of electron dense deposits within the glomerular basement membrane, compares with the updated classification based on the presence or absence of immunoglobulin deposition. As part B of the figure highlights, the

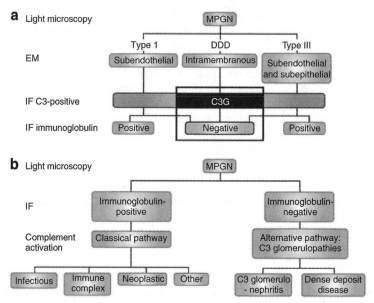

FIGURE 1.—The classification of membranoproliferative glomerulonephritis (MPGN) and C3 glomerulopathies (C3G) can overlap if based on electron microscopic findings. (a) MPGN-based and C3G-based
classifications of glomerular disease overlap, and are confusing because these two classifications are driven
by different starting points—findings on electron microscopy (EM) for MPGN and on immunofluorescence
(IF) for C3G. As a general rule, MPGN I and MPGN III are immune complex diseases characterized by sub-
endothelial or subendothelial/subepithelial densities resolved by EM; however, examples of
immunoglobulin-negative 'MPGN I' and 'MPGN III' have been recognized for decades. These types of
pathology fall under the umbrella of C3G and are often called C3 glomerulonephritis (C3GN). MPGN II
or dense deposit disease (DDD, the preferred name) is another type of C3G. (b) A simpler classification
is driven by findings on IF, and classifies MPGN as immunoglobulin-positive or -negative. The terms
MPGN I and MPGN III are not used, thereby avoiding unnecessary confusion. Immunoglobulin-positive
MPGN suggests classical pathway (CP) activation and a concerted effort should be made to identify the
underlying cause of antigenemia. Immunoglobulin-negative C3-positive MPGN is due to dysregulation
of the alternative pathway (AP) and terminal complement complex (TCC). Depending on the relative degree
of dysregulation, the EM picture can resemble DDD or C3GN. Non-MPGN C3 glomerulopathies are also
seen (see Table 2, light microscopy). (Reprinted with permission from Macmillan Publishers Ltd: Kidney
International. Sethi S, Nester CM, Smith RJH. Membranoproliferative glomerulonephritis and C3 glomerulopathy: resolving the confusion. *Kidney Int.* 2012;81:434-441, Copyright 2012.)

updated classification makes more sense from a pathophysiologic perspective.
MPGN disease with immunoglobulin deposition suggests the classical pathway
of complement activation, whereas the alternative pathway of complement activation likely drives immunoglobulin-negative cases. The extensive differential diagnosis provided in Table 1 should be considered when presented with a case of
immunoglobulin-associated MPGN. Segregating cases of MPGN in this way
has the potential to aid in selecting patients for trials of different anticomplement
therapeutics that may be developed.

M. L. Smith, MD

TABLE 1.—Immunoglobulin-Positive MPGN

Antigenic Stimulus	Associated Systemic Disease
Infectious	Viral: hepatitis B and C; HIV
	Bacterial: endocarditis; shunt nephritis; abscesses
	Protozoal: malaria; schistosomiasis
	Others: mycoplasma; mycobacterial
Autoimmune diseases	Systemic lupus erythematosus
	Scleroderma
	Sjögren's syndrome
	Mixed cryoglobulinemia
Monoclonal immunoglobulins and paraproteinemias	MGUS
	Leukemias
	Lymphomas
	Myeloma
Miscellaneous	Liver disease—hepatitis; cirrhosis
	Carcinoma
	Sarcoidosis
	Drugs
	'Idiopathic'

Abbreviations: MGUS, monoclonal gammopathy of undetermined significance; MPGN, membranoproliferative glomerulonephritis.

The Banff 2009 Working Proposal for Polyomavirus Nephropathy: A Critical Evaluation of Its Utility as a Determinant of Clinical Outcome

Masutani K, Shapiro R, Basu A, et al (Univ of Pittsburgh Med Ctr, PA)
Am J Transplant 12:907-918, 2012

Clinical outcome in BK virus nephropathy (BKVN) was examined in relation to clinical and histologic parameters with reference to the Banff Working Proposal 2009, which emphasizes tubular injury and viral load. Seventy one patients were evaluated in three eras: (i) Era-I: No BKV PCR performed (n = 36), (ii) Era-II: PCR performed for rising creatinine (n = 24) and (iii) Era III: PCR performed for routine screening (n = 11). Six of seventy-one (8.4%) patients were classified as Class A, 46/71 (64.8%) as Class B and 19/71 (26.8%) as Class C. Banff class A never occurred in Era-I. It is a heterogeneous class that includes biopsies with inflammation that have hitherto been included in Class B. Higher inflammation, but not tubular injury, nor histologic viral load correlated with worse creatinine at 3 months. On long-term follow-up, class C associated with graft loss (hazard ratio 2.45, $p = 0.03$). Clearance of viremia was associated with better graft survival at 5 years (46.0% vs. 25.0%). Viruria clearance was infrequent (15.6%). In conclusion, the clinical utility of the Banff Working Proposal 2009 derives from scoring of fibrosis and not extent of tubular injury or viral cytopathic effect. The proposal is not superior to existing schemas that include assessment of inflammation,

TABLE 1.—Salient Features of Histologic Grading Systems Applied to Study Patients

	Banff Working Proposal[1]	University of Maryland[3]	American Society of Transplantation[3]
Class A	Variable number of virus infected cells with no or minimal injury to tubular epithelial cells.	Variable number of virus infected cells with any degree of tubular injury but no or negligible inflammation	Virus infection and cytopathic effect in <25% of biopsy, with no/negligible inflammation specified to be <10% of tissue
Class B	Tubular epithelial cell necrosis or lysis with denudation of basement membrane across a length of more than 2 cells[2]	Variable number of virus infected cells with any degree of tubular injury and significant inflammation affecting less than 25% (pattern B1), 25–50% (pattern B2) or >50% (pattern B3) of the core biopsy	Essentially similar to University of Maryland, except that B1, B2, B3 are assigned progressively increasing degrees of cytopathic effect, atrophy and fibrosis
Class C	Any degree of tubular injury with interstitial fibrosis affecting >50% of cortex	Variable number of infected cells with any degree of tubular injury and tubular atrophy/fibrosis affecting >50% of core biopsy	Same as University of Maryland System

[1] The Banff Working Proposal was conceived during the 10th Banff Conference on Allograft Pathology in 2009 (10,11). This proposal describes Stages A, B and C to different evolutionary stages of the disease. To avoid confusion with other Banff Schemas where the term stage refers specifically to degrees of fibrosis, we suggest that the terms class A, B and C would be more appropriate. A detailed description of the Banff working proposal is available at: http://www.uncnephropathology.org/documents/BanffDraftforPolyomavirusNephropathyStaging.pdf

[2] A rather conspicuous feature of the Working Proposal is that the degree of inflammation is not taken into account in the staging of disease.

[3] The University of Maryland (8) and AST (4) schema are essentially identical, except that the AST schema specifically defines "no or negligible inflammation" in the Maryland system as inflammation affecting <10% of the sampled core. The Maryland system proposes a straight-forward sub-categorization of class B into categories B1 thru B3 based on percentage area affected by inflammation and atrophy. Sub-classification of class B in the AST schema assigns progressively increasing amounts of viral cytopathic effect to subclass B1, B2 and B3. However, this stipulation makes it difficult to apply the classification to many biopsies where inflammation and fibrosis are out of proportion to the degree of viral cytopathic effect.

which is a well-known prognostic marker in other renal allograft diseases (Table 1).

▶ At the 2009 Banff Conference on Allograft Pathology, the Banff Working Group proposed a new working classification for polyoma virus infection that places an emphasis on the histologic changes of acute tubular injury. The goal of the proposal was to be able to improve the ability to predict clinical outcomes. Table 1 highlights how the Banff Working Group proposal compares with 2 other existing histologic grading systems for polyoma virus infection. The primary difference is in class B in which the Banff proposal does not include a component of interstitial inflammation. It is worth noting that proactive screening of allograft recipients for BK virus polymerase chain reaction has had a significant impact on decreasing the progression of serum creatinine level increase at the 3-month mark (comparison of era 1 with era 3). These data support what most transplant nephrologists inherently know already: the degree of interstitial fibrosis and tubular atrophy is the primary predictor of graft outcome, regardless of the cause. A polyoma virus—specific grading system is not likely to gain widespread acceptance.

M. L. Smith, MD

Multilocular Cystic Renal Cell Carcinoma: Similarities and Differences in Immunoprofile Compared With Clear Cell Renal Cell Carcinoma
Williamson SR, Halat S, Eble JN, et al (Indiana Univ School of Medicine, Indianapolis; Ochsner Med Ctr, New Orleans, LA; et al)
Am J Surg Pathol 36:1425-1433, 2012

Multilocular cystic renal cell carcinoma (RCC) is an uncommon renal neoplasm composed of thin fibrous septa lining multiple cystic spaces and associated with an excellent prognosis. Clear cells with generally low-grade nuclear features line the cystic spaces and may be present within the fibrous septa, although solid mass-forming areas are by definition absent. Despite the excellent prognosis, molecular-genetic alterations are similar to those of clear cell RCC. Immunohistochemical staining characteristics, however, have not been well elucidated. We studied 24 cases of multilocular cystic RCC, classi-fied according to the 2004 World Health Organization System. Immunohis-tochemical analysis was performed using an automated immunostainer for CD10, cytokeratin 7 (CK7), α-methylacyl-CoA-racemase, epithelial membrane antigen (EMA), cytokeratin CAM 5.2, carbonic anhydrase IX (CA-IX), estrogen/progesterone receptors, smooth muscle actin, PAX-2, and vimentin. Twenty-four cases of grade 1 to 2 clear cell RCC were stained for comparison. Multilocular cystic RCC and control cases of clear cell RCC showed the following results, respectively: CD10 (63%, 96%), CK7 (92%, 38%), a-methylacyl-CoA-racemase (21%, 67%), vimentin (58%, 33%), estrogen receptor (8%, 8%), CAM 5.2 (100%, 96%), EMA, CAIX, PAX-2 (all 100%), and progesterone receptor (0%). Smooth muscle actin highlighted myofibroblastic cells within the septa of multilocular cystic

TABLE 1.—Summary of Immunohistochemical Staining Properties in Multilocular Cystic RCC and Clear Cell RCC

Antibody	Staining Characteristics	MLCRCC (N = 24) (%)	Clear Cell RCC (N = 24) (%)	Fisher Exact (P)
CD10	Negative	37	4	<0.05
	Focal	38	17	
	Diffuse	25	79	
CK7	Negative	8	62	<0.01
	Focal/patchy	29	38	
	Diffuse	63	0	
AMACR	Negative	79	33	NS
	Focal/weak	21	67	
	Diffuse	0	0	
EMA	Negative	0	0	NS
	Patchy	8	62	
	Diffuse	92	38	
CAM 5.2	Negative	0	4	NS
	Patchy	13	58	
	Diffuse	88	38	
CA-IX	Negative	0	0	NS
	Patchy	0	4	
	Diffuse	100	96	
PAX-2	Negative	0	8	NS
	Nuclear expression	100	92	
SMA	Negative in clear cells	100	100	NS
	Positive in clear cells	0	0	
Vimentin	Negative in clear cells	42	67	NS
	Positive in clear cells	58	33	
ER	Negative	92	92	NS
	Focal faint nuclear	8	8	
	Diffuse strong nuclear	0	0	
PR	Negative	100	100	NS
	Focal faint nuclear	0	0	
	Diffuse strong nuclear	0	0	

CAM 5.2 indicates cytokeratin CAM 5.2; MLCRCC, multilocular cystic RCC; NS, not significant; SMA, smooth muscle actin.

RCC and the fine capillary vascular network of clear cell RCC. In summary, multilocular cystic RCC showed expression of common clear cell RCC markers CA-IX, EMA, and PAX-2, supporting the hypothesis that multilocular cystic RCC is a subtype of clear cell RCC. In contrast to clear cell RCC, tumors less frequently expressed CD10 (63% and often focal vs. 96% and diffuse) and more frequently expressed CK7 (92%), often diffusely (63%). Coexpression of CA-IX and CK7 represents a point of overlap with the recently described clear cell papillary RCC, which also may show a prominent cystic architecture. However, the latter lacks mutation of the *VHL* gene and deletion of chromosome 3p by molecular methodologies (Table 1).

▶ This is a retrospective case-control study designed to compare the immunohistochemical expression between conventional clear cell renal cell carcinoma and multilocular cystic renal cell carcinoma. Table 1 shows the immunohistochemical expression comparison. Staining characteristics were qualitatively evaluated and defined as negative, focal (less than 75% tumor cells staining), and diffuse (greater than 75% tumor cells staining). Although there were statistically significant differences in expression of CD10 and CK7, the differences were not sufficient to suggest the possibility of using immunohistochemistry to distinguish between these 2 entities. Perhaps the most important finding is that careful hematoxylin and eosin examination remains the most robust way to make an accurate diagnosis of multilocular cystic renal cell carcinoma. The overlap of immunohistochemical expression supports the molecular findings suggesting multilocular cystic and clear cell renal cell carcinomas have similar origins. Although this is one of the largest studies to date, further characterization of the immunoprofile of multilocular cystic renal cell carcinoma is required.

M. L. Smith, MD

Clinicopathologic Correlations in Multiple Myeloma: A Case Series of 190 Patients With Kidney Biopsies

Nasr SH, Valeri AM, Sethi S, et al (Mayo Clinic, Rochester, MN; Columbia Univ, NY)
Am J Kidney Dis 59:786-794, 2012

Background.—Renal involvement is common in multiple myeloma. In this study, we examined kidney biopsy findings in patients with multiple myeloma and correlated them with their clinical renal and hematologic characteristics.

Study Design.—Case series.

Setting & Participants.—190 Mayo Clinic patients with multiple myeloma who underwent kidney biopsy between 1997-2011 were identified from our kidney biopsy database. Patients had an established diagnosis of multiple myeloma or multiple myeloma was diagnosed shortly after the results of kidney biopsy, which prompted bone marrow biopsy.

Predictors.—Myeloma cast nephropathy (MCN), AL amyloidosis, and monoclonal immunoglobulin deposition disease (MIDD).

Outcomes & Measurements.—Renal morphologic changes, clinical renal and hematologic characteristics at kidney biopsy, renal and patient outcomes.

Results.—Paraprotein-associated lesions were seen in 73% of patients; non−paraprotein-associated lesions, in 25%; and no pathology, in 2%. The most common paraprotein-associated lesions were MCN (33%), MIDD (22%), and amyloidosis (21%). The most common non−paraprotein-associated lesions were acute tubular necrosis (9%), hypertensive arteriosclerosis (6%), and diabetic nephropathy (5%). Patients with MIDD were younger than those with MCN or amyloidosis. Urine paraprotein size and bone marrow plasma cell percentage were higher in MCN than amyloidosis or MIDD. Nephrotic syndrome was more common in amyloidosis than MIDD. Percentage of albuminuria was highest in amyloidosis and lowest in MCN. Median kidney survival from kidney biopsy was 20, 30, and 51 months for MCN, amyloidosis, and MIDD, respectively ($P = 0.2$).

TABLE 1.—Kidney Biopsy Findings

Pathologic Diagnosis	No. of Patients (%)
Paraprotein-associated renal lesions	
Myeloma cast nephropathy	62 (33)
Monoclonal immunoglobulin deposition disease	41 (22)
Amyloidosis	40 (21)
Fibrillary glomerulonephritis	2 (1)
Immunotactoid glomerulopathy	1 (0.5)
Light chain proximal tubulopathy	1 (0.5)
Interstitial infiltration by malignant plasma cells	2 (1)
Non−paraprotein-associated renal lesions	
Glomerular	
Diabetic glomerulosclerosis	9 (5)
Focal segmental glomerulosclerosis	5 (3)
Postinfectious glomerulonephritis	3 (2)
Membranous glomerulopathy	2 (1)
Minimal change disease	2 (1)
Membranoproliferative glomerulonephritis	1 (0.5)
Anti−glomerular basement membrane disease	1 (0.5)
Thin basement membrane disease	1 (0.5)
Smoking-related glomerulopathy	1 (0.5)
Tubulointerstitial	
Acute tubular necrosis	17 (9)
Chronic tubulointerstitial nephritis/ nephropathy	3 (2)
Acute interstitial nephritis	1 (0.5)
Oxalate nephropathy	1 (0.5)
Nephrocalcinosis	1 (0.5)
Vascular	
Arterionephrosclerosis	12 (6)
Thrombotic microangiopathy	1 (0.5)
Normal biopsy	3 (2)

Median patient survival from multiple myeloma diagnosis was 44, 58, and 62 months for MCN, amyloidosis, and MIDD, respectively ($P = 0.4$).

Limitations.—Retrospective nature.

Conclusions.—The spectrum of renal lesions in multiple myeloma is more heterogeneous than previously reported. Clinical features favoring amyloidosis over MIDD include older age, absence of kidney failure, presence of nephrotic syndrome, absence of hematuria, and >50% albuminuria (Table 1).

▶ This study is the largest systematic review of renal biopsy findings in patients with multiple myeloma (MM). The breakdown of findings in kidney biopsies is shown in Table 1 and highlights an impressive spectrum of findings seen in biopsies from patients with MM. The authors note that only 1 case of light chain proximal tubulopathy was identified in this series; this is usually an early renal manifestation and typically seen in the setting of monoclonal gammopathy of undetermined significance, an entity not included in this cohort. Although it was reasonable to include patients whose diagnosis of MM was near the time of renal biopsy (time frame not given), it should be recognized that some patients with undiagnosed MM and a kidney biopsy that did not show paraprotein-associated disease on biopsy may have been missed. Therefore, if any, the bias would be toward there being an increased number of non-paraprotein-related renal disease. The clinical features favoring different paraprotein-related disease should be helpful in guiding our clinical colleagues, especially when a biopsy may be contraindicated, as the authors suggest.

M. L. Smith, MD

Histologic Tumor Necrosis Is an Independent Prognostic Indicator for Clear Cell and Papillary Renal Cell Carcinoma

Pichler M, Hutterer GC, Chromecki TF, et al (Med Univ of Graz, Austria)
Am J Clin Pathol 137:283-289, 2012

Histologic tumor necrosis (TN) has been reported to indicate a poor prognosis for different human cancers. In papillary renal cell carcinoma (RCC), data regarding the prognostic impact of TN are conflicting. We retrospectively studied the pathology records of 2,333 consecutive patients who underwent nephrectomy from 1984 to 2006 at a single tertiary academic center. In multivariate analyses regarding clear cell RCC, the presence of histologic TN was an independent negative prognostic factor for metastasis-free (hazard ratio [HR], 2.32; confidence interval [CI], 1.86-2.9; $P < .001$) and overall (HR, 1.52; CI, 1.31-1.76; $P < .001$) survival. Regarding papillary RCC, the presence of histologic TN represented an independent predictor of metastasis-free (HR, 5.22; CI, 2.2-12.5; $P < .001$) and overall (HR, 1.69; CI, 1.11-2.58; $P = .015$) survival. Our findings suggest that the presence of TN is an independent predictor of

---

TABLE 3.—Multivariate Analysis of Clinicopathologic Parameters for the Prediction of Metastasis-Free and Overall Survival in Patients With Papillary Renal Cell Carcinoma

Parameter	Metastasis-Free Survival		Overall Survival	
	HR (95% CI)	*P*	HR (95% CI)	*P*
Age at operation (y)		.79		.002
≤65	1 (reference)		1 (reference)	
>65	0.89 (0.4-1.99)		1.95 (1.27-3)	
Sex		.03		.06
Female	1 (reference)		1 (reference)	
Male	3 (1.12-8.2)		1.56 (0.97-2.53)	
T stage		<.001		.04
pT1-2	1 (reference)		1 (reference)	
pT3-4	9 (2.65-30)		1.59 (1.02-2.51)	
Tumor grade		.005		<.001
G1 + G2	1 (reference)		1 (reference)	
G3 + G4	3.68 (1.47-9.22)		3.28 (1.99-5.4)	
Presence of tumor necrosis		<.001		.015
No	1 (reference)		1 (reference)	
Yes	5.22 (2.17-12.54)		1.69 (1.11-2.58)	
Vascular invasion		.009		.004
Absent	1 (reference)		1 (reference)	
Present	2.92 (1.29-6.6)		1.99 (1.23-3.2)	

CI, confidence interval; HR, hazard ratio.

clinical outcome in clear cell and papillary RCC. Thus, histologic TN might be a reliable prognostic indicator and should, therefore, routinely be examined during pathologic analysis of RCC specimens (Table 3).

▶ This retrospective multivariate analysis of 1891 clear cell renal cell carcinomas and 248 papillary renal cell carcinomas found tumor necrosis to be an independent negative prognostic marker. Tumor necrosis was defined as the presence of coagulative necrosis identified microscopically with homogenous clusters and sheets of degenerating and dead tumor cells. The importance of tumor necrosis in papillary renal cell carcinoma is less established than in clear cell renal cell carcinoma.[1,2] The multivariate analysis for the cases of papillary renal cell carcinoma in this study is given in Table 3 and shows that, in addition to tumor necrosis, male sex, higher stage, higher grade, and vascular invasion are also prognostic predictors. One of the deficiencies of this article includes the retrospective nature of the review in which tumor necrosis was specifically being sought out. Furthermore, there was no analysis of the amount or percentage of necrosis present, a feature that has been suggested to be important for prognostic significance. Finally, although the authors state a minimum of 3 hematoxylin and eosin–stained slides of each tumor were reviewed, studies have shown a significant amount of histologic variability when all sections of a given renal cell carcinoma are reviewed. Larger multi-institutional studies are required for definitive characterization of the prognosis of tumor necrosis in papillary carcinoma of the kidney.

M. L. Smith, MD

References

1. Kim H, Cho NH, Kim DS, et al. Renal cell carcinoma in South Korea: a multicenter study. *Hum Pathol.* 2004;35:1556-1563.
2. Sengupta S, Lohse CM, Leibovich BC, et al. Histologic coagulative tumor necrosis as a prognostic indicator of renal cell carcinoma aggressiveness. *Cancer.* 2005;104: 511-520.

Chromophobe Renal Cell Carcinoma: The Impact of Tumor Grade on Outcome

Cheville JC, Lohse CM, Sukov WR, et al (Mayo Clinic, Rochester, MN)
Am J Surg Pathol 36:851-856, 2012

It has been reported that Fuhrman grading is not appropriate for chromophobe renal cell carcinoma (RCC). The objective of this study was to determine whether nucleolar grading and the recently described chromophobe RCC grading system by Paner and colleagues provide prognostic information. Pathologic features of 185 patients with chromophobe RCC treated surgically between 1970 and 2006 were reviewed, including nucleolar grade, chromophobe RCC grade, the 2010 TNM groupings, sarcomatoid differentiation, and coagulative tumor necrosis. Cancer-specific (CS) survival was estimated using the Kaplan-Meier method, and associations

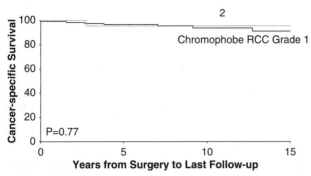

FIGURE 9.—Associations of chromophobe RCC grade with CS survival for 155 patients with TNM stage grouping I or II nonsarcomatoid chromophobe RCC. (Reprinted from Cheville JC, Lohse CM, Sukov WR, et al. Chromophobe renal cell carcinoma: the impact of tumor grade on outcome. *Am J Surg Pathol.* 2012;36:851-856, with permission from Lippincott Williams & Wilkins.)

with CS survival were evaluated using Cox proportional hazard regression models. Twenty-three patients died from RCC at a mean of 3.0 years after surgery (median 1.3; range 0 to 16) with estimated CS rates (95% confidence interval) of 89% (84 to 94), 86% (81 to 92), and 85% (78 to 91) at 5, 10, and 15 years after surgery. Univariate associations with CS survival included the 2010 TNM stage groupings, sarcomatoid differentiation, coagulative tumor necrosis, chromophobe RCC grade, and nucleolar grade (all $P < 0.001$). These last 4 features remained significantly associated with CS survival after adjusting for the 2010 TNM stage groupings. When the analysis was restricted to the 155 patients with nonsarcomatoid TNM stage groupings I and II chromophobe RCC, only stage grouping (I vs. II) was significantly associated with CS survival ($P = 0.03$). Although the chromophobe RCC grading system described by Paner and colleagues and nucleolar grade are associated with CS survival in chromophobe RCC, they add no additional prognostic information once TNM stage and sarcomatoid differentiation are assessed (Fig 9).

▶ There is currently no consensus on the appropriate grading of chromophobe renal cell carcinoma. Recent publications have indicated a novel chromophobe renal cell carcinoma grading system that remains an independent predictor of renal cell carcinoma—related death, metastasis, and recurrence.[1] Others have shown no association between chromophobe renal cell carcinoma grade and outcomes.[2] These prior 2 conflicting articles included over 300 patients combined. This article adds an additional 185 patients to the analysis and further supports the lack of predictive value of the chromophobe grade after excluding sarcomatoid histology and restricting to TNM stage grouping I and II (Fig 9). They also found the nucleolar grade, a modification of the Fuhrman grading system, also did not add predictive value. Urologists have also begun to publish studies about the potential usefulness of the chromophobe renal cell carcinoma grading system.[3] This article, in combination with the others, suggests there is no data-driven consensus yet and further multi-institutional studies are required before a decision can be made. In the era of evidence-based medicine, it may be reasonable to report both grading systems as additional data are accumulated and analyzed.

M. L. Smith, MD

References

1. Paner GP, Amin MB, Alvarado-Cabrero I, et al. A novel tumor grading scheme for chromophobe renal cell carcinoma: prognostic utility and comparison with Fuhrman nuclear grade. *Am J Surg Pathol.* 2010;34:1233-1240.
2. Przybycin CG, Cronin AM, Darvishian F, et al. Chromophobe renal cell carcinoma: a clinicopathologic study of 203 tumors in 200 patients with primary resection at a single institution. *Am J Surg Pathol.* 2011;35:962-970.
3. Finley DS, Shuch B, Said JW, et al. The chromophobe tumor grading system is the preferred grading scheme for chromophobe renal cell carcinoma. *J Urol.* 2011; 186:2168-2174.

12 Head and Neck

Associations Between Salivary Gland Histopathologic Diagnoses and Phenotypic Features of Sjögren's Syndrome Among 1,726 Registry Participants
Daniels TE, for the Sjögren's International Collaborative Clinical Alliance Research Groups (Univ of California, San Francisco; et al)
Arthritis Rheum 63:2021-2030, 2011

Objective.—To examine associations between labial salivary gland (LSG) histopathology and other phenotypic features of Sjögren's syndrome (SS).

Methods.—The database of the Sjögren's International Collaborative Clinical Alliance (SICCA), a registry of patients with symptoms of possible SS as well as those with obvious disease, was used for the present study. LSG biopsy specimens from SICCA participants were subjected to protocol-directed histopathologic assessments. Among the 1,726 LSG specimens exhibiting any pattern of sialadenitis, we compared biopsy diagnoses against concurrent salivary, ocular, and serologic features.

Results.—LSG specimens included 61% with focal lymphocytic sialadenitis (FLS; 69% of which had focus scores of ≥ 1 per 4 mm^2) and 37% with nonspecific or sclerosing chronic sialadenitis (NS/SCS). Focus scores of ≥ 1 were strongly associated with serum anti-SSA/ SSB positivity, rheumatoid

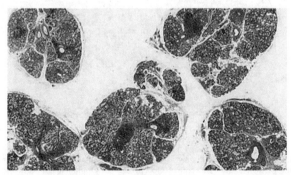

FIGURE 1.—Hematoxylin and eosin–stained labial salivary glands exhibiting focal lymphocytic sialadenitis. Approximately 10 focal lymphocytic infiltrates can be seen in this image. Under the microscope, there was a total glandular area of 24 mm^2, yielding a focus score of 2 foci per 4 mm^2. Original magnification × 2. (Reprinted from Daniels TE, for the Sjögren's International Collaborative Clinical Alliance Research Groups. Associations between salivary gland histopathologic diagnoses and phenotypic features of Sjögren's syndrome among 1,726 registry participants. *Arthritis Rheum.* 2011;63:2021-2030, with permission from Arthritis & Rheumatism and John Wiley and Sons.)

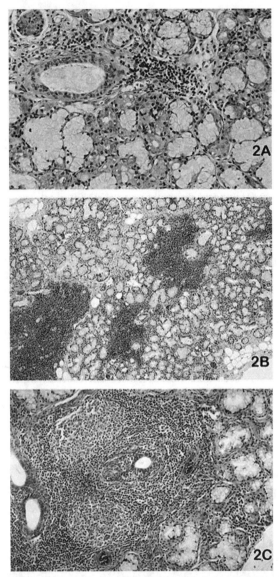

FIGURE 2.—Hematoxylin and eosin–stained labial salivary glands (LSGs) exhibiting focal lymphocytic sialadenitis (FLS). **A**, LSG with a small lymphocytic aggregate that is minimally sized (> 50 cells) for inclusion in a focus score calculation. Original magnification × 100. **B**, LSG with 4 variously sized lymphocytic foci. Note the normalappearing acini immediately adjacent to the lymphocyte aggregates, a characteristic feature of FLS. The entire specimen had a focus score of 3 foci per 4 mm^2. Original magnification × 16. **C**, LSG with 2 prominent lymphocytic germinal centers and ductal hyperplasia within a large lymphocytic focus. Original magnification × 40. (Reprinted from Daniels TE, for the Sjögren's International Collaborative Clinical Alliance Research Groups. Associations between salivary gland histopathologic diagnoses and phenotypic features of Sjögren's syndrome among 1,726 registry participants. *Arthritis Rheum.* 2011;63:2021-2030, with permission from Arthritis & Rheumatism and John Wiley and Sons.)

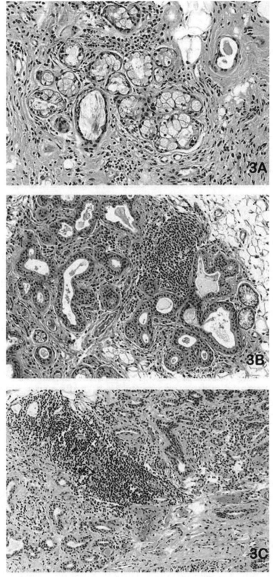

FIGURE 3.—Hematoxylin and eosin–stained labial salivary glands exhibiting nonspecific chronic sialadenitis (NSCS) and sclerosing chronic sialadenitis (SCS). These patterns do not represent the salivary component of Sjögren's syndrome, and all of these specimens are from participants who were negative for anti-SSA/SSB and rheumatoid factor. **A,** NSCS and SCS with scattered lymphocytes and plasma cells and prominent interstitial fibrosis. Original magnification × 100. **B,** SCS with duct dilation, interstitial fibrosis, and a prominent lymphocytic infiltrate, but without adjacent normal-appearing acini. Original magnification × 50. **C,** SCS with severe interstitial fibrosis, a lymphocytic aggregate, many duct-like structures, and no normal-appearing acini. Original magnification × 50. (Reprinted from Daniels TE, for the Sjögren's International Collaborative Clinical Alliance Research Groups. Associations between salivary gland histopathologic diagnoses and phenotypic features of Sjögren's syndrome among 1,726 registry participants. *Arthritis Rheum.* 2011;63:2021-2030, with permission from Arthritis & Rheumatism and John Wiley and Sons.)

factor, and the ocular component of SS, but not with symptoms of dry mouth or dry eyes. Those with positive anti-SSA/SSB were 9 times (95% confidence interval [95% CI] 7.4—11.9) more likely to have a focus score of ≥ 1 than were those without anti-SSA/SSB, and those with an unstimulated whole salivary flow rate of < 0.1 ml/minute were 2 times (95% CI 1.7—2.8) more likely to have a focus score of ≥ 1 than were those with a higher flow rate, after controlling for other phenotypic features of SS.

Conclusion.—Distinguishing FLS from NS/SCS is essential in assessing LSG biopsies, before determining focus score. A diagnosis of FLS with a focus score of ≥ 1 per 4 mm^2, as compared to FLS with a focus score of < 1 or NS/SCS, is strongly associated with the ocular and serologic components of SS and reflects SS autoimmunity (Figs 1-3).

▶ This is a large-scale and very interesting prospective cohort study on Sjögren syndrome from the 2011 Sjögren International Collaborative Clinical Alliance (SICCA) that confirms the importance of distinguishing focal lymphocytic sialadenitis associated with Sjögren syndrome from nonspecific or sclerosing chronic sialadenitis (Figs 1-3) and further discusses the criteria for diagnosis. The authors state that a labial salivary gland (LSG) biopsy can yield histopathologic information about the extent and nature of the disease process that is specific for diagnosing the salivary component of Sjögren syndrome in a manner that is not achieved by other methods (parotid flow rates, sialographic imaging, etc), and that the lack of uniformity of reporting these cases could be overcome by following the protocol indicated in this article and on the SICCA website.[1] Review of the article and the website is of great help to those pathologists who are not quite familiar with the best scoring methods in this reasonably common biopsy in general practice of pathology. The article mainly affirms, as seen from the abstract, that an LSG biopsy focus with a focus score equal to or higher than 1 is the best method for diagnosing its salivary gland component.

M. S. Said, MD, PhD

Reference

1. Sjögren International Collaborative Clinical Alliance (SICCA). Questionnaires, forms & protocols: Labial salivary glands - histopathological assessment for general application. http://sicca.ucsf.edu. Accessed August 31, 2012.

Clinicopathological characterization of mammary analogue secretory carcinoma of salivary glands
Chiosea SI, Griffith C, Assaad A, et al (Univ of Pittsburgh Med Ctr, PA; Virginia Mason Med Ctr, Seattle, WA)
Histopathology 2012 [Epub ahead of print]

Aims.—Mammary analogue secretory carcinoma (MASC) is a recently described tumour with *ETV6* translocation. We aimed to characterize the clinical significance of recognizing MASC.

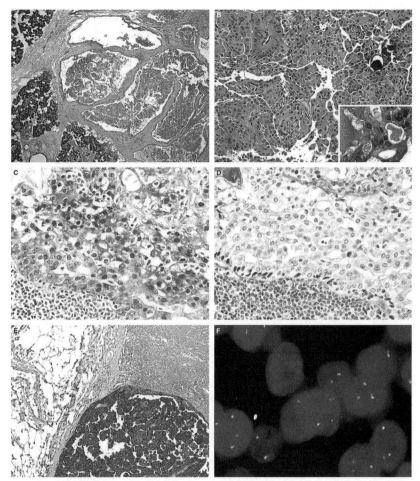

FIGURE 2.—Morphological, immunohistochemical and molecular features of prototypical mammary analogue secretory carcinoma (MASC). A, Well-circumscribed papillary cystic neoplasm (H&E). B, Solid and papillary architecture; note psammoma body in the right upper corner (H&E). Inset: intraluminal mucicarmine positive secretions. C, Positive S100 immunohistochemistry. D, p63 immunohistochemistry highlights peripheral layer of residual basal cells. E, Mammaglobin positivity in a lymph node deposit of MASC. F, *ETV6* fluorescence *in-situ* hybridization (FISH) showing one fused (yellow) and one split (red and green) signal indicative of *ETV6* translocation. For interpretation of the references to color in this figure legend, the reader is referred to web version of this article. (Reprinted from Chiosea SI, Griffith C, Assaad A, et al. Clinicopathological characterization of mammary analogue secretory carcinoma of salivary glands. *Histopathology*. 2012 [Epub ahead of print], with permission from Blackwell Publishing Limited.)

Methods and Results.—Thirty-six patients with MASC (27 identified retrospectively and nine prospectively) are presented. Historically, MASC mimicked other salivary tumours, as follows: 14 of 37 (37.8%) adenocarcinoma, not otherwise specified, 11 of 89 (12.4%) acinic cell carcinomas (AciCC), one of five (20%) mucin-producing signet ring adenocarcinomas, and one of 165 (0.6%) mucoepidermoid carcinomas. Demographically, MASC affected males more commonly (1.4:1). The average age at diagnosis

TABLE 1.—Clinicopathological Features of Patients with Mammary Analogue Secretory Carcinoma, n = 36

Feature	Overall	Consult	In-House	Site Distribution of Original Diagnoses		
				Overall	Consult	In-house
Gender, men/women	21/15	16/12	5/3			
Average age, years*	45.7	46.1	43.2			
Anatomical site Parotid gland	26	20	6	AciCC-10; ANOS-9; MASC-5; MEC-1; SigAdeno-1	AciCC-8; ANOS-7; MASC-4; SigAdeno-1	AciCC-2; ANOS-2; MASC-1; MEC-1;
Submandibular gland	3	2	1	ANOS-3	ANOS-2	ANOS-1
Soft palate	3	2	1	MASC-2; ANOS-1	MASC-2	ANOS-1
Buccal mucosa	2	2	0	MASC-2	MASC-2	N/A
Base of tongue	1	1	0	ANOS-1	ANOS-1	N/A
Upper lip	1	1	0	AciCC-1	AciCC-1	N/A
T stage†						
1	21	18	3			
2	5	3	2			
3	4	3	1			
4	2	1	1			
N stage‡						
0	14	12	2			
1	3	1	2			
2b	1	0	1			

AciCC, Acinic cell carcinoma; ANOS, adenocarcinoma, not otherwise specified; MASC, mammary analogue secretory carcinoma (all cases originally diagnosed as MASC were identified prospectively); MEC, mucoepidermoid carcinoma; SigAdeno, signet ring adenocarcinoma; NA, not applicable.
*Age was unknown for one in-house patient.
†T stage was unknown for four patients, one in-house and three consult patients.
‡Lymph nodes were not sampled in 18 cases, 15 consult cases and three in-house cases.

was 45.7 years. Parotid gland was the most common site of involvement (26 of 36, 72.2%), although other head and neck sites, including the base of tongue, were affected. Of 18 patients with neck dissection, lymph node involvement was identified in four patients (four of 18, 22.2%). Survival analysis of MASC cases presented here, combined with those reported previously, revealed a mean disease-free survival for patients with MASC of 92 months [$n = 29$; 95% confidence interval (CI) 71–115 months], compared with a mean DFS of 121 months for patients with AciCC ($n = 38$; 95% CI 92–149, $P = 0.43$).

Conclusions.—Although perhaps slightly more aggressive, MASC clinical outcome mimics that of AciCC (Fig 2, Table 1).

▶ Skálová et al[1] were the first group to describe the rare new entity of mammary analogue secretory carcinoma of the salivary glands (MASC) in 16 patients, elaborate on its morphologic and genetic features (contains the ETV6-NTRK3 Fusion gene), and note that its features are strongly reminiscent of secretory breast carcinoma (hence the name MASC). This article deals with a larger series of 36 patients and mostly confirms the previous findings of Skálová et al (Fig 2 and Table 1). It also adds nonparotid sites (mainly the tongue and submandibular gland) as sites of occurrence in addition to having a more well-defined disease-free survival mean. The article concluded that MASC has similar outcome data to its main mimicker acinic cell carcinoma. Although Skálová et al were the first to show the presence of the ETV6-NTRK3 Fusion gene in the salivary glands, the authors discuss the possible clinical implications of this findings in more detail in the current article and note the potential value in future therapeutic strategies for patients in more advanced disease stages with this tumor (use of tyrosine kinase inhibitors and insulin-like growth factor receptor inhibitors).

M. S. Said, MD, PhD

Reference

1. Skálová A, Vanecek T, Sima R, et al. Mammary analogue secretory carcinoma of salivary glands, containing the ETV6-NTRK3 fusion gene: a hitherto undescribed salivary gland tumor entity. *Am J Surg Pathol.* 2010;34:599-608.

IgG4+ Plasma Cells in Sclerosing Variant of Mucoepidermoid Carcinoma

Tian W, Yakirevich E, Matoso A, et al (Warren Alpert Med School at Brown Univ, Providence, RI)
Am J Surg Pathol 36:973-979, 2012

IgG4-related sclerosing disease is a recently described syndrome with unique histologic features characterized by intense lymphoplasmacytic infiltrates with increased IgG4+ plasma cells and dense stromal sclerosis. The disease spectrum frequently includes benign inflammatory diseases, such as autoimmune pancreatitis, cholangitis, and chronic sclerosing sialadenitis (CSS). Mucoepidermoid carcinoma (MEC) is the most common primary malignancy in the salivary gland. The rare sclerosing variant of MEC is

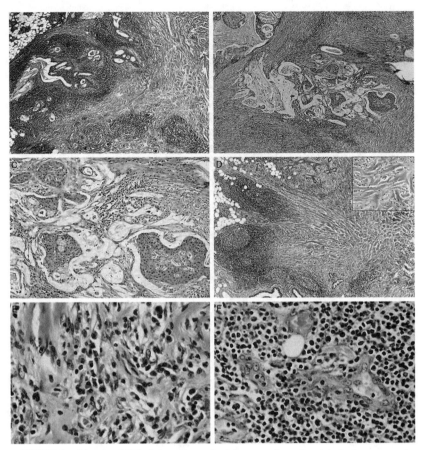

FIGURE 1.—Sclerosing MEC of the salivary gland (hematoxylin and eosin). A, Low-power view showing sclerosing MEC with central sclerosis with peripheral tumor nests surrounded by a dense lymphoplasmacytic infiltrate. Adjacent salivary gland (upper left corner) contains no inflammation. B, MEC nests surrounded by pools of mucin, reactive fibrosis, and chronic inflammation. C, Details of (B) demonstrating tumor nests composed of squamous, intermediate, and mucus-secreting cells surrounded by pools of mucin. D, Keloid-type dense collagen fibrosis in a background inflammatory infiltrate, more pronounced at the periphery of the tumor with lymphoid follicle formation. Inset: Details of keloid-like area. E, Inflammatory infiltrate consists predominantly of plasma cells, lymphocytes, and a few eosinophils. F, Venulitis with prominent chronic inflammatory infiltrate and reactive endothelial cells. (Reprinted from Tian W, Yakirevich E, Matoso A, et al. IgG4+ plasma cells in sclerosing variant of mucoepidermoid carcinoma. *Am J Surg Pathol.* 2012;36:973-979, with permission from Lippincott Williams & Wilkins.)

characterized by dense stromal sclerosis and lymphoplasmacytic infiltrates. Our goal was to further characterize lymphoplasmacytic infiltrates with respect to IgG4 expression. Six sclerosing MECs from our pathology service over the past 20 years were selected. In addition, 11 regular MECs with lymphoplasmacytic infiltrates, 4 CSS cases, and 12 nonsclerosing chronic sialadenitis cases were evaluated. None of the sclerosing MEC patients had IgG4-related sclerosing disease. The absolute number of IgG4+ plasma cells was significantly increased in sclerosing MEC as compared with the regular type (75 vs. 20 per image field; $P < 0.05$). Furthermore, the

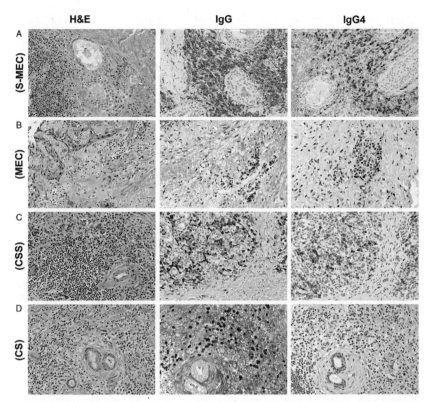

FIGURE 2.—Immunohistochemistry study of IgG4 and IgG in S-MEC, MEC, CSS, and CS. A, S-MEC, with significantly increased IgG4$^+$ plasma cells in a background of increased IgG$^+$ plasma cells. B, regular MEC has few IgG4$^+$ plasma cells in a background of IgG$^+$ plasma cells. C, CSS with lymphoplasmacytic infiltrates surrounding atrophic salivary gland ducts has significantly increased IgG4$^+$ plasma cells in a background of increased IgG$^+$ plasma cells. D, regular CS has very few IgG4$^+$ plasma cells in a background of mildly increased IgG$^+$ plasma cells. S-MEC indicates sclerosing mucoepidermoid carcinoma. (Reprinted from Tian W, Yakirevich E, Matoso A, et al. IgG4$^+$ plasma cells in sclerosing variant of mucoepidermoid carcinoma. *Am J Surg Pathol.* 2012;36:973-979, with permission from Lippincott Williams & Wilkins.)

TABLE 2.—Mean (Range) of IgG4$^+$ and IgG$^+$ Plasma Cell Counts

	S-MEC (n = 6)	MEC (n = 11)	CSS (n = 4)	CS (n = 12)
IgG4	75 (18-190)	20 (3-42)	52 (7-108)	3.4 (0-11)
IgG	172 (54-279)	108 (23-212)	88 (37-152)	74 (7-288)

S-MEC indicates sclerosing MEC.

proportion of IgG4$^+$/IgG$^+$ plasma cells was markedly elevated in sclerosing MEC as compared with the regular type (46.5% vs. 17%; $P < 0.05$). In CSS, IgG4$^+$/IgG$^+$ ratio was significantly increased as compared with nonsclerosing chronic sialadenitis (54% vs. 6.73%; $P < 0.01$). This study is the first to demonstrate increased IgG4 plasma cells in sclerosing MEC. The association of elevated IgG4$^+$ plasma cells with increased fibrosis in the sclerosing variant of MEC suggests a role of IgG4$^+$ plasma cells in fibrogenesis and may be a new concept related to sclerosis in cancer (Figs 1 and 2, Table 2).

▶ More head and neck lesions show features in common with the immunoglobulin (Ig) G4 sclerosing diseases (ie, IgG4-related system disease [RSD]) are being defined to probably include in the list of these prolific diseases whose most famous participant has been the entity of "autoimmune pancreatitis" or to see if such similarities are tenuous without solid ground of inclusion in these processes. In this context, chronic sclerosing sialadenitis (ie, Küttner's tumor) is another important head and neck participant of these entities that has been characterized by increased IgG4 content with increased fibrosis[1] and is considered by some authors as a true participant of IgG4-RSD. The orbital area, lacrimal glands, thyroid glands, and sinonasal area have also been the site of pathologic changes of similar nature. In this article, the authors review a series of 6 cases to add to the 16 already included in the world literature of the "sclerosing variant of mucoepidermoid carcinoma" and describe its most important features (see Figs 1 and 2) and demonstrate, as mentioned in the abstract, elevated IgG4 plasma cells (Table 2) and significant fibrosis. However, they also mention that malignancy in the background of IgG4RSD is uncommon and mention studies that showed increased IgG4 in various cancers in the body.[2] In conclusion, although the article showed similar morphologic changes to those seen in the IgG4RSDs, it could not definitively conclude that these were secondary to an IgG4RSD process and proposed that it could be the immune response to the tumor that have induced IgG4 increase and subsequent fibrosis. Although some of the IgG4-related processes are proven in the head and neck region, others, such as the sclerosing variant of mucoepidermoid carcinoma remains unestablished and probably an unlikely participant despite the morphologic similarities. More studies are most likely needed to further prove that contention.

M. S. Said, MD, PhD

References

1. Kitagawa S, Zen Y, Harada K, et al. Abundant IgG4-positive plasma cell infiltration characterizes chronic sclerosing sialadenitis (Küttner's tumor). *Am J Surg Pathol*. 2005;29:783-791.
2. Strehl JD, Hartmann A, Agaimy A. Numerous IgG4-positive plasma cells are ubiquitous in diverse localised non-specific chronic inflammatory conditions and need to be distinguished from IgG4-related systemic disorders. *J Clin Pathol*. 2011;64:237-243.

Angiomatoid change in polyps of the nasal and paranasal regions: an underrecognized and commonly misdiagnosed lesion—report of 45 cases
Hadravsky L, Skalova A, Kacerovska D, et al (Charles Univ in Prague, Plzeň, Czech Republic; et al)
Virchows Arch 460:203-209, 2012

We present 45 patients with angiomatoid polyps of the nasal and paranasal regions (APNPRs), which are underrecognized lesions which may

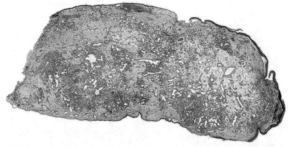

FIGURE 1.—Scanning magnification of polyp with angiomatoid change. (Reprinted from Hadravsky L, Skalova A, Kacerovska D, et al. Angiomatoid change in polyps of the nasal and paranasal regions: an underrecognized and commonly misdiagnosed lesion—report of 45 cases. *Virchows Arch.* 2012;460:203-209, with permission from Springer-Verlag.)

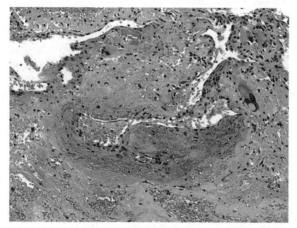

FIGURE 3.—Postthrombotic changes with stromal atypias. (Reprinted from Hadravsky L, Skalova A, Kacerovska D, et al. Angiomatoid change in polyps of the nasal and paranasal regions: an underrecognized and commonly misdiagnosed lesion—report of 45 cases. *Virchows Arch.* 2012;460:203-209, with permission from Springer-Verlag.)

cause considerable diagnostic difficulties. There were 32 men and 13 women in our series. The average age at diagnosis was 49 years in men and 54.3 years in women. Locations were known in 41 cases and included the nasal septum (14), maxillary sinus (12), ethmoid sinuses (5), lateral wall of the nasal cavity (5), sphenoid sinus (1), and nasal cavity, not otherwise specified (4). X-ray or computed tomography was performed in 19 cases and revealed bone erosions/deviations in four cases. Initial misdiagnoses submitted by referring pathologists were reported in 20/32 of the consultation cases. Our study confirms that APNPRs are benign lesions which often recur and sometimes multiple recurrences are seen. APNPRs sometimes cause severe changes of the skeletal bones especially in recurrent lesions. Awareness of the above described features and familiarity with the clinical

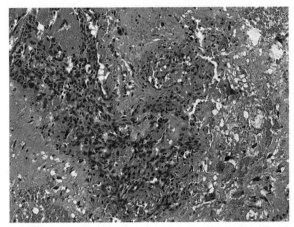

FIGURE 4.—Proliferation of capillaries with atypias simulating angiosarcoma and mucous spillage into the stroma. (Reprinted from Hadravsky L, Skalova A, Kacerovska D, et al. Angiomatoid change in polyps of the nasal and paranasal regions: an underrecognized and commonly misdiagnosed lesion—report of 45 cases. *Virchows Arch.* 2012;460:203-209, with permission from Springer-Verlag.)

presentation of APNPRs is the best way to avoid a misdiagnosis (Figs 1, 3, and 4).

▶ This is a nice and informative systematic study on the somewhat unfamiliar and often misdiagnosed entity of angiomatoid nasal polyps and their features encountered and concluded from the study of 45 patients. The major causes of misdiagnosis as mentioned in the study are the secondary changes that a nasal polyp can undergo if left undiscovered or untreated including thrombosis with infarction, postinfarction cellular atypia mimicking sarcomatous change, vascular proliferation, reparative changes, associated reactive bone changes, and pseudoepitheliomatous hyperplasia of the overlying epithelium (Figs 1, 3, and 4). In their analysis, the authors mention that the thin stalk is unmatched by the growth of the polyp through the sinus ostium and into the nasal cavity and that kinking or obstructing of the stalk as it emerges from the ostium predisposes to the infarction with the ensuing changes both morphologically and in the patient symptoms (epistaxis, nasal obstruction, mucus or pus discharge). The major differential diagnosis of these lesions as encountered in the consultations of the authors includes a variety of sometimes alarming initial impressions including angiosarcomas, hemangiopericytomas, and nasopharyngeal angiofibromas with the possible ensuing unwarranted aggressive management highlighting the importance of awareness of this entity.

M. S. Said, MD, PhD

Malignant tumors of the sinonasal tract in the pediatric population

Yi JS, Cho GS, Shim MJ, et al (Univ of Ulsan College of Medicine, Seoul, South Korea)

Acta Oto-Laryngol 132:S21-S26, 2012

Conclusion.—Sarcoma and lymphoma comprised 75% of 20 cases of pediatric sinonasal malignancies. As regards treatment, all 20 patients received chemotherapy and 6 patients (30%) underwent surgery. The overall 5-year survival rate was 52%, with favorable outcome for solid tumors compared with lymphoma.

Objective.—We aimed to investigate the clinical features and treatment outcomes of sinonasal malignancies in 20 pediatric patients.

Methods.—Clinical features were evaluated and tumors were staged according to the staging system for each histologic type.

Results.—The 20 patients consisted of 12 males and 8 females, ranging in age from 1 to 16 years, with a median age of 9.6 years at diagnosis. More than half of the patients presented with nasal obstruction as the primary symptom, and mean symptom duration to diagnosis was 5.4 months. Primary tumor sites included the paranasal sinuses alone in four patients, the nasal cavity alone in eight, and both in eight. Eight tumors were sarcomas and seven were lymphomas. The remaining tumors included three olfactory neuroblastomas and two primitive neuroectodermal tumors. The main treatment modality was chemotherapy rather than surgery. The overall survival rate was 52%, and patients with solid tumors survived significantly longer than those with lymphoma ($p = 0.02$) (Table 1).

▶ Reports on the pediatric sinonasal malignancies are rather limited. In 2008, a retrospective study by Benoit et al[1] described 16 pediatric patients from the Boston area between 1991 and 2006 and found that the most common malignancy was rhabdomyosarcoma (37.5%) followed by esthesioneuroblastoma (25%), non-rhabdomyosarcoma soft-tissue tumors (6.25% fibrosarcoma, neurofibrosarcoma, high-grade sarcoma, MFH, malignant PNST), malignant tumors of bone and cartilage (18.75%), hematolymphoid tumors (6.25%), and Ewing sarcoma/primitive neuroectodermal tumors (6.25%). The current article is describing 20 pediatric Korean patients and thus may give some insight into the regional variations, if present, as well as enriching somewhat scarce data on the subject. The results are shown in Table 1 and show that hematolymphoid tumors followed closely by rhabdomyosarcoma predominate the types of malignancies present, making the hematolymphoid population more prominent than the ones in the previous article by Hydarusky et al. Both articles have shown that most of the cases presented at an advanced stage, thus highlighting the necessity of vigilance and care when dealing with what can seem like everyday symptoms for a child. Although many instances may represent a passing short-term illness, others, though rare, can have a more serious underlying cause and emphasize long-term surveillance to avoid recurrences that can occur after a relatively long time in some cases.[1]

M. S. Said, MD, PhD

TABLE 1.—Clinical Manifestation and Treatment Outcomes of the 20 Pediatric Patients with Sinonasal Malignancy

Tumor	Age at diagnosis (Years)	Presenting Symptom	Symptom Duration (Months)	Location	Stage	Lymph Node Metastasis	Distant Metastasis	Treatment	Outcome	Follow-up (Months)
BCL	11	NO	4	MS, ES	IV	Peritoneum	Lung	CTx	DOD	7
BCL	15	Facial swelling	5	NC + MS	II	–	–	CTx	DOD	11
NKTL	5	NO	8	NC	I	–	Bone	CTx + RTx	DOD	13
NKTL	12	NO	2	NC	II	Cervical	–	CTx + RTx	NED	8
NKTL	16	NO	18	NC	IV	–	Peritoneum	CTx + RTx	DOD	23
NKTL	11	NO	17	NC	IV	–	–	CTx + RTx	DOD	22
NKTL	15	Rhinorrhea	25	NC + MS, ES	II	–	–	CTx	NED	37
RMS	13	Exophthalmos	1	NC + MS, ES	IV	Cervical	Lung	CTx + RTx	REC	10
RMS	6	NO	0.5	NC	III	Cervical	–	*Surgery + RTx + CTx	NED	27
RMS	12	Exophthalmos	1	NC + ES	III	–	–	RTx + CTx	NED	20
RMS	4	Epistaxis	0.5	NC	II	–	–	RTx + CTx	NED	115
RMS	15	Facial swelling	1	MS	IV	–	–	RTx + CTx	NED	133
RMS	10	Facial swelling	1	NC	II	–	–	*Surgery + RTx + CTx	NED	40
FS	1	Facial swelling	2	NC + MS	I	–	–	†Surgery + CTx	NED	125
FS	9	NO	4	ES, MS	I	–	–	‡Surgery + CTx	NED	68
ON	9	Headache	3	NC + MS, ES, SS	C	–	–	*Surgery + RTx + CTx	DOD	18
ON	3	NO	4	NC + MS	C	–	–	*Surgery + CTx	DOD	21
ON	10	NO	2	MS, ES, SS	D	Cervical	–	RTx + CTx	DOD	17
PNET	3	NO	8	NC	I	–	–	CTx	NED	14
PNET	11	Exophthalmos	1	NC + MS, ES	II	–	–	RTx + CTx	NED	82

BCL, B-cell lymphoma; CTx, chemotherapy; DOD, died of disease; ES, ethmoid sinus; FS, fibrosarcoma; MS, maxillary sinus; NC, nasal cavity; NED, no evidence of disease; NKTL, NK/T-cell lymphoma; NO, nasal obstruction; ON, olfactory neuroblastoma; PNET, primitive neuroectodermal tumor; REC, recurrence; RMS, rhabdomyosarcoma; RTx, radiation therapy; SS, sphenoid sinus.

*Endoscopic excision.

†Wide excision.

‡Excision via open rhinoplasty approach.

Reference

1. Benoit M, Bhattacharyya N, Faquin W, Cunningham M. Cancer of the nasal cavity in the pediatric population. *Pediatric.* 2008;121:e141-e145.

Fungal Rhinosinusitis: A Retrospective Microbiologic and Pathologic Review of 400 Patients at a Single University Medical Center

Montone KT, Livolsi VA, Feldman MD, et al (Perelman School of Medicine at the Univ of Pennsylvania, Philadelphia; et al)
Int J Otolaryngol 2012:1-9, 2012

Fungal Rhinosinusitis (FRS) is a well known entity, but only in more recent times have the types of FRS been more fully defined. In this study, we evaluate the diagnosis of FRS in a single medical center. Cases were divided into 2 main categories, non-invasive and invasive. Non-invasive FRS included fungus ball (FB) and allergic fungal rhinosinusitis (AFRS). Invasive FRS included acute invasive fungal rhinosinusitis (AIFRS), chronic invasive fungal rhinosinusitis (CIFRS), and chronic invasive granulomatous fungal rhinosinusitis (CGFRS). Fungal culture data, if available was reviewed. 400 patients with FRS were identified. 87.25% were noninvasive (45% AFRS, 40% FB, and 2% combined AFRS and FB and 12.5% were invasive 11% AIFRS 1.2% CIFRS 0.5% CGFRS. One patient (0.25%) had combined FB/CGFRS. *Aspergillus sp.* or dematiaceous species were the most common fungi isolated in AFS while *Aspergillus sp.* was most

TABLE 1.—Classification of Fungal Rhinosinusitis

	Histopathologic Criteria
Non-invasive FRS	
Fungus ball (FB)	An entangled mass on fungi with Minimal surrounding inflammatory reaction or surrounding fibrinous necrotic exudate containing fungal forms; no tissue invasion or granulomatous reaction is present
Allergic fungal rhinosinusitis (AFRS)	The presence of eosinophilic mucin (mucinous material admixed with eosinophils, acute inflammatory cells, eosinophilic debris, and Charcot-Leyden crystals; sparse fungi or positive fungal cultures; no tissue invasion present)
Mixed FB/AFRS	The presence of features of both AFRS and FB
Invasive FRS	
Acute (AIFRS)	Invasion of fungal forms into submucosal with frequent angioinvasion and necrosis in a patient with symptoms of less than one-month duration
Chronic (CIFRS)	Invasion of fungal forms into submucosal often with surrounding chronic inflammation and fibrosis in patient with long-standing symptoms (>3-month duration)
Chronic granulomatous (CGFRS)	Invasion of fungal forms into submucosal often with surrounding chronic inflammation, fibrosis, and granuloma production in patient with long-standing symptoms (>3-month duration)
Mixed Non-invasive/invasive FRS	A mixture of either of the invasive and non-invasive categories

TABLE 3.—Clinical Summary of FRS Patients

Diagnosis	Avg. Age (Range)	M : F	No.	No. with Cultures (% Positive)	Most Common Isolates (%)
FB	55 (18–90)	1 : 2	161	107 (51%)	*Aspergillus sp.* (66%)
AFRS	45 (18–88)	1.2 : 1	180	142 (89%)	Dematiaceous fungi (36%) *Aspergillus sp.* (35%)
AIFRS	54 (24–82)	1.5 : 1	44	27 (67%)	*Aspergillus sp.* *Rhizopus sp.*
CIFRS	48 (21–65)	1 : 1	4	2 (100%)	*C. albicans* *Scedosporium apiospermium*
CGFRS	58 (50–66)	1 : 1	2	1 (100%)	*A. flavus*

common in FB and AIFRS. In our experience, most FRS is non-invasive. In our patient population, invasive FRS is rare with AIFRS representing >90% of cases. Culture data supports that a variety of fungal agents are responsible for FRS, but *Aspergillus sp.* appears to be one of the most common organisms in patients with FRS (Tables 1 and 3).

▶ Fungal rhinosinusitis is a common diagnostic entity in the usual practice of almost all pathologists. This is a current US-based large series of 400 patients with rhinosinusitis who were classified according to the histologic criteria shown in Table 1, and their clinical summary is shown in Table 3. The article also highlighted some of the world geographic diversity in the subtype incidence variations that are seen with these infections, noting, for example, that in India, the incidence of chronic granulomatous fungal rhinosinusitis was far more prevalent than in the United States, whereas fungal ball formations were less encountered in India than in the United States.[1] Interestingly, however, the cause for these world regional variations is not completely understood. The authors also note the interesting debate involving and relating to chronic rhinosinusitis (usually treated by antibiotics) to an inflammatory reaction to fungi.[2] *Aspergillus* species remain the most commonly isolated fungus in different types of fungal rhinosinusitis worldwide.

M. S. Said, MD, PhD

References

1. Das A, Bal A, Chakrabarti A, Panda N, Joshi K. Spectrum of fungal rhinosinusitis; histopathologist's perspective. *Histopathology.* 2009;54:854-859.
2. Ebbens F, Fokkens W. The mold conundrum in chronic rhinosinusitis: where do we stand today? *Curr Allergy Asthma Rep.* 2008;8:93-101.

Trends in sinonasal cancer in The Netherlands: More squamous cell cancer, less adenocarcinoma: A population-based study 1973–2009
Kuijpens JHLP, Louwman MWJ, Peters R, et al (VGZ Health Insurance Company, Eindhoven, The Netherlands; Comprehensive Cancer Centre South (IKZ), Eindhoven, The Netherlands; ArboUnie Occupational Health Service, Eindhoven, The Netherlands; et al)
Eur J Cancer 2012 [Epub ahead of print]

Background.—Cancer of the nasal cavity or the paranasal sinuses (sinonasal cancer) is rare. Sinonasal cancer has been associated with various occupational risk factors such as exposure to dust of hard wood and leather. Also, a relationship with smoking habits has been suggested. We studied the long term trends in incidence to evaluate a putative effect of past preventive measures or changes in risk factors.

Design.—A retrospective population-based descriptive study.

Objective.—To interpret the long term trends in incidence of sinonasal cancer in The Netherlands.

Methods.—Data of all 3329 patients >15 years registered during 1989–2009 by the Netherlands Cancer Registry (NCR) were analysed, by data of 447 patients registered by the Eindhoven Cancer Registry (ECR) during 1973–2009 were analysed separately. Information on patients and tumour characteristics was obtained from both registries. The incidence was calculated per 1,000,000 person years and standardised using the European Standard Population.

Results.—Squamous cell carcinoma (SCC) was the most prominent histological type (48%), followed by adenocarcinoma (15%) and melanoma (8%). SCC was more frequently located in the nasal cavity or sinus maxillaris, but adenocarcinoma was more located in the ethmoid sinus. The male incidence increased during 1973–1995 with a peak of 15/1,000,000/year, decreasing since then to 11/1,000,000/year due to a declining incidence of both SCC and adenocarcinoma. In females the incidence remained stable around 5/1,000,000/year up to 2006 and increased to 7.5/1,000,000 in 2009 as a result of more SCC. The male/female ratio for SCC decreased from 2.7 to 2.0, and for adenocarcinoma from 3.4 to 2.8 since 1989.

Conclusions.—The higher incidence in males and the different trends in incidence in males and females may reflect differences in previous exposure to risk factors. Adenocarcinoma, related to occupational exposures, tend to decline. The trends in both male and female sinonasal SCC are comparable with the trends in lung cancer (Table 1).

▶ In addition to continuous research efforts to define the variable etiologies of head and neck cancers, large epidemiologic studies are of immense importance in defining many aspects of these diseases, including the type of population they occur in, their variable trends over the years, and the effectiveness of preventative measures taken by local or national health organizations or governments, to name a few. Unfortunately, many of these studies tend to be present in the developed parts of the world and are not prevalent in many parts of the developing

TABLE 1.—Histology and Topography of 3329 Patients with Sinonasal Cancer Registered by The Netherlands Cancer Registry (NCR), 1989–2009

	Squamous Cell Carcinoma N (%)	Adenocarcinoma N (%)	Olfactorius Neuroblastoma N (%)	Melanoma N (%)	Other/Unknown N (%)	Total N (%)
Nasal cavity	1124 (55.8)	192 (9.5)	85 (4.2)	213 (10.6)	401 (19.9)	2015 (100)
Maxillary sinus	345 (46.4)	109 (14.7)	1 (0.1)	18 (2.4)	271 (36.4)	744 (100)
Ethmoidal sinus	67 (17.9)	163 (43.6)	24 (6.4)	12 (3.2)	108 (28.9)	374 (100)
Frontal and sphenoid sinus	26 (31.7)	16 (19.5)	3 (3.7)	3 (3.7)	34 (41.5)	82 (100)
Multiple locations and not specified	34 (29.8)	25 (21.9)	2 (1.8)	10 (8.8)	43 (37.7)	114 (100)
All locations	1596 (47.9)	505 (15.2)	115 (3.5)	256 (7.7)	857 (25.7)	3329 (100)

countries, probably in many occasions because of lack of adequate resources. This is an example of a significant study conducted in the Netherlands and involves prevalence of sinonasal carcinoma in the country. Probably one of the important aspects of the study is that it highlights the effect of preventative measures or other social trends and factors on the prevalence of certain types of cancer, in this case sinonasal adenocarcinoma. This study has concluded that its decrease in The Netherlands was due to government implementation of exposure levels to wood dust within its wood industries in addition to the fact that many leather-processing industries have moved to other low-income countries from The Netherlands. Additionally, there are fewer people working in the wood and leather industries, thus decreasing the number of people exposed to leather dust. Similarly, squamous cell carcinoma showed a decreasing trend in men, probably related to both smoking habits and industrial exposure; the increasing trend of squamous cell carcinoma in the female population could be indicative of a change of social habits with increased smoking in that population. Specific recent or current long-term retrospective national epidemiologic trend studies of sinonasal cancer are not readily available in the current US medical literature.

M. S. Said, MD, PhD

Head and neck paragangliomas: clinical and molecular genetic classification
Offergeld C, Brase C, Yaremchuk S, et al (Albert-Ludwigs-Univ, Freiburg, Germany; Friedrich-Alexander-Univ of Erlangen-Nürnberg, Germany; Inst of Otolaryngology of the Academy of Med Science of Ukraine, Kiev, Ukraine; et al)
Clinics 67:19-28, 2012

Head and neck paragangliomas are tumors arising from specialized neural crest cells. Prominent locations are the carotid body along with the vagal, jugular, and tympanic glomus. Head and neck paragangliomas are slowly growing tumors, with some carotid body tumors being reported to exist for many years as a painless lateral mass on the neck. Symptoms depend on the specific locations. In contrast to paraganglial tumors of the adrenals, abdomen and thorax, head and neck paragangliomas seldom

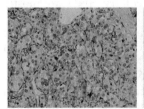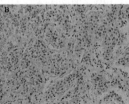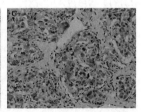

FIGURE 3.—Histology and immunostaining of head and neck paragangliomas. (A) Demonstration of sustentacular cells by S-100 protein in an HNP. The delicate net of sustentacular cells is surrounding the so-called Zellballen of chief cells (x200). (B) Complete immunohistochemical negativity for SDHB strongly suggesting a SDHB germline mutation (×200). (C) Immunohistochemical demonstration of SDHB protein in tumor cells, virtually excluding a germline mutation in *SDHB* (×200). (Reprinted from Offergeld C, Brase C, Yaremchuk S, et al. Head and neck paragangliomas: clinical and molecular genetic classification. *Clinics.* 2012;67:19-28, with permission from Clinics.)

TABLE 1.—The Shamblin Classification of Carotid Body Tumors

Class	Tumor Characteristics
I	Splaying of the carotid bifurcation with little attachment to the carotid vessels; complete resection with very little morbidity
II	Partial surrounding of internal and external carotid artery; complete resection more challenging
III	Complete surrounding of the carotid vessels; complete resection often requires major vessel reconstruction

TABLE 2.—Classification of Jugulotympanic Paragangliomas According to Fisch and Mattox

Class	Location and Extension of Paraganglioma
A	Paragangliomas that arise along the tympanic plexus on promontory
B	Paragangliomas with invasion of the hypotympanon; cortical bone over jugular bulb intact
C_1	Paragangliomas with erosion of the carotid foramen
C_2	Paragangliomas with destruction of the vertical carotid canal
C_3	Paragangliomas with involvement of the horizontal portion of the carotid canal; foramen lacerum intact
C_4	Paragangliomas with invasion of the foramen lacerum and cavernous sinus
De $_{1/2}$	Paragangliomas with intracranial but extradural extension; $De_{1/2}$ according to displacement of the dura (De_1 = less than 2 cm, De_2 = more than 2 cm)
Di $_{1/2/3}$	Paragangliomas with intracranial and intradural extension; $Di_{1/2/3}$ according to depth of invasion into the posterior cranial fossa (Di_1 = less than 2 cm, Di_2 = between 2 and 4 cm, Di_3 = more than 4 cm)

release catecholamines and are hence rarely vasoactive. Petrous bone, jugular, and tympanic head and neck paragangliomas may cause hearing loss. The internationally accepted clinical classifications for carotid body tumors are based on the Shamblin Class I–III stages, which correspond to postoperative permanent side effects. For petrous-bone paragangliomas in the head and neck, the Fisch classification is used. Regarding the molecular genetics, head and neck paragangliomas have been associated with nine susceptibility genes: *NF1, RET, VHL, SDHA, SDHB, SDHC, SDHD, SDHAF2 (SDH5)*, and *TMEM127*. Hereditary HNPs are mostly caused by mutations of the SDHD gene, but *SDHB* and *SDHC* mutations are not uncommon in such patients. Head and neck paragangliomas are rarely associated with mutations of VHL, RET, or NF1. The research on *SDHA, SDHAF2* and *TMEM127* is ongoing. Multiple head and neck paragangliomas are common in patients with *SDHD* mutations, while malignant head and neck paraganglioma is mostly seen in patients with SDHB mutations. The treatment of choice is surgical resection. Good postoperative results can be expected in carotid body tumors of Shamblin Class I and II, whereas operations on other carotid body tumors and other head and neck paragangliomas frequently result in deficits of the cranial nerves adjacent to the tumors. Slow growth and the tendency of

TABLE 3.—Molecular Classification of Head and Neck Paragangliomas (HNPs)

Syndrome	VHL	PGL1	PGL2	PGL3	PGL4	TMEM127
MIM ID	193300	168000	60650	605373	115310	613903
Inheritance	Autosomal Dominant	Autosomal Dominant with parent-of-origin effect	Autosomal Dominant with parent-of-origin effect	Autosomal Dominant	Autosomal Dominant	Autosomal dominant
Gene name	VHL	SDHD	SDHAF2	SDHC	SDHB	TMEM127
Protein function	An ubiquitin ligase protein; it plays a role in the oxygensensing pathway	One of two membraneanchoring subunits of complex II (SDH)	Mitochondrial assembly factor for complex II—interacts directly with SDHA	One of two membraneanchoring subunits of complex II (SDH)	The iron-sulfur protein that form together with SDHA, the main catalytic domain of complex II	Endosomal trafficking?; mTOR regulation?
Locus	3p25-26	11q23	11q13.1	1q21	1p36	2q11
Age at diagnosis of Pheochromocytoma mean and range, in years	22 (5–67)	27 (5–65)	unknown	Extremely rare	34 (12–66)	43 (34–54)
Exons (n)/amino acids (n)	3/213	4/159	4/166	6/169	8/280	3/238
HNP (%)	0,5	41	73–86	100	8	1–2
Age at diagnosis HNP Median (range, in years)	23 (7–39)	40 (12–74)	45 (15–65)	46 (13–73)	42 (9–75)	34
Pheo risk (%)	10–34	53	0	<3	28	25
PG Abdominal extraadrenal (%)	17	59	0	0	62	1–2
Multifocality (%)	56	55	0	9	11	33
Malignant (%)	4%	0	0	0	32	5
Clinical Phenotype	Sympathetic Noradrenergic	Parasympathetic, occasionally noradrenergic	Parasympa thetic	Parasympa thetic	Noradrenergic	Sympathetic Noradrenergic
Associated tumors	Eye and CNS hemangioblastomas, clear cell renal cancer, islet cell tumors, endolymphatic sac tumors of the inner ear	Rarely Papillary thyroid cancer, GIST	GIST	GIST	Rarely renal cell cancer GIST	

Adapted from Bausch et al. (73), Hensen et al. (74) and Neumann and Eng (75).
Editor's Note: Please refer to original journal article for full references.
CNS = central nervous system; GIST = gastrointestinal stromal tumor, mTOR = mammalian target of rapamycin; PGL = Paraganglioma syndrome; SDHAF2 = succinate dehydrogenase complex assembly factor 2;
TMEM127 = transmembrane protein 127.

hereditary head and neck paragangliomas to be multifocal may justify less aggressive treatment strategies (Fig 3, Tables 1-3).

▶ This is an interesting multi-institutional review article that updates the reader on different aspects of head and neck paragangliomas, which are quite a frequent diagnosis encountered in that location by the practicing pathologists. Paragangliomas have a similar histologic picture (Fig 3), regardless of where they are found, in the various head and neck sites. Although they are mostly benign, it remains a difficult task to define the histologic difference between benign and malignant paragangliomas, and lymph node metastasis remains possibly the only way of ascertaining malignancy with certainty. The article reviews some of the clinical schemes used to classify paragangliomas in different sites (Tables 1 and 2) and the surgical/treatment outcomes based on these classifications. The article also reviews the molecular/genetic classification, which is a useful update (Table 3) dealing with the 9 different susceptibility genes of the paraganglial tumors, including some more recently described in ongoing research (see abstract). The authors point out that a thorough genotype-phenotype study for different head and neck paragangliomas is currently lacking and note that patients with mutations of SDHB, SDHC, and SDHD genes may develop tumors in the carotid body, and vagal, jugular, and tympanic paraganglia (see also Table 3 and Fig 3). The authors also point out the study by Van Nederveen et al, which showed the potential of using immunohistochemical staining against SDHB as a screening/selection tool for further genetic study (Fig 3).[1]

M. S. Said, MD, PhD

Reference

1. van Nederveen FH, Gaal J, Favier J, et al. An immunohistochemical procedure to detect patients with paraganglioma and pheochromocytoma with germline SDHB, SDHC, or SDHD gene mutations: a retrospective and prospective analysis. *Lancet Oncol.* 2009;10:764-771.

Helicobacter pylori **infection of the larynx may be an emerging risk factor for laryngeal squamous cell carcinoma**

Gong H, Shi Y, Zhou L, et al (Fudan Univ, Shanghai, China; Nanhui Central Hosp, Shanghai, China)
Clin Transl Oncol 2012 [Epub ahead of print]

Introduction.—Several studies have implicated *Helicobacter pylori* as a risk factor in laryngeal cancer, but other studies disagree. It is fundamental that the relationship between *Helicobacter pylori* and laryngeal cancer be verified in order to provide evidence of ways to prevent the initiation and development of this carcinoma.

Materials and Methods.—In total, 81 patients with laryngeal squamous cell carcinoma and 75 control subjects were enrolled in a case—control study. Semi-nested polymerase chain reaction techniques were applied to detect *Helicobacter pylori* in the laryngeal mucosa and enzymelinked

TABLE 2.—*H. pylori* Infection was Tested by SN-PCR and ELISA Methods within Case and Control Groups

| | *H. pylori* Positive | | *H. pylori* Negative | | | |
	N	%	N	%	Total	p^*
SN-PCR						<0.001
Cases	58	71.6	23	28.4	81	
Controls	19	25.3	56	74.7	75	
ELISA						0.79
Cases	63	77.8	18	22.2	81	
Controls	57	76.0	18	24.0	75	

*p value were tested from Pearson Chi-Square test.

TABLE 3.—Colonization of *H. pylori* in Normal and Tumor Tissues of Positive *H. pylori* Infection LSCC cases

| | *H. pylori* Positive | | *H. pylori* Negative | | | |
	N	%	N	%	Total	p^*
Normal tissues	27	46.6	0	0.0	27	<0.001
Tumor tissues	8	13.8	0	0.0	8	
N and T^a	23	39.7	23	100	46	

*p value was tested from Exact test.
[a]Normal and tumor tissues.

TABLE 4.—Logistic Regression Analyses Estimating Risk Factors for LSCC

| | Cases | | Controls | | p^* Crude OR 95% CI | $p^†$ Adjusted OR 95% CI | $p^‡$ Adjusted OR 95% CI |
	N	%	N	%			
H. pylori infection					<0.001	<0.001	<0.001
No infection	23	28.4	56	74.7	7.43	7.15	8.12
Infection	58	71.6	19	25.3	3.46−16.13	3.29−15.53	3.07−21.45

Binary logistical regression method: forward LR.
*Variable included the individual risk factor with *H. pylori* infection.
†Variables included age, sex, tobacco smoking, alcohol drinking, and *H. pylori* infection.
‡Variables included sex, age, marriage status, education experience, salary income, occupation status, smoking, drinking, and *H. pylori* infection.

immunosorbent assays were used to detect serum antibodies against *Helicobacter pylori*. Risk factors associated with laryngeal carcinoma were analyzed using logistic regression models.

Results.—The presence of *Helicobacter pylori* in the larynx was higher in patients with laryngeal cancer than in control subjects (71.6 vs. 25.3%, $p < 0.001$). Among patients with laryngeal carcinoma, rates of *Helicobacter pylori* infection were higher in normal laryngeal tissues than in tumor tissues. After adjusting for confounding factors, regression analysis indicated that the microbe was an independent risk factor for laryngeal cancer (OR = 7.15, 95% CI [3.29, 15.53], $p < 0.001$).

Conclusions.—This study suggests that *Helicobacter pylori* is present in the mucosa of the larynx. The microorganism may be an independent risk factor for laryngeal squamous cell carcinoma. The laryngeal mucosa thus provides a reservoir for the bacteria possibly, and is a likely staging place for its transmission to other areas (Tables 2-4).

▶ The etiology of laryngeal cancer has been related classically to smoking and alcohol consumption and more recently to a possible role of human papilloma virus (HPV) involvement. *Helicobacter pylori* bacterium, known for its implication in gastric carcinoma and lymphoma initiation, has been studied more recently as a contributing factor to this significant type of cancer with mixed reviews and studies, some of which are supportive and others are not.[1,2] It is also worth noting that various studies have discussed *H pylori* implications in more benign head and neck entities (eg, otitis media, chronic rhinosinusitis, nasal polyps, etc).[3] The study, through the results shown in Tables 2-4, reaches the conclusion that by the use of 2 logistic regression models to exclude the influence of other potentiating agents (smoking and alcohol), *H pylori* infection was accompanied by an 8-fold increase in the risk of laryngeal squamous cell carcinoma independent of these factors. The authors also theorize that in a similar fashion to initiation of gastric malignancy, the secreted proteins from *H pylori* affect gastric mucosal defenses, and they similarly are involved in at least the cooperative initiation of laryngeal cancer to a mucosa that can also be the result of the effects of smoking, alcohol consumption, or the HPV effect. This is an interesting study and it potentially supports those who find a role for *H pylori* in initiating laryngeal squamous cell carcinoma. However, I could not help noticing that although the study corrected for most of the risk factors to reach its conclusion, there was no mention of how they excluded the potential effect of HPV or at least the HPV status of their patient population, at least from my understanding, from their counted risk factors or of HPV as an emerging and important potential factor or cofactor in influencing laryngeal and oropharyngeal squamous cell carcinoma. I think future studies should carefully consider the potential role of HPV in addition to the more proven and significant factors such as smoking and alcohol intake when investigating an emerging factor or cofactor such as *H pylori* and more carefully define it.

M. S. Said, MD, PhD

References

1. Rezaii J, Tavakoli H, Esfandiari K, et al. Association between *Helicobacter pylori* infection and laryngohypopharyngeal carcinoma: a case-control study and review of the literature. *Head Neck.* 2008;30:1624-1627.
2. Nurgalieva ZZ, Graham DY, Dahlstrom KR, Wei Q, Sturgis EM. A pilot study of *Helicobacter pylori* infection and risk of laryngopharyngeal cancer. *Head Neck.* 2005;27:22-27.
3. Grandis JR, Perez-Perez GI, Yu VL, Johnson JT, Blaser MJ. Lack of serologic evidence for *Helicobacter pylori* infection in head and neck cancer. *Head Neck.* 1997;19:216-218.

FoxP3 expression is associated with aggressiveness in differentiated thyroid carcinomas

Cunha LL, Morari EC, Nonogaki S, et al (Univ of Campinas (Unicamp), São Paulo, Brazil; Adolfo Lutz Inst, São Paulo, Brazil; et al)
Clinics 67:483-488, 2012

Objectives.—Forkhead box P3 (FoxP3) expression has been observed in human cancer cells but has not yet been reported in thyroid cells. We investigated the prognostic significance of both FoxP3 expression and intratumoral FoxP3⁺ lymphocyte infiltration in differentiated thyroid carcinoma cells.

Methods.—We constructed a tissue microarray with 385 thyroid tissues, including 266 malignant tissues (from 253 papillary thyroid carcinomas and 13 follicular carcinomas), 114 benign lesions, and 5 normal thyroid tissues.

Results.—We determined the expression of FoxP3 in both tumor cells and tumor-infiltrating lymphocytes using immunohistochemical techniques. Cellular expression of FoxP3 was evident in 71% of benign and 91.9% of malignant tissues. The nuclear and cytoplasmic expression patterns were quantified separately. A multivariate logistic regression analysis indicated that cytoplasmic FoxP3 expression is an independent risk factor for thyroid malignancy. Cytoplasmic FoxP3 staining was inversely correlated with

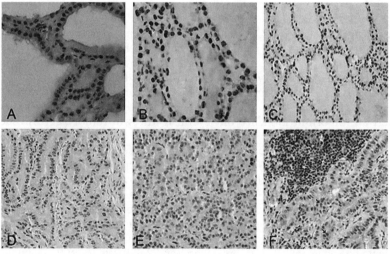

FIGURE 1.—Different levels of FoxP3 expression in various thyroid tissues and lesions. (A) Normal thyroid tissues showed the lowest FoxP3 staining. (B) Goiter lesions presented with intermediate FoxP3 immunostaining. In contrast to the normal thyroid, the goiter cells exhibited increased cytoplasmic and nuclear staining. (C) Follicular adenoma cells demonstrated pronounced cytoplasmic and nuclear FoxP3 immunostaining. (D) Papillary thyroid carcinomas showed strong FoxP3 expression. In particular, increased cytoplasmic expression is evident. (E) Follicular thyroid carcinoma tissues showed faint immunostaining. (F) A papillary thyroid carcinoma with FoxP3⁺ tumor cells and FoxP3⁺ lymphocytes. The white arrows show regulatory T lymphocytes infiltrating the malignant tissue. The black arrows show papillary thyroid carcinoma cells with both cytoplasmic and nuclear FoxP3 staining. Magnification = 400x. (Reprinted from Cunha LL, Morari EC, Nonogaki S, et al. FoxP3 expression is associated with aggressiveness in differentiated thyroid carcinomas. *Clinics.* 2012;67:483-488, with permission from Clinics.)

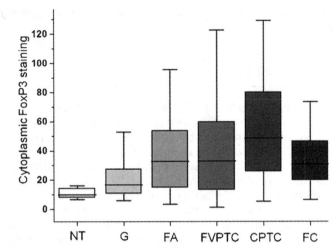

FIGURE 2.—Cytoplasmic FoxP3 immunostaining in different thyroid tissues. This boxplot of the immunohistochemical quantification data provides evidence of progressive FoxP3 staining in different stages of tumor evolution. Computer-generated numerical values that represent the intensity and extent of the brown (FoxP3) staining are plotted on the y-axis. Abbreviations: NT = normal thyroid; G = goiter; FA = follicular adenoma; FVPTC = follicular variant of papillary thyroid carcinoma; CPTC = classic papillary thyroid carcinoma; FC = follicular carcinoma. (Reprinted from Cunha LL, Morari EC, Nonogaki S, et al. FoxP3 expression is associated with aggressiveness in differentiated thyroid carcinomas. *Clinics.* 2012;67:483-488, with permission from Clinics.)

patient age. Nuclear FoxP3 staining was more intense in younger patients and in tumors presenting with metastasis at diagnosis. FoxP3$^+$ lymphocytes were more frequent in tumors smaller than 2 cm, those without extrathyroidal invasion, and in patients with concurrent chronic lymphocytic thyroiditis.

Conclusions.—We demonstrated FoxP3 expression in differentiated thyroid carcinoma cells and found evidence that this expression may exert an important influence on several features of tumor aggressiveness (Figs 1 and 2).

▶ The expression of FoxP3 in the thyroid gland has been investigated before in the regulatory T (treg) lymphocyte—associated tumor cells of papillary carcinoma cases[1] and was reviewed in the Year Book of 2010. This article deals with the expression of this interesting marker not only in the T-regulatory lymphocytes but also in the thyroid gland normal follicular cells and their different derivative neoplasms (ie, follicular adenoma, follicular carcinoma, and classic papillary carcinoma and its follicular variant). Figs 1 and 2 illustrate the authors' findings that the cytoplasmic expression is increased in hyperplastic conditions and more significantly increased in tumorous thyroid conditions in contrast to the normal tissue that has the lowest levels of expression. The authors also mention that Foxp3 nuclear expression is increased in the tumors presenting with metastasis, although their log-rank analysis could not validate FoxP3 as a reliable prognostic marker. Although on many occasions the diagnosis of thyroid cancers can be a straightforward task, they can present diagnostic challenges and difficulties in making definitive decisions, and indeed genuine differences exist in diagnostic opinions. During the last two editions of the YEAR BOOK we reviewed different genetic and immunohistochemical markers that are currently used or may have a future use in helping with this task and providing potential value in explaining the evolution and prognosis of these tumors. The data presented in this article, if they stands the test of time and other group validations and scrutiny, can provide a marker to neoplastic changes in the thyroid gland and additional studies may indeed help to determine that. The findings of this article were also interesting because of the authors' review of their 253 components of papillary carcinoma and that they showed more expression in the small tumors and for the presence of concurrent tumors in the absence of extrathyroidal extension. The authors commented that this finding is in contrast to the findings of French et al,[1] whose studies revealed more association with lymph node metastasis. However, there are differences in methodology and case selection; for example, French et al selected cases that did not show evidence of associated chronic lymphocytic thyroiditis.

M. S. Said, MD, PhD

Reference

1. French JD, Weber ZJ, Fretwell DL, Said S, Klopper JP, Haugen BR. Tumor-associated lymphocytes and increased FoxP3+ regulatory T cell frequency correlate with more aggressive papillary thyroid cancer. *J Clin Endocrinol Metab.* 2010;95: 2325-2333.

Villous Papillary Thyroid Carcinoma: a Variant Associated with Marfan Syndrome

Winer DA, Winer S, Rotstein L, et al (Univ Health Network, Toronto, Ontario, Canada)
Endocr Pathol 2012 [Epub ahead of print]

Background.—Marfan syndrome (MFS) is a hereditary autosomal dominant disorder of the extracellular matrix usually associated with mutations in the fibrillin-1 (FBN1) gene. Patients with MFS usually have skeletal, ocular, and cardiovascular manifestations, such as tall slender stature, arachnodactyly, scoliosis, pectus excavatum or carinatum, ectopia lentis, and aortic dilatation or dissection. No relationship has been noted between MFS and papillary thyroid carcinoma (PTC), the most common endocrine malignancy. Distinct genetic events are associated with PTC, producing numerous variants. Several biomarkers are predictive of aggressive or invasive behavior in PTC. EMT is a trans-differentiation program in which epithelial cells lose cell adhesion, reorganize their cytoskeleton, and exhibit increased mobility. It may promote early invasive behavior in cancer and is strongly induced by TGF-β. A unique histologic villous growth pattern of PTC was found in a patient with MFS.

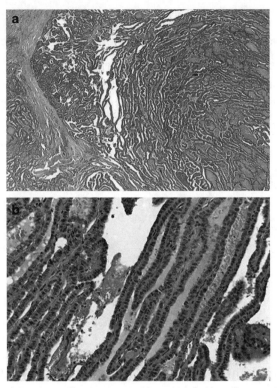

FIGURE 1.—a—b Invasive papillary carcinoma with a unique florid papillary growth pattern characterized by long villous fronds (hematoxylin and eosin). (Reprinted from Winer DA, Winer S, Rotstein L, et al. Villous papillary thyroid carcinoma: a variant associated with marfan syndrome. *Endocr Pathol.* 2012;[Epub ahead of print], with permission from Springer Science+Business Media, LLC.)

Case Report.—Man, 46, with a known history of MFS had a left thyroid mass found on routine physical examination. His sister and two nephews had MFS, and he had already tested positive for the known familial mutation in the FBN1 gene. The patient also reported insulin resistance, remote tonsillectomy, and mild aortic root enlargement visible on echocardiogram. He had no exposure to ionizing radiation or family history of thyroid cancer and was taking no medications. Physical examination revealed he was tall with marfanoid habitus and a firm mass in the left thyroid. Laboratory tests found normal thyroid-stimulating hormone (TSH) levels, normal free T4 levels, and negative anti-thyroid peroxidase and anti-thyroglobulin antibodies. Ultrasound revealed a mass in the left upper pole of the thyroid measuring $3.0 \times 2.9 \times 2.6$ cm. The results of needle biopsy were suspicious for PTC.

Total thyroidectomy with paratracheal node sampling was performed. Gross examination confirmed the nodule in the left

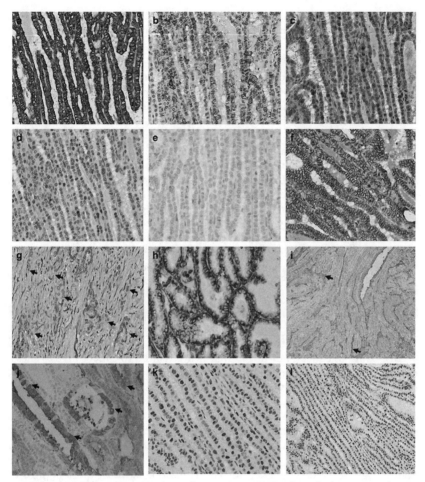

FIGURE 2.—The tumor is positive for cytokeratin 19 (a), HBME-1 (b), and galectin-3 (c) with prominent nuclear expression of cyclin D1 (d) and loss of nuclear p27 (e). The tumor exhibits variable expression of Ecadherin, with central regions maintaining strong membranous staining (f), whereas the invasive fronts show either weak expression or loss of E-cadherin (g, *arrows*). Expression of vimentin (h) is consistent with widespread changes of epithelial–mesenchymal transition. Staining for TGF-β (i) confirms the presence of abundant cytokine present in the stroma of this tumor (*arrows*), as well as within the tumor cell cytoplasm (j, *arrows*). Phosphorylated SMAD3 (k) and p21 (l) are strongly reactive in tumor cell nuclei, consistent with prominent TGF-β signal activation. (Reprinted from Winer DA, Winer S, Rotstein L, et al. Villous papillary thyroid carcinoma: a variant associated with marfan syndrome. *Endocr Pathol.* 2012;[Epub ahead of print], with permission from Springer Science+Business Media, LLC.)

upper pole of the thyroid. Histologic analysis revealed the lesion was a widely invasive papillary carcinoma with a unique florid papillary growth pattern marked by long villous fronds. Extensive invasive growth with focal involvement of the surgical resection margin was noted. Vascular invasion characterized by intravascular tumor cells with adherent thrombus and microscopic lymph node metastasis were noted in one paratracheal node. No unequivocal evidence of extrathyroidal extension was found in the surgical specimen.

Additional molecular and immunohistochemical tests revealed nuclear staining for TTF-1 and cytoplasmic positivity for thyroglobulin, indicating thyroid origin. The tumor strongly stained positively for markers of malignancy associated with PTC and showed prominent nuclear expression of cyclin D1 and loss of nuclear p27—indicating an aggressive profile. Staining for E-cadherin and vimentin yielded variable expression of E-cadherin, central regions with strong membranous expression, and weak expression or loss at invasive fronts. The center and periphery of the tumor demonstrated regional expression of vimentin, which is characteristic of widespread EMT changes. Abundant cytokine was noted in tumor stroma and focally in tumor cytoplasm. Tumor cells stained for phosphorylated SMAD3 showed prominent TGF-? signal activation. Genetic analysis found BRAF gene mutation consistent with prominent papillary tumor architecture.

Conclusions.—This documents the first case of PTC found in a patient with MFS. The histologic pattern of the tumor is unique and may be related to the environment in which it developed. MFS is not considered predisposing to cancer, but its hallmarks are related to cancer invasiveness. Further studies will be needed to determine if this is a new variant of PTC, villous PTC, associated with MFS (Figs 1 and 2).

▶ This is an interesting article illustrating the features of what could prove to be a new morphologic appearance of papillary thyroid carcinoma. Being the most common type of thyroid cancer, papillary thyroid carcinoma exhibits a number of morphologic variants, some purely morphologic without much departure from the expected clinical behavior and some predictive of more aggressive behavior for the tumor cells. The authors, in their discussion, hypothesize on the causes of the unusual morphology, in that it could be caused by the combination of *BRAF* mutation, altered transforming growth factor-β signaling, and the weak connective tissue integrity seen in Marfan syndrome, and relate their other findings to it, as seen in the abstract. They also mention in their discussion the relation of the cribriform morular variant of papillary thyroid carcinoma to familial adenomatous polyposis (FAP) as an example of a variant of a morphology/distinct genetic syndrome linkage. Although the incidence of FAP far exceeds that of Marfan syndrome in general, let alone the copresence of papillary carcinoma, it is an observation worth recording in the literature and may prove more valid in the future if other cases present themselves in a recurring constant observation, even in rare instances as with Marfan syndrome. Although this is the first description of this morphology, it also brings to mind the presence of the elongated compressed thinned follicles seen in the tall cell variant in some cases, while here we see the elongated thinned crowded villous papillary forms (and maybe also elongated follicles) that in some fashion both appear on a somewhat similar morphologic continuum.

M. S. Said, MD, PhD

Human Papillomavirus-16 Infection in Advanced Oral Cavity Cancer Patients Is Related to an Increased Risk of Distant Metastases and Poor Survival

Lee L-A, Huang C-G, Liao C-T, et al (Chang Gung Memorial Hosp and Chang Gung Univ, Taoyuan, Taiwan)

PLoS ONE 7:e40767, 2012

Background.—Human papillomavirus (HPV) is an oncogenic virus causing oropharyngeal cancers and resulting in a favorable outcome after the treatment. The role of HPV in oral cavity squamous cell carcinoma (OSCC) remains ambiguous.

Objective.—This study aimed to examine the effect of HPV infection on disease control among patients with OSCC following radical surgery with radiation-based adjuvant therapy.

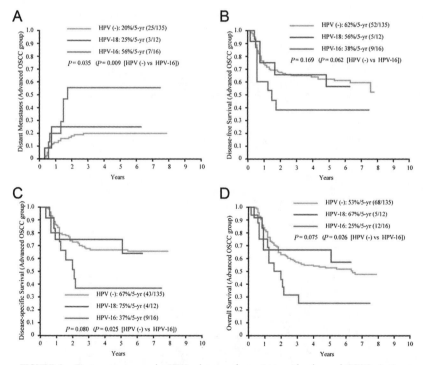

FIGURE 2.—Five-year outcomes by HPV subgroups for patients with advanced OSCC. A, time to distant metastases; B, DFS; C, DSS; D, OS. (Reprinted from Lee L-A, Huang C-G, Liao C-T, et al. Human papillomavirus-16 infection in advanced oral cavity cancer patients is related to an increased risk of distant metastases and poor survival. *PLoS One.* 2012;7:e40767, © National Center for Biotechnology Information.)

TABLE 1.—HPV Statuses and 5-Year Control and Survival Rates in Advanced OSCC Patients (n = 173)

Characteristics (n, %)	Local Control (5-yr %, n Event)	P	Neck Control (5-yr %, n Event)	P	Distant Metastases (5-yr %, n Event)	P	Disease-Free Survival (5-yr %, n Event)	P	Disease-Specific Survival (5-yr %, n Event)	P	Overall Survival (5-yr %, n Event)	P
Solitary HPV-16		0.774		0.726		0.007		0.058		0.025		0.028
No (157, 91)	84 (23)		82 (28)		19 (28)		62 (61)		68 (50)		53 (80)	
Yes (16, 9)	87 (2)		77 (3)		56 (7)		38 (9)		37 (9)		25 (12)	
Solitary HPV-18		0.797		0.416		0.685		0.955		0.996		0.602
No (161, 93)	86 (23)		81 (30)		20 (32)		60 (65)		66 (55)		46 (87)	
Yes (12, 7)	83 (2)		92 (1)		25 (3)		58 (5)		67 (4)		58 (5)	
HPV-16 and/or HPV-18		0.378		0.634		0.031		0.125		0.057		0.088
No (143, 83)	86 (20)		81 (27)		18 (25)		62 (55)		69 (45)		49 (73)	
Yes (30, 17)	83 (5)		87 (4)		43 (10)		50 (15)		53 (14)		37 (19)	
High-risk HPV		0.361		0.653		0.147		0.188		0.078		0.073
No (137, 79)	86 (19)		81 (26)		18 (25)		61 (53)		69 (43)		50 (69)	
Yes (36, 21)	83 (6)		86 (5)		28 (10)		53 (17)		56 (16)		36 (23)	
HPV		0.512		0.528		0.230		0.352		0.158		0.113
No (135, 78)	86 (19)		81 (26)		19 (25)		61 (53)		68 (43)		50 (68)	
Yes (38, 22)	84 (6)		87 (5)		27 (10)		55 (17)		58 (16)		37 (24)	

HPV: human papillomavirus. OSCC: oral squamous cell carcinoma. n: patient number. W-M: Well-moderate.

Patients and Method.—We prospectively followed 173 patients with advanced OSCC (96% were stage III/IV) who had undergone radical surgery and adjuvant therapy between 2004 and 2006. They were followed between surgery and death or up to 60 months. Surgical specimens were examined using a PCR-based HPV blot test. The primary endpoints were the risk of relapse and the time to relapse; the secondary endpoints were disease-free survival, disease-specific survival, and overall survival.

Results.—The prevalence of HPV-positive OSCC was 22%; HPV-16 (9%) and HPV-18 (7%) were the genotypes most commonly encountered. Solitary HPV-16 infection was a poor predictor of 5-year distant metastases (hazard ratio, 3.4; 95% confidence interval, 1.4–8.0; $P = 0.005$), disease-free survival ($P = 0.037$), disease-specific survival ($P = 0.006$), and overall survival ($P = 0.010$), whereas HPV-18 infection had no impact on 5-year outcomes. The rate of 5-year distant metastases was significantly higher in the HPV-16 or level IV/V metastasis group compared with both the extracapsular spread or tumor depth ≥11-mm group and patients without risk factors ($P < 0.001$).

Conclusions.—HPV infections in advanced OSCC patients are not uncommon and clinically relevant. Compared with HPV-16-negative advanced OSCC patients, those with a single HPV-16 infection are at higher risk of distant metastases and poor survival despite undergoing radiation-based adjuvant therapy and require a more aggressive adjuvant treatment and a more thorough follow-up (Fig 2, Table 1).

▶ The role of human papillomavirus (HPV) infections as an etiologic factor in head and neck cancers continues to be characterized after decades of regarding smoking and alcohol use as the 2 main contributing agents to oral cancer. This article adds the results of an interesting study on the effect of oncogenic HPV high-risk "subtype" infection on the prognosis of oral cancer, namely HPV-16 and -18 (see Table 1, Fig 2). HPV-16 and -18 are high-risk HPV types and are the most prevalent types in female cervix cancers and are actually 2 of the major HPV subtype components of the current HPV vaccine for prevention of cervical cancer in women, as is well-known. The study shows the prevalence of these 2 subtypes in 173 patients with advanced oral squamous cell carcinoma and supplies the important conclusion indicated in the abstract with solitary HPV-16's (and not HPV-18's) relationship to a poorer prognostic outcome as enumerated in the abstract. Such findings should impact the aggressiveness of the therapeutic protocols for these patients and may indicate or highlight the necessity for differential HPV high-risk typing when testing tumor tissue. The conclusion of the study shows that solitary HPV-16 infection in patients with advanced oral squamous cell carcinoma requires priority adjuvant treatment and follow-up because of increased risk of early metastasis and death. In addition, the study also showed that the level of region IV/V metastasis, extracapsular extension, and tumor depth of more than 11 mm are independent risk factors for 5-year distant metastasis in advanced oral squamous cell carcinoma.

M. S. Said, MD, PhD

13 Neuropathology

Chronic Traumatic Encephalopathy: A Potential Late Effect of Sport-Related Concussive and Subconcussive Head Trauma
Gavett BE, Stern RA, McKee AC (Boston Univ, MA)
Clin Sports Med 30:179-188, 2011

Chronic traumatic encephalopathy (CTE) is a form of neurodegeneration believed to result from repeated head injuries. Originally termed *dementia pugilistica* because of its association with boxing, the neuropathology of CTE was first described by Corsellis in 1973 in a case series of 15 retired boxers. CTE has recently been found to occur after other causes of repeated head trauma, suggesting that any repeated blows to the head, such as those that occur in American football, hockey, soccer, professional wrestling, and physical abuse, can also lead to neurodegenerative changes. These changes often include cerebral atrophy, cavum septi pellucidi with fenestrations, shrinkage of the mammillary bodies, dense tau immunoreactive inclusions (neurofibrillary tangles, glial tangles, and neuropil neurites), and, in some cases, a TDP-43 proteinopathy. In association with these pathologic changes, disordered memory and executive functioning, behavioral and personality disturbances (eg, apathy, depression, irritability, impulsiveness, suicidality), parkinsonism, and, occasionally, motor neuron disease are seen in affected individuals. No formal clinical or pathologic diagnostic criteria for CTE currently exist, but the distinctive neuropathologic profile of the disorder lends promise for future research into its prevention, diagnosis, and treatment.

▶ Although this is a review article summarizing current knowledge related to chronic traumatic encephalopathy (CTE), I believe it is 10 pages worth reading on this topic for several reasons. First, the authors of this review perform research in this area, so they are experts on CTE at the laboratory level. Second, the authors make a point of emphasizing the distinctive gross and microscopic neuropathologic features of this disease that clearly separate it from Alzheimer's disease and other neurodegenerative diseases, even though it may be considered a tau protein—associated disease. Third, awareness of these distinctive pathologic features is necessary to recognize them at autopsy and, thus, provide clinical staff caring for the patient and the patient's family with complete and accurate cause of death information. Because the incidence and prevalence of CTE are unknown because of the infrequency of autopsy performance, accurate recognition of this disorder is especially important.

D. M. Grzybicki, MD, PhD

Inflammatory Cortical Demyelination in Early Multiple Sclerosis

Lucchinetti CF, Popescu BFG, Bunyan RF, et al (Mayo Clinic College of Medicine, Rochester, MN; et al)

N Engl J Med 365:2188-2197, 2011

Background.—Cortical disease has emerged as a critical aspect of the pathogenesis of multiple sclerosis, being associated with disease progression and cognitive impairment. Most studies of cortical lesions have focused on autopsy findings in patients with long-standing, chronic, progressive multiple sclerosis, and the noninflammatory nature of these lesions has been emphasized. Magnetic resonance imaging studies indicate that cortical damage occurs early in the disease.

Methods.—We evaluated the prevalence and character of demyelinating cortical lesions in patients with multiple sclerosis. Cortical tissues were obtained in passing during biopsy sampling of white-matter lesions. In most cases, biopsy was done with the use of stereotactic procedures to diagnose suspected tumors. Patients with sufficient cortex (138 of 563 patients screened) were evaluated for cortical demyelination. Using immunohistochemistry, we characterized cortical lesions with respect to demyelinating activity, inflammatory infiltrates, the presence of meningeal inflammation, and a topographic association between cortical demyelination and meningeal inflammation. Diagnoses were ascertained in a subgroup of 77 patients (56%) at the last follow-up visit (at a median of 3.5 years).

Results.—Cortical demyelination was present in 53 patients (38%) (104 lesions and 222 tissue blocks) and was absent in 85 patients (121 tissue blocks). Twenty-five patients with cortical demyelination had definite multiple sclerosis (81% of 31 patients who underwent long-term follow-up), as did 33 patients without cortical demyelination (72% of 46 patients who underwent long-term follow-up). In representative tissues, 58 of 71 lesions (82%) showed CD3+ T-cell infiltrates, and 32 of 78 lesions (41%) showed macrophage-associated demyelination. Meningeal inflammation was topographically associated with cortical demyelination in patients who had sufficient meningeal tissue for study.

Conclusions.—In this cohort of patients with early-stage multiple sclerosis, cortical demyelinating lesions were frequent, inflammatory, and strongly associated with meningeal inflammation. (Funded by the National Multiple Sclerosis Society and the National Institutes of Health.)

▶ Historically, multiple sclerosis (MS) has been characterized as an inflammatory, demyelinating, white matter disease; however, recent neuropathologic studies have reported the additional existence of demyelinating cortical gray matter lesions in patients with this disease. The presence of cortical lesions has been associated with the clinically expected cognitive or discrete neurologic deficits and correlates with prognosis. Before the publication of this article, cortical demyelination primarily has been described in patients with long-standing MS and as lacking associated inflammation. These authors describe the presence of cortical inflammation and demyelination as well as meningeal inflammation in a subset of brain tissues from patients undergoing stereotactic biopsy procedures for suspected tumor. These patients were subsequently diagnosed with early MS. Because cortical involvement in MS is known to correlate with prognosis, these findings may support the clinical usefulness of the identification of cortical inflammatory demyelinating lesions in patients with MS at the time of initial onset.

D. M. Grzybicki, MD, PhD

Differential analysis of glioblastoma multiforme proteome by a 2D-DIGE approach

Collet B, Guitton N, Saïkali S, et al (Centre Régional de Lutte contre le Cancer, Rennes, France; High-Throughput Proteomics Platform Biogenouest, Rennes, France; CHU Pontchaillou, Rennes, France; et al)
Proteome Sci 9:16, 2011

Background.—Genomics, transcriptomics and proteomics of glioblastoma multiforme (GBM) have recently emerged as possible tools to discover therapeutic targets and biomarkers for new therapies including immunotherapy. It is well known that macroscopically complete surgical excision, radiotherapy and chemotherapy have therapeutic limitations to improve survival in these patients. In this study, we used a differential proteomic-based technique (2D-Difference Gel Electrophoresis) coupled with matrix-assisted laser desorption/ionization-time of flight (MALDI-TOF) mass spectrometry to identify proteins that may serve as brain tumor antigens in new therapeutic assays. Five samples of patients presenting a GBM and five samples of microscopically normal brain tissues derived from brain epileptic surgery specimen were labeled and run in 2D-PAGE (Two-Dimensional Polyacrylamide Gel Electrophoresis) with an internal pool sample on each gel. Five gels were matched and compared with DIA (Difference In-gel Analysis) software. Differential spots were picked, in-gel digested and peptide mass fingerprints were obtained.

Results.—From 51 protein-spots significantly up-regulated in GBM samples, mass spectrometry (MS) identified twenty-two proteins. The differential expression of a selected protein set was first validated by western-blotting, then tested on large cohorts of GBM specimens and non-tumor tissues, using immunohistochemistry and real-time RT-PCR.

Conclusions.—Our results confirmed the importance of previously described proteins in glioma pathology and their potential usefulness as biological markers but also revealed some new interesting targets for future therapies.

▶ A large body of proteomics literature exists that focuses on the identification of glioblastoma multiforme (GBM)—associated proteins useful for diagnosis or clinical management. The search for clinically important tumor protein targets is motivated by both high interobserver variability for histopathologic diagnosis and a persistent lack of other feasible molecular targets useful for therapies resulting in widespread improvement in the outcomes of patients with GBM.

This article by Collet et al is a good example of the type of proteomics study currently populating this body of literature.

The authors performed a case-control study with 5 samples of patient GBM tissue and 5 samples of microscopically normal tissue from patients who had cortical excisions secondary to a seizure disorder. Comparison of tissue proteins present in the 2 samples was performed using 2-dimensional difference gel electrophoresis together with matrix-assisted laser desorption/ionization time-of-flight mass spectrometry. Their results are important because they not only confirm the upregulation of multiple proteins in GBM tissues that previously have been reported (eg, HSP 27 and Mn-SOD) but also describe the upregulation of proteins not previously reported (eg, alkaline dehydrogenase) that warrant further investigation as potential therapeutic targets.

The major limitations of the study are that it is a single-center study with examination of a small number of specimens, and this is the major limitation of many of the currently published proteomics studies related to GBM. These limitations, together with the lack of standardized methods, have resulted in relatively inconsistent or invalidated information. In response to these limitations, the National Cancer Institute has developed the Proteome Characterization Centers, a collaborative aimed at providing validated, comprehensive genomic and proteomic information about multiple tumor types (including GBM) and developing and improving proteomic technologies.[1]

D. M. Grzybicki, MD, PhD

Reference

1. Kalinina J, Peng J, Ritchie JC, Van Meir EG. Proteomics of gliomas: Initial biomarker discovery and evolution of technology. *Neuro Oncol.* 2011;13:926-942.

A yeast functional screen predicts new candidate ALS disease genes
Couthouis J, Hart MP, Shorter J, et al (Univ of Pennsylvania School of Medicine, Philadelphia; et al)
Proc Natl Acad Sci U S A 108:20881-20890, 2011

Amyotrophic lateral sclerosis (ALS) is a devastating and universally fatal neurodegenerative disease. Mutations in two related RNA-binding proteins, TDP-43 and FUS, that harbor prion-like domains, cause some forms of ALS. There are at least 213 human proteins harboring RNA recognition motifs, including FUS and TDP-43, raising the possibility that additional RNA-binding proteins might contribute to ALS pathogenesis. We performed a systematic survey of these proteins to find additional candidates similar to TDP-43 and FUS, followed by bioinformatics to predict prion-like domains in a subset of them. We sequenced one of these genes, *TAF15*, in patients with ALS and identified missense variants, which were absent in a large number of healthy controls. These disease-associated variants of TAF15 caused formation of cytoplasmic foci when expressed in primary cultures of spinal cord neurons. Very similar to TDP-43 and FUS, TAF15 aggregated in vitro and conferred neurodegeneration in *Drosophila*, with the ALS-linked variants having a more severe effect than wild type. Immunohistochemistry of post-mortem spinal cord tissue revealed mislocalization of TAF15 in motor neurons of patients with ALS. We propose that aggregation-prone RNA-binding proteins might contribute very broadly to ALS pathogenesis and the genes identified in our yeast functional screen, coupled with prion-like domain prediction analysis, now provide a powerful resource to facilitate ALS disease gene discovery.

▶ Amyotrophic lateral sclerosis (ALS), as well as other neurodegenerative diseases, has been shown to be associated with an accumulation of misfolded proteins in neurons and glia in the central nervous system. Spreading of mis-folded protein conformations present in Alzheimer's disease, similar to the mech-anism of infectious prions, was demonstrated approximately 2 decades ago. Since that time, a significant amount of evidence has been generated supporting the idea that multiple neurodegenerative diseases, including ALS, progress clin-ically and neuropathologically via a mechanism similar to prions. In addition, it is now clear that the accumulation of 2 RNA binding proteins (FUS and TDP-43), which have domains similar to prions, is responsible for the development of ALS in some patients.

The findings reported in this article by Couthouis et al are important for 2 major reasons. First, they describe another RNA-binding protein, TAF-15, which demonstrates characteristics similar to FUS and TDP-43 both in vitro and in vivo, thus making it a good candidate for involvement in the pathogenesis of ALS. Second, the investigators describe methods for screening and testing candidate proteins that will most likely be highly useful for identifying additional proteins potentially involved in the pathogenesis of ALS as well as with the path-ogenesis of other neurodegenerative diseases known to involve accumulations of misfolded proteins.

D. M. Grzybicki, MD, PhD

Progression of Tau Pathology in Cholinergic Basal Forebrain Neurons in Mild Cognitive Impairment and Alzheimer's Disease

Vana L, Kanaan NM, Ugwu IC, et al (Northwestern Univ, Chicago, IL; Michigan State Univ, Grand Rapids; et al)
Am J Pathol 179:2533-2550, 2011

Tau is a microtubule-associated protein that forms neurofibrillary tangles (NFTs) in the selective vulnerable long projection neurons of the cholinergic basal forebrain (CBF) in Alzheimer's disease (AD). Although CBF neurode-generation correlates with cognitive decline during AD progression, little is known about the temporal changes of tau accumulation in this region. We investigated tau posttranslational modifications during NFT evolution within the CBF neurons of the nucleus basalis (NB) using tissue from subjects with no cognitive impairment, mild cognitive impairment, and AD. The pS422 anti-body was used as an early tau pathology marker that labels tau phosphory-lated at Ser422; the TauC3 antibody was used to detect later stage tau pathology. Stereologic evaluation of NB tissue immunostained for pS422 and TauC3 revealed an increase in neurons expressing these tau epitopes during disease progression. We also investigated the occurrence of pretangle tau events within cholinergic NB neurons by dual staining for the cholinergic cell marker, p75[NTR], which displays a phenotypic down-regulation within CBF perikarya in AD. As pS422+ neurons increased in number, p75[NTR]+ neurons decreased, and these changes correlated with both AD neuropathology and cognitive decline. Also, NFTs developed slower in the CBF compared with previously examined cortical regions. Taken together, these results suggest that changes in cognition are associated with pretangle events within NB cholinergic neurons before frank NFT deposition.

▶ The clinical diagnosis of mild cognitive impairment (MCI) was generated out of neurology memory clinics and has become a common diagnosis among elderly patients in the United States. It is used to characterize patients who are single-domain impaired and thus do not fit the minimum criteria for Alzheimer's disease (AD). Most patients with clinical MCI have memory loss and do progress to AD, although not all follow this clinical course. Characterization of the neuropathologic correlates of MCI is important in order to better understand its pathogenesis and its potential relationship to AD.

This article by Vana et al is important because it describes the progression of both tau pathological characteristics in cholinergic basal forebrain neurons (CBF) and cognitive changes from normal brains to patients with MCI and finally to patients with AD. They show that phosphorylated tau, present in CBF but not yet forming neurofibrillary tangles (NFT), is associated with declining cognition. Therefore, the initial accumulation of phosphorylated tau appears to be toxic for CBF and to correlate with MCI, rather than the presence or volume of NFT. These findings provide information that may be useful for development of MCI and AD therapies aimed at posttranslational phosphorylated tau.

D. M. Grzybicki, MD, PhD

Association of *LRRK2* exonic variants with susceptibility to Parkinson's disease: a case—control study
Ross OA, on behalf of the Genetic Epidemiology Of Parkinson's Disease (GEO-PD) Consortium (Mayo Clinic, Jacksonville, FL; et al)
Lancet Neurol 10:898-908, 2012

Background.—The leucine-rich repeat kinase 2 gene (*LRRK2*) harbours highly penetrant mutations that are linked to familial parkinsonism. However, the extent of its polymorphic variability in relation to risk of Parkinson's disease (PD) has not been assessed systematically. We therefore assessed the frequency of *LRRK2* exonic variants in individuals with and without PD, to investigate the role of the variants in PD susceptibility.

Methods.—*LRRK2* was genotyped in patients with PD and controls from three series (white, Asian, and Arab—Berber) from sites participating in the Genetic Epidemiology of Parkinson's Disease Consortium. Genotyping was done for exonic variants of LRRK2 that were identified through searches of literature and the personal communications of consortium members. Associations with PD were assessed by use of logistic regression models. For variants that had a minor allele frequency of $0 \cdot 5\%$ or greater, single variant associations were assessed, whereas for rarer variants information was collapsed across variants.

Findings.—121 exonic *LRRK2* variants were assessed in 15 540 individuals: 6995 white patients with PD and 5595 controls, 1376 Asian patients and 962 controls, and 240 Arab—Berber patients and 372 controls. After exclusion of carriers of known pathogenic mutations, new independent risk associations were identified for polymorphic variants in white individuals (M1646T, odds ratio $1 \cdot 43$, 95% CI $1 \cdot 15 - 1 \cdot 78$; $p = 0 \cdot 0012$) and Asian individuals (A419V, $2 \cdot 27$, $1 \cdot 35 - 3 \cdot 83$; $p = 0 \cdot 0011$). A protective haplotype (N551K-R1398H-K1423K) was noted at a frequency greater than 5% in the white and Asian series, with a similar finding in the Arab—Berber series (combined odds ratio $0 \cdot 82$, $0 \cdot 72 - 0 \cdot 94$; $p = 0 \cdot 0043$). Of the two previously reported Asian risk variants, G2385R was associated with disease ($1 \cdot 73$, $1 \cdot 20 - 2 \cdot 49$; $p = 0 \cdot 0026$), but no association was noted for R1628P ($0 \cdot 62$, $0 \cdot 36 - 1 \cdot 07$; $p = 0 \cdot 087$). In the Arab—Berber series, Y2189C showed potential evidence of risk association with PD ($4 \cdot 48$, $1 \cdot 33 - 15 \cdot 09$; $p = 0 \cdot 012$).

Interpretation.—The results for *LRRK2* show that several rare and common genetic variants in the same gene can have independent effects on disease risk. LRRK2, and the pathway in which it functions, is important in the cause and pathogenesis of PD in a greater proportion of patients with this disease than previously believed. These results will help discriminate those patients who will benefit most from therapies targeted at LRRK2 pathogenic activity.

▶ Previous studies have shown that variations in the gene LRRK2 are significantly associated with Parkinson's disease, both familial and sporadic forms. LRRK2 codes for an enzyme with both kinase and GTPase activities. A pathogenic mechanism involving toxic levels of enzyme activity in dopaminergic neurons underpins current therapeutic investigations aimed at the development of an effective kinase inhibitor.

This study by multiple international members of the Genetic Epidemiology of Parkinson's Disease Consortium is important because, due to the large nature of the study, the investigators were able to validate previously proposed risk-associated mutations, provide evidence for a lack of risk association for variants previously proposed to have associations, and identify new variants with independent risk associations. That ethnic variability could also be demonstrated is both scientifically and clinically significant. A key characteristic of their sampling method that may be important for understanding risk associations contributed by specific variants is that, because of the lack of complete clinical information for every patient, their sample likely included patients with both familial and sporadic forms of the disease.

D. M. Grzybicki, MD, PhD

Simulated brain biopsy for diagnosing neurodegeneration using autopsy-confirmed cases

Venneti S, Robinson JL, Roy S, et al (Univ of Pennsylvania, Philadelphia)
Acta Neuropathol 122:737-745, 2011

Risks associated with brain biopsy limit availability of tissues and the role of brain biopsy in diagnosing neurodegeneration is unclear. We developed a simulated brain biopsy paradigm to comprehensively evaluate potential accuracy of detecting neurodegeneration in biopsies. Postmortem tissue from the frontal, temporal and parietal cortices and basal ganglia from 73 cases including Alzheimer's disease (AD), Lewy body disease (LBD), frontotemporal lobar degeneration-TDP43 (FTLD-TDP), multiple system atrophy (MSA), Pick's disease (PiD), corticobasal degeneration (CBD) and progressive supranuclear palsy (PSP) were evaluated using H&E and immunostains. Brain biopsy was simulated in a blinded manner by masking each slide with opaque tape except for an area measuring 10 mm in diameter. Diagnoses obtained from frontal cortex only or all 4-brain regions were then compared with autopsy diagnoses. Diagnostic sensitivity in frontal cortex was highest in FTLD-TDP (88%), AD (80%) and LBD (79%); intermediate for MSA (71%), CBD (66%) and PiD (66%) and lowest for PSP (0%) (average 64%). Specificity was 43%. Sensitivities were enhanced with all 4-brain regions: FTLD-TDP (100%), AD (80%), LBD (100%), MSA (100%), CBD (83%), PiD (100%) and PSP (88%) (average 92%). Specificity was 71%. Simulated brain biopsy addressed limitations of standard brain biopsies such as tissue availability and lack of autopsy confirmation of diagnoses. These data could inform efforts to establish criteria for biopsy diagnosis of neurodegenerative disorders to guide care of individuals who undergo biopsy for enigmatic causes of cognitive impairment or when evidence of an underlying neurodegenerative disease may influence future therapy.

▶ This study by Venneti et al reveals important information about the current probabilities of accurately diagnosing neurodegenerative diseases on brain biopsy. Based on the length of the authors' discussion and their exhaustive consideration of all the limitations of the study, it appears that reviewers focused on the fact that this is not a clinical effectiveness study aimed at the simulation of diagnostic performance in day-to-day practice. However, despite this limitation, I believe the information is important because it provides data related to an emerging challenge in neuropathology practice. As the US population continues to age and therapies for neurodegeneration are developed, it will become more and more important for neuropathologists to provide accurate (although likely limited) diagnostic information to clinicians about the presence of neurodegenerative diseases during life.

D. M. Grzybicki, MD, PhD

14 Cytopathology

Preoperative Diagnosis of Benign Thyroid Nodules with Indeterminate Cytology
Alexander EK, Kennedy GC, Baloch ZW, et al (Brigham and Women's Hosp and Harvard Med School, Boston; Veracyte, South San Francisco, CA; Univ of Pennsylvania, Philadelphia; et al)
N Engl J Med 367:705-715, 2012

Background.—Approximately 15 to 30% of thyroid nodules evaluated by means of fine-needle aspiration are not clearly benign or malignant. Patients with cytologically indeterminate nodules are often referred for diagnostic surgery, though most of these nodules prove to be benign. A novel diagnostic test that measures the expression of 167 genes has shown promise in improving preoperative risk assessment.

Methods.—We performed a 19-month, prospective, multicenter validation study involving 49 clinical sites, 3789 patients, and 4812 fine-needle aspirates from thyroid nodules 1 cm or larger that required evaluation. We obtained 577 cytologically indeterminate aspirates, 413 of which had corresponding histopathological specimens from excised lesions. Results of a central, blinded histopathological review served as the reference standard. After inclusion criteria were met, a gene-expression classifier was used to test 265 indeterminate nodules in this analysis, and its performance was assessed.

Results.—Of the 265 indeterminate nodules, 85 were malignant. The gene-expression classifier correctly identified 78 of the 85 nodules as suspicious (92% sensitivity; 95% confidence interval [CI], 84 to 97), with a specificity of 52% (95% CI, 44 to 59). The negative predictive values for "atypia (or follicular lesion) of undetermined clinical significance," "follicular neoplasm or lesion suspicious for follicular neoplasm," or "suspicious cytologic findings" were 95%, 94%, and 85%, respectively. Analysis of 7 aspirates with false negative results revealed that 6 had a paucity of thyroid follicular cells, suggesting insufficient sampling of the nodule.

Conclusions.—These data suggest consideration of a more conservative approach for most patients with thyroid nodules that are cytologically indeterminate on fine-needle aspiration and benign according to gene-expression classifier results. (Funded by Veracyte.)

▶ Alexander and colleagues show the potential value of ancillary testing using a microarray assay described as a gene-expression classifier for cytologically indeterminate fine needle aspiration specimens (Fig 1 in the original article). The authors point out that from 15% to 30% of aspirates yield indeterminate results,

271

including the diagnoses of atypia (or follicular lesion) of undetermined signifi-cance, follicular neoplasm or suspicious for follicular neoplasm, and suspicious for malignancy and that many patients with these diagnoses undergo surgical excision to prove that they have a benign condition. In the current situation, why do so many patients have these cytologic diagnoses? Although the authors may consider that the diagnosis of follicular neoplasm or suspicious for follicular neoplasm is nondiagnostic, the general nature of these lesions is one in which a cytopathologist cannot definitively determine if malignancy is present. These lesions often are adenomas (with some being cellular hyperplastic nodules) that cannot be distinguished by a follicular carcinoma because the features of capsular or vascular invasion cannot be assessed by fine-needle aspiration. However, the root cause for the classification of aspirates into the other 2 cate-gories is less well understood, although poor specimen quality is a contributing factor. Even though some investigative teams have proposed the use of specimen adequacy schema (rather than the binary system of nondiagnostic and diag-nostic), the use of these schema has not been widely adopted, perhaps because clinicians (who perform a large number of the aspirations) would take their busi-ness elsewhere if they received less than optimal diagnoses. The use of molecular testing may become an important tool to adjudicate specific thyroid gland fine-needle aspiration diagnoses. For additional reading, please see reference list.[1,2]

S. S. Raab, MD

References

1. Moses W, Weng J, Sansano I, et al. Molecular testing for somatic mutations improves the accuracy of thyroid fine-needle aspiration biopsy. *World J Surg.* 2010;34:2589-2594.
2. Lewis CM, Chang KP, Pitman M, Faquin WC, Randolph GW. Thyroid fine-needle aspiration biopsy: variability in reporting. *Thyroid.* 2009;19:717-723.

Fine-Needle Aspiration Cytology of Sclerosing Adenosis of the Breast: A Retrospective Review of Cytologic Features in Conjunction With Corresponding Histologic Features and Radiologic Findings

Kundu UR, Guo M, Landon G, et al (The Univ of Texas MD Anderson Cancer Ctr, Houston)
Am J Clin Pathol 138:96-102, 2012

We retrospectively reviewed 25 fine-needle aspiration cases of sclerosing adenosis of the breast in conjunction with histologic features of the paired core-needle biopsy and radiologic findings. The original cytologic diagnoses were benign (n = 19), focally atypical (n = 3), and suspicious for carcinoma (n = 3). The frequent features, although not specific, were low-to-moderate cellularity, bland epithelial cells that focally formed cohesive groups/tubules or occasionally discohesive clusters or individual cells, and fragments of dense fibrous stroma. Some tubules had an angulated configuration. Myoe-pithelial cells were present in all cases but were scant or absent in small epithelial groups. These cytologic features closely reflected the histologic appearances (ie, compressed and attenuated tubules and sclerotic stroma), but may cause overinterpretation on cytologic smears, especially when angulated tubules, discohesive or individual epithelial cells, scanty myoepithelial cells, and nuclear atypia are noted concurrently. Familiarity with its cytologic features may prevent false-positive diagnosis. Histologic confirmation is recommended for difficult cases.

▶ In North America, the replacement of breast fine-needle aspiration (FNA) by core biopsy has occurred for a variety of reasons, one of which is the assumed higher FNA error frequency (compared with core biopsy). The presumed risk is that a FNA false-negative diagnosis will lead to a delay in diagnosis if a core biopsy is not performed anyway. Kundu et al report the possibility of the opposite problem—that of a FNA false-positive diagnosis—because 6 of 25 cases of breast-sclerosing adenosis were called atypical or suspicious for cancer. These data are important for high-volume performers of breast FNA. The question in North America is if breast FNA will ever be used again as a primary triage tool. I believe that breast FNA may have a large impact on clinical practice if it is incorporated into a 1-stop clinic in which women may have a FNA diagnosis followed by same-day scheduling with care providers who initiate treatment protocols. In this scenario, the importance of the FNA is related to the immediacy of the diagnosis, which plays a larger role than accuracy. Clinicians in 1-stop clinics also may perform core biopsies, which later are correlated with the cytopathology diagnosis (interestingly, if there is not a question of fixation time for biomarkers, core tissues also could be processed in short periods). If the breast biopsy care process is not changed in North America, I do not see breast FNA as growing again as a cytopathology subspecialty. I think the article by Kundu et al has much more meaning in an environment in which breast FNA is used frequently. For additional reading, please see reference list.[1-3]

S. S. Raab, MD

References

1. Taşkin F, Köseoğlu K, Unsal A, Erkuş M, Ozbaş S, Karaman C. Sclerosing adenosis of the breast: radiologic appearance and efficiency of core needle biopsy. *Diagn Interv Radiol.* 2011;17:311-316.
2. Ogawa Y, Kato Y, Nakata B, et al. Diagnostic potential and pitfalls of ultrasound-guided fine-needle aspiration cytology for breast lesions. *Surg Today.* 1998;28:167-172.
3. Cangiarella J, Waisman J, Shapiro RL, Simsir A. Cytologic features of tubular adenocarcinoma of the breast by aspiration biopsy. *Diagn Cytopathol.* 2001;25:311-315.

American Cancer Society, American Society for Colposcopy and Cervical Pathology, and American Society for Clinical Pathology Screening Guidelines for the Prevention and Early Detection of Cervical Cancer
Saslow D, Solomon D, Lawson HW, et al (American Cancer Society, Atlanta, GA; Natl Insts of Health, Rockville, MD; Emory Univ School of Medicine, Atlanta, GA; et al)
Am J Clin Pathol 137:516-542, 2012

An update to the American Cancer Society (ACS) guideline regarding screening for the early detection of cervical precancerous lesions and cancer is presented. The guidelines are based on a systematic evidence review, contributions from 6 working groups, and a recent symposium cosponsored by the ACS, the American Society for Colposcopy and Cervical Pathology, and the American Society for Clinical Pathology, which was attended by 25 organizations. The new screening recommendations address age-appropriate screening strategies, including the use of cytology and high-risk human papillomavirus (HPV) testing, follow-up (eg, the management of screen positives and screening intervals for screen negatives) of women after screening, the age at which to exit screening, future considerations regarding HPV testing alone as a primary screening approach, and screening strategies for women vaccinated against HPV16 and HPV18 infections.

Cervical cancer screening has successfully decreased cervical cancer incidence and mortality. The American Cancer Society (ACS) guideline for the early detection of cervical cancer was last reviewed and updated in 2002; for the first time, those recommendations incorporated human papillomavirus (HPV) DNA testing. Since that time, numerous studies have been published that support changes to recommended age-appropriate screening as well as the management of abnormal screening results, as summarized in Table 1.

▶ Saslow et al report the current American Cancer Society (ACS) screening guidelines, which are endorsed by a number of pathology and clinical societies. For the practicing cytopathologist, this article serves as a great reference to answer clinical questions regarding clinical follow-up for women with various Pap test Bethesda System categories of diagnosis, high-risk human papilloma virus (HPV) test results, and clinical scenarios. Of note, the ACS currently does not recommend that screening practices should change on the basis of HPV vaccination status. The section entitled "Recommendations for Future Research" highlights the main factors that will determine the future of gynecologic cytology practice in North America, at least as viewed by the ACS. In my opinion, the recommendations are conservative, as the pathology and clinical societies wait for additional evidence from high-risk HPV testing and vaccination studies. For example, a large number of individuals believe that additional data are necessary to show that HPV testing alone (with its lower specificity) is an acceptable alternative to cotesting (as harm also results from this lower specificity). How policy and decision makers will use future study data to alter guidelines will be interesting because competing quality metrics of safety, patient centeredness, and efficiency will need to be discussed. Future decisions on policy will involve stakeholders outside of medical experts in pathology and gynecology. Members of the medical field generally do not receive formal training in addressing policy decision making because front-line patient care is separated from policy making. Our medical societies often are our instrument for influencing these policies and our pathology societies will play a critical role in this decision-making process. For further reading, please see reference list.[1-3]

S. S. Raab, MD

References

1. Kinney W, Stoler MH, Castle PE. Special commentary: patient safety and the next generation of HPV DNA tests. *Am J Clin Pathol.* 2010;134:193-199.

2. Elbasha EH, Dasbach EJ, Insinga RP. Model for assessing human papillomavirus vaccination strategies. *Emerg Infect Dis*. 2007;13:28-41.
3. Schiffman M, Castle PE, Jeronimo J, Rodriguez AC, Wacholder S. Human papillomavirus and cervical cancer. *Lancet*. 2007;370:890-907.

Practice Patterns in Cervical Cancer Screening and Human Papillomavirus Testing

Tatsas AD, Phelan DF, Gravitt PE (The Johns Hopkins Univ School of Medicine, Baltimore, MD; Johns Hopkins Bloomberg School of Public Health, Baltimore, MD)
Am J Clin Pathol 138:223-229, 2012

The use of human papillomavirus DNA testing plus Papanicolaou (Pap) testing (cotesting) for cervical cancer screening in women 30 years and older has been recommended since 2006. However, few studies have detailed the adoption of such cotesting in clinical practice. We examined the trends in monthly percentage of Pap tests ordered as cotests in our laboratory over a 2.5-year period and used joinpoint regression to identify periods in which there was a change in the average monthly proportion of cotests. Cotesting of patients 30 years and older increased from 15.9% in January 2008 to 39.4% in June 2010. In patients aged 18 to 29 years, cotesting initially increased, but showed a downward trend in the last 14 months of the study, ending at 7.7% in June 2010. Our study highlights increased adoption of age-appropriate cotesting as well as the persistence of age-inappropriate cotesting.

▶ Tatsas et al report on how cytopathology laboratory data may be used to track clinical practice patterns of cotesting high-risk human papilloma virus DNA and Pap results. These patterns presumably reflect practice adherence to clinical guidelines based on clinical effectiveness studies and consensus opinion. Although Tatsas et al show that laboratories are able to track these practice patterns, is a future role of the laboratory to perform this tracking as a quality check on clinical practices? I think pathologists have a tremendous future in ensuring that quality practice standards are met. With the introduction of robust information technology systems, laboratory professionals could assess cotesting practices (such as cervical cancer screening practices) and other testing practices (such as test over, under, or misordering). An important link to be made for this article is the one between clinical outcomes and cost with guideline adherence. I believe that our pathology societies should assist laboratories in becoming the data champions and assessors in health care, which would extend the pathologist's role outside of the laboratory. In some ways, clinical practice has become so complex that not all practitioners are aware of current guidelines and the laboratory through its information system could assist these practices. Paying for this added quality (in addition to limiting test overordering) would benefit the patient and the practice. For additional reading, please see reference list.[1,2]

S. S. Raab, MD

References

1. Shirts BH, Jackson BR. Informatics methods for laboratory evaluation of HPV ordering patterns with an example from a nationwide sample in the United States, 2003-2009. *J Pathol Inform.* 2010;1:26.
2. Lee JW, Berkowitz Z, Saraiya M. Low-risk human papillomavirus testing and other nonrecommended human papillomavirus testing practices among U.S. health care providers. *Obstet Gynecol.* 2011;118:4-13.

Follow-up Outcomes in a Large Cohort of Patients With Human Papillomavirus—Negative ASC-H Cervical Screening Test Results

Cohen D, Austin RM, Gilbert C, et al (Univ of Pittsburgh Med Ctr, PA)
Am J Clin Pathol 138:517-523, 2012

Limited follow-up data are available on patients with cervical cytology results of atypical squamous cells, cannot exclude a high-grade intraepithelial lesion (ASC-H), who test negative for high-risk human papillomavirus (hrHPV). Between June 2005 and December 2010, 885 patients were identified with ThinPrep results of Hybrid Capture 2 (HC2) hrHPV-negative cervical ASC-H liquid-based cytology and follow-up histopathology or cytology results extending to September 2011. Of the 885 patients with available follow-up results, 549 (62.0%) had at least 1 histopathologic result during the entire follow-up period, whereas 336 (38.0%) had only cytologic follow-up documented. In an average follow-up period of 29 months, 14 (1.6%) of 885 patients with HPV-negative ASC-H results showed evidence of high-grade cervical intraepithelial neoplasia (CIN2/3). No cases of invasive cervical cancer were diagnosed. Four of 14 patients with HPV-negative ASC-H results with follow-up diagnoses of CIN2/3 had a history of earlier CIN2/3 diagnoses before HPV-negative ASC-H results. Follow-up of patients with HPV-negative ASC-H results using methods specified in this study yielded low rates of detectible CIN2/3 and no diagnoses of cervical cancer. Triage of study patients with HPV-negative ASC-H results to routine HPV and cytology cotesting at 1 year was a safe follow-up option.

▶ Similar to the data of women who have atypical squamous cells of undetermined significance (ASC-US) and high-risk human papillomavirus (HPV)−, Cohen et al show that the women who have high-grade intraepithelial lesion (ASC-H) and high-risk HPV− are of low risk to have high-grade cervical intraepithelial neoplasia (CIN2) + on follow-up. This finding is not a surprise, but this study raises more important issues regarding 2001 Bethesda System categorical use and HPV results for quality control. In the ALTS study (a seminal work guiding the 2001 Bethesda System participants), the group of patients who had ASC-H had an 84% frequency of high-risk HPV (or 16% HPV−) and a 59% frequency of CIN2 + on histologic follow-up. Cohen et al reported that for the 67-month study period, the high-risk HPV + frequency in ASC-H women was 54.3%. In 2006, Cibas et al reported that at their institution, the frequency of ASC-US high-risk HPV+ ranged from 29.6% to 61.8% (mean: 45.8%). The reported ASC-H frequency of women who had a high-risk HPV+ frequency by Cohen et al fell within this range. This may mean that the population of women with ASC-H studied by Cohen et al most likely is not the same as that reported in the ALTS study informing the 2001 Bethesda System. This may reflect real-world use of the diagnostic category of ASC-H. Some labs may use the high-risk HPV+ frequency as a quality assurance measure to benchmark practice use of ASC-H to national standards. If cotested, women with high-risk HPV− are treated the same (eg, normal screening) regardless of whether they have ASC-US or ASC-H and all high-risk HPV+ women are recommended for colposcopic examination, then why separate ASC? For additional reading, please see reference list.[1,2]

S. S. Raab, MD

References

1. Cibas ES, Zou KH, Crum CP, Kuo F. Using the rate of positive high-risk HPV test results for ASC-US together with the ASC-US/SIL ratio in evaluating the performance of cytopathologists. *Am J Clin Pathol.* 2008;129:97-101.
2. Sherman ME, Castle PE, Solomon D. Cervical cytology of atypical squamous cells cannot exclude high-grade squamous intraepithelial lesion (ASC-H): characteristics and histologic outcomes. *Cancer.* 2006;108:298-305.

Comparison of ultrasound-guided core biopsy versus fine-needle aspiration biopsy in the evaluation of salivary gland lesions

Douville NJ, Bradford CR (Univ of Michigan, Ann Arbor)
Head Neck 2012 [Epub ahead of print]

Ultrasound-guided core biopsy provides many benefits compared with fine-needle aspiration cytology and has begun to emerge as part of the diagnostic work-up for a salivary gland lesion. Although the increased potential for tumor-seeding and capsule rupture has been extensively discussed, the safety of this procedure is widely accepted based on infrequent reports of tumor-seeding. In fact, a review of the literature shows only 2 cases of salivary tumor seeding following biopsy with larger-gauge needle characteristics, with 2 reported cases of salivary tumor seeding following fine-needle aspiration cytology. However, the follow-up interval of such studies (<7 years) is substantially less than the 20-year follow-up typically necessary to detect remote recurrence. Studies on tumor recurrence of pleomorphic adenoma, the most common salivary gland lesion, suggest that as many as 16% of tumor recurrences occur at least 10 years following initial surgery, with average time to recurrence ranging anywhere from 6.1 to 11.8 years postoperatively. Despite the benefits of ultrasound-guided core biopsy over fine-needle aspiration biopsy, which include both improved consistency and diagnostic accuracy, current studies lack adequate patient numbers and follow-up duration to confirm comparable safety profile to currently accepted fine-needle aspiration cytology. In this report we: (1) compare the relative benefits of each procedure, (2) review evidence regarding tumor seeding in each procedure, (3) discuss time course and patient numbers necessary to detect tumor recurrence, and (4) describe how these uncertainties should be factored into clinical considerations.

▶ Douville and Bradford compare the strengths and weaknesses of the techniques of ultrasound-guided core biopsy and fine-needle aspiration biopsy of the salivary gland. This manuscript helps to highlight the marked heterogeneity of the cytopathology literature regarding fine-needle aspiration in general and for salivary gland specifically. The accuracy and ability to perform ancillary testing is highly operator- and institution-dependent. For example, fine-needle aspiration may be performed with or without ultrasound guidance; by pathologists, clinicians, or radiologists; and depending on the operator, cell blocks for immunohistochemical analysis may be easily obtained (not obtaining these cells blocks is cited as a limitation of fine-needle aspiration). Because the cytopathology literature contains articles that report salivary gland diagnostic accuracy under a number of conditions, it is difficult to determine if core biopsy would be a better technique, which also would have an accuracy that would depend on a number of variables. These data reflect the variability of practice, indicating that in the current state, the quality of technique will be institution-specific. Articles such as these provide the clinician view of "general" cytopathology services, which may not accurately portray individual practice. For additional reading, please see reference list.[1,2]

S. S. Raab, MD

References

1. Schmidt RL, Hall BJ, Wilson AR, Layfield LJ. A systematic review and meta-analysis of the diagnostic accuracy of fine-needle aspiration cytology for parotid gland lesions. *Am J Clin Pathol.* 2011;136:45-59.
2. Novoa E, Gürtler N, Arnoux A, Kraft M. Role of ultrasound-guided core-needle biopsy in the assessment of head and neck lesions: a meta-analysis and systematic review of the literature. *Head Neck.* 2012;34:1497-1503.

Risk of Cervical Precancer and Cancer Among HIV-Infected Women With Normal Cervical Cytology and No Evidence of Oncogenic HPV Infection

Keller MJ, Burk RD, Xie X, et al (Albert Einstein College of Medicine, Bronx, NY; et al)
JAMA 308:362-369, 2012

Context.—US cervical cancer screening guidelines for human immunodeficiency virus (HIV)—uninfected women 30 years or older have recently been revised, increasing the suggested interval between Papanicolaou (Pap) tests from 3 years to 5 years among those with normal cervical cytology (Pap test) results who test negative for oncogenic human papillomavirus (HPV). Whether a 3-year or 5-year screening interval could be used in HIV-infected women who are cytologically normal and oncogenic HPV—negative is unknown.

Objective.—To determine the risk of cervical precancer or cancer defined cytologically (high-grade squamous intraepithelial lesions or greater [HSIL+]) or histologically (cervical intraepithelial neoplasia 2 or greater [CIN-2+]), as 2 separate end points, in HIV-infected women and HIV-uninfected women who at baseline had a normal Pap test result and were negative for oncogenic HPV.

Design, Setting, and Participants.—Participants included 420 HIV-infected women and 279 HIV-uninfected women with normal cervical cytology at their enrollment in a multi-institutional US cohort of the Women's Interagency HIV Study, between October 1, 2001, and September 30, 2002, with follow-up through April 30, 2011. Semiannual visits at 6 clinical sites included Pap testing and, if indicated, cervical biopsy. Cervicovaginal lavage specimens from enrollment were tested for HPV DNA using polymerase chain reaction. The primary analysis was truncated at 5 years of follow-up.

Main Outcome Measure.—Five-year cumulative incidence of cervical precancer and cancer.

Results.—No oncogenic HPV was detected in 369 (88% [95% CI, 84%-91%]) HIV-infected women and 255 (91% [95% CI, 88%-94%]) HIV-uninfected women with normal cervical cytology at enrollment. Among these oncogenic HPV—negative women, 2 cases of HSIL + were observed; an HIV-uninfected woman and an HIV-infected woman with a CD4 cell count of 500 cells/μL or greater. Histologic data were obtained from 4 of the 6 clinical sites. There were 6 cases of CIN-2 + in 145 HIV-uninfected women (cumulative incidence, 5% [95% CI, 1%-8%]) and 9 cases in 219 HIV-infected women (cumulative incidence, 5% [95% CI, 2%-8%]). This included 1 case of CIN-2 + in 44 oncogenic HPV—negative HIV-infected women with CD4 cell count less than 350 cells/μL (cumulative incidence, 2% [95% CI, 0%-7%]), 1 case in 47 women with CD4 cell count of 350 to 499 cells/μL (cumulative incidence, 2% [95% CI, 0%-7%]), and 7 cases in 128 women with CD4 cell count of 500 cells/μL or greater (cumulative incidence, 6% [95% CI, 2%-10%]). One HIV-infected and 1 HIV-uninfected woman had CIN-3, but none had cancer.

Conclusion.—The 5-year cumulative incidence of HSIL + and CIN-2 + was similar in HIV-infected women and HIV-uninfected women who were cytologically normal and oncogenic HPV—negative at enrollment.

► The data provided by Keller et al fills a gap in the cervical cancer screening literature by showing that HIV-infected women with high-risk human papillomavirus—with negative cytology may have the same follow-up as HIV-noninfected women with the same testing results. This is a nice analysis. For additional reading, please see reference list.[1,2]

S. S. Raab, MD

References

1. Stout NK, Goldhaber-Fiebert JD, Ortendahl JD, Goldie SJ. Trade-offs in cervical cancer prevention: balancing benefits and risks. *Arch Intern Med.* 2008;168: 1881-1889.

2. Moyer VA. Screening for cervical cancer: U.S. preventive services task force recommendation statement. *Ann Intern Med.* 2012;156:880-891.

Trends in Pancreatic Pathology Practice Before and After Implementation of Endoscopic Ultrasound-Guided Fine-Needle Aspiration: An Example Of Disruptive Innovation Effect?

Eltoum IA, Alston EA, Roberson J (Univ of Alabama at Birmingham)
Arch Pathol Lab Med 136:447-453, 2012

Context.—Little has been reported on changes in pancreatic pathology practice after implementation of endoscopic ultrasound-guided fine-needle aspiration (EUS-FNA).

Objectives.—We assessed the impact of EUS-FNA on cytologic diagnosis replacing histologic diagnosis for pancreatic disease and determined whether it fulfills Christensen criteria of a disruptive innovation effect.

Design.—Pattern of utilization during 20 years, diagnostic categories, and diagnostic accuracy of pancreatic cytology were compared before and after implementation of EUS-FNA. The disruptive effect of cytology relevant to biopsy was assessed by comparing the utilization trends and the accuracy of diagnosis over time.

Results.—The mean annual volume (standard deviation) of cytologic specimens increased from 24 (11) to 231 (10) after implementation of EUS-FNA, and that of histologic specimens increased from 97 (42) to 377 (148). The average percentage of annual cases managed by following cytology alone was 19% (10) before versus 51% (8) after implementation. The percentage managed by histology alone was 56% before versus 23% after implementation. Non—endoscopic ultrasound-guided fine-needle aspiration cytology decreased from 36% to 1%. Needle biopsies decreased from 7% to 1%, and other biopsy types from 29% to 9%. Unsatisfactory (7% versus 1%), atypical (16% versus 4%), and suspicious (16% versus 3%) diagnoses were significantly reduced. The accuracy of cytologic diagnosis significantly improved: the sensitivity (confidence interval) and specificity (confidence interval) for cancer diagnosis were 55% (38%—70%) and 78% (58%—89%) before versus 88% (84%—91%) and 96% (93%—98%) after implementation, respectively.

Conclusions.—Endoscopic ultrasound-guided fine-needle aspiration improved the accuracy of cytologic diagnosis, reduced the number of indeterminate diagnoses, and replaced the need for tissue biopsy. Given its cost and simplicity as compared with tissue biopsy, this trend represents a disruptive innovation effect.

▶ Eltoum and colleagues report the disruptive nature of endoscopic ultrasound-guided pancreatic fine-needle aspiration (EUS-FNA). In some institutions, pancreatic EUS-FNA has largely replaced core (or open) biopsy technology (Fig 6 in the original article). Although I agree that cost and convenience were large drivers of this change, the heavy burden fell on improving both the sample quality (radiology) and the interpretive ability (diagnosis). The accuracy of histology still may be higher, but EUS-FNA is sufficiently high to serve as a diagnostic triage test (at least in the hand of the Eltoum et al). An interesting aspect of this change would be to learn the core drivers of practice that led to adoption. Obviously, an EUS-FNA—trained radiologist would have to pioneer the change in an institution. Eltoum et al show that the number of cytology procedures markedly increased after introduction of the EUS-FNA service, and a detailed cost comparison was not performed. Presumably, the increase in the number of FNAs benefited the patients, but the questions of potential overtesting and cost burdens cannot be addressed. The challenge for cytopathologists and cytotechnologists has been in learning a new field of diagnosis and recognizing the pitfalls. The field of diagnostic pancreatic cytology is not an easy one, and the assessment of harm associated with pancreatic EUS-FNS errors is still unknown. For some institutions, the teamwork-based practice involving immediate interpretation and feedback to the radiologist probably is a key component that has led to improved samples and diagnostic interpretation. Thus, the adoption of pancreatic EUS-FNA requires a number of system changes (eg, specialized expertise in radiology and cytopathology) that need to be further characterized to assess potential barriers to adoption. For further reading, please see reference list.[1,2]

S. S. Raab, MD

References

1. Queneau PE, Sauvé G, Koch S, et al. The impact on clinical practice of endoscopic ultrasonography used for the diagnosis and staging of pancreatic adenocarcinoma. *JOP.* 2001;2:98-104.
2. Danneels E. Disruptive technology reconsidered: a critique and research agenda. *J Prod Innovat Manag.* 2004;21:246-258.

Atypia of Undetermined Significance and Nondiagnostic Rates in The Bethesda System for Reporting Thyroid Cytopathology Are Inversely Related

VanderLaan PA, Renshaw AA, Krane JF (Brigham and Women's Hosp and Harvard Med School, Boston, MA; Baptist Hosp of Miami, FL)
Am J Clin Pathol 137:462-465, 2012

There is substantial variation in the reported rates of different diagnostic categories in The Bethesda System for Reporting Thyroid Cytopathology (TBS). Specifically, the relationship between the nondiagnostic (ND) and atypia of undetermined significance (AUS) categories has not been closely examined previously. Data from published series in the literature and from 2 separate hospitals with more than 15,000 thyroid aspirates were reviewed. The AUS and ND rates were consistently negatively correlated when analyzed by year, aspirator, and cytologist. The strongest correlation was with cytologists ($P < .0003$). Absolute ND rates decreased by 1% for every 3.5% increase in AUS, implying the existence of a discrete population of cases that cytologists will classify as ND or AUS. As such, AUS and ND are not independent variables. Awareness of this relationship may be useful for laboratories and individual cytopathologists for refining the use of TBS (Fig 3).

▶ VanderLaan et al show that at least for one institution, the Bethesda System diagnoses for thyroid gland fine-needle aspiration of atypia of undetermined significance (AUS) and nondiagnostic (ND) are negatively correlated at a level of statistical significance (Fig 3). In a sense, these diagnoses represent failures in practice, as a definitive diagnosis was not reached. For the ND category, insufficient material is present (or too much artifact is present), and root causes include failures in the aspiration process (in turn, caused by a number of system problems including technology and training), preparation, and interpretation (although this may be less frequent). The use of the AUS category is probably not well understood, and a hypothesis is that some AUS diagnoses may arise from borderline insufficient specimens. However, other root causes include failures in processing technique and cytopathologist cognitive processes. Although VanderLaan and colleagues evaluate the relationship of specimen quality and diagnostic category, their evaluation is not deep enough. The authors do not do a direct analysis of specimen quality in the AUS cases and only rely on evaluating data of cytologist, aspirator, and preparatory technique. VanderLaan et al even comment on the fact that other laboratories show a low ND and AUS frequency and state that it is unclear how this was achieved. These laboratories may be performing best practices! Clearly, there is a lack of understanding of how process differences (such as immediate interpretation or aspiration and diagnostic expertise) may explain a lower number of process failures. It is possible that the AUS cases arise from 2 separate populations: (1) cases that are borderline ND (and called ND by some cytopathologists) and (2) cases that are adequate and difficult to classify (for perhaps a number of reasons). If the number of borderline ND specimens is decreased by improving sample quality, then the

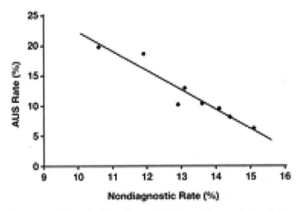

FIGURE 3.—Atypia of undetermined significance (AUS) vs nondiagnostic rate, Brigham and Women's Hospital, Boston, MA, by cytologist. $y = -3.22x + 54.6$; $R^2 = 0.91$; $P < .0003$. (Reprinted from Vander-Laan PA, Renshaw AA, Krane JF. Atypia of undetermined significance and nondiagnostic rates in the Bethesda system for reporting thyroid cytopathology are inversely related. *Am J Clin Pathol.* 2012;137:462-465, © [2012] American Society for Clinical Pathology.)

negative correlation between ND and AUS may disappear. A conclusion I make from these data is that we do not fully understand many of the processes that affect diagnostic interpretation. For additional reading, see reference list.[1,2]

S. S. Raab, MD

References

1. Abele JS, Levine RA. Diagnostic criteria and risk-adapted approach to indeterminate thyroid cytodiagnosis. *Cancer Cytopathol.* 2010;118:415-422.
2. Luu MH, Fischer AH, Pisharodi L, Owens CL. Improved preoperative definitive diagnosis of papillary thyroid carcinoma in FNAs prepared with both ThinPrep and conventional smears compared with FNAs prepared with ThinPrep alone. *Cancer Cytopathol.* 2011;119:68-73.

Low-Grade Squamous Intraepithelial Lesion, Cannot Exclude High-Grade Squamous Intraepithelial Lesion: A Category With an Increased Outcome of High-Grade Lesions: Use as a Quality Assurance Measure
Nishino HT, Wilbur DC, Tambouret RH (Harvard Med School, Boston, MA)
Am J Clin Pathol 138:198-202, 2012

"Low-grade squamous intraepithelial lesion (LSIL), cannot exclude high-grade squamous intraepithelial lesion" (LSIL-H) is an increasingly used, equivocal interpretive category in gynecologic cytology. In an effort to evaluate its potential usefulness as a measure of quality assurance, we studied patterns of use of the LSIL-H diagnosis compared with "LSIL" and "high-grade squamous intraepithelial lesion" (HSIL) with corresponding histologic outcomes for 10 cytopathologists in our practice. In our laboratory, while the overall rate of associated cervical intraepithelial neoplasia 2 or greater on histologic follow-up for LSIL-H was intermediate between that of LSIL and HSIL, the outcomes for individual cytopathologists varied widely. Monitoring this particular utilization-outcome data with periodic confidential feedback to individual cytopathologists offers an opportunity for practice improvement within a laboratory and serves as an additional measure of quality assurance. These data may be useful for establishing and/or realigning the diagnostic criteria for this equivocal cytologic interpretation endorsed by a pathology practice.

▶ It is not surprising that the frequency of CIN 2+ follow-up for women who have a Pap test diagnosis of high-grade squamous intraepithelial lesion (LSIL-H) lies between the frequency of cervical intraepithelial neoplasia (CIN) 2+ follow-up for women with low-grade squamous intraepithelial lesion (LSIL) and the women with high-grade squamous intraepithelial lesion (HSIL). In Table 2 in the original article, Nishino et al summarize the literature showing follow-up for women with LSIL-H providing perspective of the clinical significance of this diagnosis. First, the utility of this diagnosis depends on factors in addition to the probability of a CIN 2+ lesion being present. For some clinicians, this is a confusing diagnosis, because "cannot exclude HSIL" implies that the clinicians have to exclude HSIL. If the colposcopic diagnosis comes back as CIN 1, will some clinicians repeat colposcopic examination because they may not have adequately sampled the lesion, or is the CIN 1 diagnosis sufficient to exclude HSIL? Does the LSIL-H diagnosis cause a biased assessment of the surgical specimen to overcall CIN 2 +? Answering these and other questions would provide greater insight as to the effect of LSIL-H on clinical care, in addition to using LSIL-H as quality assurance tool. Standardizing the use of LSIL-H may be equally challenging because of standardizing the use of atypical squamous cells of undetermined significance, and do we really want to measure a LSIL/LSIL-H ratio to determine the potential over call or under call frequency of individual cytopathologists and cytotechnologists? In Bethesda 2001, the introduction of LSIL-H was for classifying lesions of a high level of uncertainty (for HSIL) and, in my opinion, was for limited use. However, no quantification limit for categorical use was set. The introduction also opened the door for the system to express greater degrees of diagnostic uncertainty without a clear course of assessing clinical impact and meaning of this uncertainty. For additional reading, please see reference list.[1,2]

S. S. Raab, MD

References

1. Alsharif M, Kjeldahl K, Curran C, Miller S, Gulbahce HE, Pambuccian SE. Clinical significance of the diagnosis of low-grade squamous intraepithelial lesion, cannot exclude high-grade squamous intraepithelial lesion. *Cancer.* 2009;117: 92-100.
2. Owens CL, Moats DR, Burroughs FH, Gustafson KS. "Low-grade squamous intraepithelial lesion, cannot exclude high-grade squamous intraepithelial lesion" is a distinct cytologic category: histologic outcomes and HPV prevalence. *Am J Clin Pathol.* 2007;128:398-403.

15 Techniques/Molecular

Phenotypic Heterogeneity of Genomic Disorders and Rare Copy-Number Variants
Girirajan S, Rosenfeld JA, Coe BP, et al (Univ of Washington, Seattle; Signature Genomic Laboratories, Spokane, WA; et al)
N Engl J Med 367:1321-1331, 2012

Background.—Some copy-number variants are associated with genomic disorders with extreme phenotypic heterogeneity. The cause of this variation is unknown, which presents challenges in genetic diagnosis, counseling, and management.

Methods.—We analyzed the genomes of 2312 children known to carry a copy-number variant associated with intellectual disability and congenital abnormalities, using array comparative genomic hybridization.

Results.—Among the affected children, 10.1% carried a second large copy-number variant in addition to the primary genetic lesion. We identified seven genomic disorders, each defined by a specific copy-number variant, in which the affected children were more likely to carry multiple copy-number variants than were controls. We found that syndromic disorders could be distinguished from those with extreme phenotypic heterogeneity on the basis of the total number of copy-number variants and whether the variants are inherited or de novo. Children who carried two large copy-number variants of unknown clinical significance were eight times as likely to have developmental delay as were controls (odds ratio, 8.16; 95% confidence interval, 5.33 to 13.07; $P = 2.11 \times 10^{-38}$). Among affected children, inherited copy-number variants tended to co-occur with a second-site large copy-number variant (Spearman correlation coefficient, 0.66; $P < 0.001$). Boys were more likely than girls to have disorders of phenotypic heterogeneity ($P < 0.001$), and mothers were more likely than fathers to transmit second-site copy-number variants to their offspring ($P = 0.02$).

Conclusions.—Multiple, large copy-number variants, including those of unknown pathogenic significance, compound to result in a severe clinical presentation, and secondary copy-number variants are preferentially transmitted from maternal carriers. (Funded by the Simons Foundation Autism Research Initiative and the National Institutes of Health.)

▶ The finding of copy number variants (DNA with abnormal numbers of copies of parts of chromosomes) has been common in genomic analysis. It is not clear yet what these gains or losses in gene copies mean in the pathology of disease. Copy number variants have been associated with some intellectual disabilities and congenital abnormalities. Such disorders show a broad range of phenotypic heterogeneity with highly variable clinical manifestations and the pathogenic role of individual copy number variations is far from clear. Why do people with the same genetic abnormality show such different manifestations?

This is a large (n = 2312) study of affected children known to carry a primary copy number variant associated with intellectual disability and congenital abnormalities. A total of 8.7% of affected children also showed a secondary large copy number variant at multiple disparate sites. Among children with the same primary copy number variant, those with additional second-site variants had more phenotypic deficits than those with a single variant.

One more complexity is added to the genetic story, by detecting additional deletions or duplications previously undetected before extensive exome sequencing. The authors suggest the addition of another copy number mutation of unknown clinical significance may play a role in the expression of the primary abnormality in genetic neurological disease. For further reading, please see reference.[1]

A. McCullough, MD

Reference

1. Brunner HG. The variability of genetic disease. *N Engl J Med.* 2012;367: 1350-1352.

Comprehensive molecular portraits of human breast tumours
The Cancer Genome Atlas Network (Washington Univ in St Louis, MO; et al)
Nature 490:61-70, 2012

We analysed primary breast cancers by genomic DNA copy number arrays, DNA methylation, exome sequencing, messenger RNA arrays, microRNA sequencing and reverse-phase protein arrays. Our ability to integrate information across platforms provided key insights into previously defined gene expression subtypes and demonstrated the existence of four main breast cancer classes when combining data from five platforms, each of which shows significant molecular heterogeneity. Somatic mutations in only three genes (*TP53, PIK3CA* and *GATA3*) occurred at >10% incidence across all breast cancers; however, there were numerous subtype-associated and novel gene mutations including the enrichment of specific mutations in *GATA3, PIK3CA* and *MAP3K1* with the luminal A subtype. We identified two novel protein-expression-defined subgroups, possibly produced by stromal/microenvironmental elements, and integrated analyses identified specific signalling pathways dominant in each molecular subtype including a HER2/phosphorylated HER2/EGFR/phosphorylated EGFR signature within the HER2-enriched expression subtype. Comparison of basal-like breast tumours with high-grade serous ovarian tumours showed many molecular commonalities, indicating a related aetiology and similar therapeutic opportunities. The biological finding of the four main breast cancer subtypes caused by different subsets of genetic

TABLE 1.—Highlights of Genomic, Clinical and Proteomic Features of Subtypes

Subtype	Luminal A	Luminal B	Basal-like	HER2E
ER+/HER2- (%)	87	82	10	20
HER2+ (%)	7	15	2	68
TNBCs (%)	2	1	80	9
TP53 pathway	TP53 mut (12%); gain of MDM2 (14%)	TP53 mut (32%); gain of MDM2 (31%)	TP53 mut (84%); gain of MDM2 (14%)	TP53 mut (75%); gain of MDM2 (30%)
PIK3CA/PTEN pathway	PIK3CA mut (49%); PTEN mut/loss (13%); INPP4B loss (9%)	PIK3CA mut (32%) PTEN mut/loss (24%) INPP4B loss (16%)	PIK3CA mut (7%); PTEN mut/loss (35%); INPP4B loss (30%)	PIK3CA mut (42%); PTEN mut/loss (19%); INPP4B loss (30%)
RB1 pathway	Cyclin D1 amp (29%); CDK4 gain (14%); low expression of CDKN2C; high expression of RB1	Cyclin D1 amp (58%); CDK4 gain (25%)	RB1 mut/loss (20%); cyclin E1 amp (9%); high expression of CDKN2A; low expression of RB1	Cyclin D1 amp (38%); CDK4 gain (24%)
mRNA expression	High ER cluster; low proliferation	Lower ER cluster; high proliferation	Basal signature; high proliferation	HER2 amplicon signature; high proliferation
Copy number	Most diploid; many with quiet genomes; 1q, 8q, 8p11 gain; 16q loss; 11q13.3 amp (24%)	Most aneuploid; many with focal amp; 1q, 8q, 8p11 gain; 8p, 16q loss; 11q13.3 amp (51%); 8p11.23 amp (28%)	Most aneuploid; high genomic instability; 1q, 10p gain; 8p, 5q loss; MYC focal gain (40%)	Most aneuploid; high genomic instability; 1q, 8q gain; 8p loss; 17q12 focal ERRB2 amp (71%)
DNA mutations	PIK3CA (49%); TP53 (12%); GATA3 (14%); MAP3K1 (14%)	TP53 (32%); PIK3CA (32%); MAP3K1 (5%)	TP53 (84%); PIK3CA (7%)	TP53 (75%); PIK3CA (42%); PIK3R1 (8%)
DNA methylation	—	Hypermethylated phenotype for subset	Hypomethylated	—
Protein expression	High oestrogen signalling; high MYB; RPPA reactive subtypes	Less oestrogen signalling; high FOXM1 and MYC; RPPA reactive subtypes	High expression of DNA repair proteins, PTEN and INPP4B loss signature (pAKT)	High protein and phosphoprotein expression of EGFR and HER2

Percentages are based on 466 tumour overlap list. Amp, amplification; mut, mutation.

and epigenetic abnormalities raises the hypothesis that much of the clinically observable plasticity and heterogeneity occurs within, and not across, these major biological subtypes of breast cancer (Table 1).

▶ The Cancer Genome Atlas Network continues publishing large series of highly characterized malignancies by anatomic site. This report represents the most comprehensive collation of breast carcinoma genomic data to date, an amalgamation of data from six different methods from 825 patients (Agilent mRNA expression microarrays, Illumina Infinium DNA methylation chips, Affymetrix 6.0 single nucleotide polymorphism arrays, miRNA sequencing, and whole-exome sequencing, with partial data from reverse-phase protein arrays). This paper received considerable notice in the lay press. The data here are based on primary carcinomas and exclude analyses of metastases.

There is both old and new news here. The old news is the sobering data about the diverse panoply of mutations in breast carcinomas as a group. Also old is the separation of the majority of primary breast carcinomas into 4 relatively distinct genomic subtypes: luminal A, luminal B, basal-like, and HER-2 positive.

The new news? What stands out in these data is that vast genetic heterogeneity is partially defined by the genomic subtypes. Only 3 genes of a vast number of genes represented the most common mutations (> 10% incidence) across all breast cancer types: GATA3, PIK3CA, and MAP3K1. Increases in gene incidence vary considerably between subtypes, and some genomic subtypes show high-frequency mutations (eg, TP 53 mutation in 80% of basal-like tumors; Table 1). Although it seems unlikely we will find a unifying group of preserved mutations to define a particular molecular type, there are high-frequency mutations within genomic subtypes to mine for drug targeting and possible etiological mechanisms.

The diversity of the subtypes of breast carcinoma seems likely to expand (eg, with a description of subtypes of HER-2 expressing carcinomas here). Comparison of these data to previously analyzed sets of other carcinomas will likely suggest plenty of new drug trials based on molecular similarities to other carcinomas. Notably within this group of breast carcinomas, basal-like breast tumors showed many similar abnormalities to those found in high-grade serous ovarian carcinomas. Can breast cancer trials with ovarian carcinoma agents be far behind?

What does complex data like these mean to the practice of surgical pathology? Genetic typing of breast carcinomas and the genomic subtypes of breast carcinoma are part of the new lexicon of breast cancer: here to stay. We can expect plenty of requests for detailed typing in the future, further scrutiny of the performance characteristics and/or quantitation of immunohistochemical protein expression assays in fixed tissue, and husbanding of tissue resources for various genetic and/or drug targeting analyses to come.

A. McCullough, MD

ROCK Inhibitor and Feeder Cells Induce the Conditional Reprogramming of Epithelial Cells

Liu X, Ory V, Chapman S, et al (Georgetown Univ Med School, Washington, DC; Natl Inst of Allergy and Infectious Diseases, Bethesda, MD; et al)
Am J Pathol 180:599-607, 2012

We demonstrate that a Rho kinase inhibitor (Y-27632), in combination with fibroblast feeder cells, induces normal and tumor epithelial cells from many tissues to proliferate indefinitely *in vitro*, without transduction of exogenous viral or cellular genes. Primary prostate and mammary cells, for example, are reprogrammed toward a basaloid, stem-like phenotype and form well-organized prostaspheres and mammospheres in Matrigel. However, in contrast to the selection of rare stem-like cells, the described growth conditions can generate 2×10^6 cells in 5 to 6 days from needle biopsies, and can generate cultures from cryopreserved tissue and from fewer than four viable cells. Continued cell proliferation is dependent on both feeder cells and Y-27632, and the conditionally reprogrammed cells (CRCs) retain a normal karyotype and remain nontumorigenic. This technique also efficiently establishes cell cultures from human and rodent tumors. For example, CRCs established from human prostate adenocarcinoma displayed instability of chromosome 13, proliferated abnormally in Matrigel, and formed tumors in mice with severe combined immunodeficiency. The ability to rapidly generate many tumor cells from small biopsy specimens and frozen tissue provides significant opportunities for cell-based diagnostics and therapeutics (including chemosensitivity testing) and greatly expands the value of biobanking. In addition, the CRC method allows for the genetic manipulation of epithelial cells *ex vivo* and their subsequent evaluation *in vivo* in the same host.

▶ Despite the use of cell culture systems for thousands of investigations, the initiation and maintenance of cell lines that can avoid senescence and stay true to their original phenotypical characteristics has proven difficult with traditional cell culture methods. Getting a specific tumor into a cell line that could be maintained over time is a technical challenge and making a long-lasting cell line of normal tissues from the same individual patient previously technically impossible.

This article details an important advance for preparing cell cultures of tumors and normal tissues, now termed the Georgetown method. This method relies on Rho kinase inhibitor in combination with fibroblast feeder cells to promote indefinite cell culture growth of both normal and tumoral epithelial cells from an array of tissue types. Their immortalized growth and "conditional reprogramming" by this method leads to a virtually unlimited proliferation of the culture without the onset of senescence and without transformation of the cell's original phenotypic integrity. The authors also propagated and maintained normal cell lines from the same patients in normal/tumor matched pairs. Some other exciting aspects of this work include the very small volumes (as few as 4 cells) that successfully led to cultures, the propagation of cultures from frozen specimens, and the short period they report to make a cell line (as little as 6 days).

The ability to take almost any tumor in small volume with accompanying normal epithelium from the same organ from any individual patient, immortalize it, and maintain them in their original states through multiple passages seems a huge breakthrough to me. No more searching for a suitable cell line would seem necessary; just take a small biopsy of the carcinoma and set it up. No more running out of tissue and no more worrying about if the tissue has transformed through multiple cell culture passages. This method diminishes many technical challenges in the tissue limitations of studying a particular tumor. As a pathologist sometimes called on to stretch limited fresh-tissue resources for various researchers, I can breathe easier; this method has the potential to make expansion of banked tissue virtually unlimited.

If you can maintain the cell line and keep its lineage true, you can also have ample opportunity to study it, including studying it for potential therapeutic purposes. The same group in another report[1] describes the use of this method to harvest and immortalize tissue from a patient with pulmonary human papilloma virus—related papillomatosis. They obtained a small amount of tissue from a lung biopsy, established a cell line, tested with antiviral medications in vitro, and subsequently showed an in vivo response in the patient with the chosen drug.

A. McCullough, MD

Reference

1. Yuan H, Myers S, Wang J, et al. Use of reprogrammed cells to identify therapy for respiratory papillomatosis. N Engl J Med. 2012;367:1220-1227.

Comprehensive genomic characterization of squamous cell lung cancers
The Cancer Genome Atlas Research Network (The Eli and Edythe L. Broad Inst of Massachusetts Inst of Technology and Harvard Univ Cambridge; Dana-Farber Cancer Inst, Boston, MA; et al)
Nature 489:519-525, 2012

Lung squamous cell carcinoma is a common type of lung cancer, causing approximately 400 000 deaths per year worldwide. Genomic alterations in squamous cell lung cancers have not been comprehensively characterized, and no molecularly targeted agents have been specifically developed for its treatment. As part of The Cancer Genome Atlas, here we profile 178 lung squamous cell carcinomas to provide a comprehensive landscape of genomic and epigenomic alterations. We show that the tumour type is characterized by complex genomic alterations, with a mean of 360 exonic mutations, 165 genomic rearrangements, and 323 segments of copy number alteration per tumour. We find statistically recurrent mutations in 11 genes, including mutation of *TP53* in nearly all specimens. Previously unreported loss-of-function mutations are seen in the *HLA-A* class I major histocompatibility gene. Significantly altered pathways included *NFE2L2* and *KEAP1* in 34%, squamous differentiation genes in 44%, phosphatidylinositol-3-OH kinase pathway genes in 47%, and *CDKN2A* and *RB1* in 72% of tumours.

We identified a potential therapeutic target in most tumours, offering new avenues of investigation for the treatment of squamous cell lung cancers.

▶ This article is another tome from the Cancer Genome Atlas Research network to collate the diverse and numerous mutations in squamous cell carcinoma of the lung.

We are all hearing a great deal about *EGFR* and *ALK* mutations in pulmonary adenocarcinoma, and testing for these abnormalities may well be routine at your site due to the advent of targeted therapy for these malignancies. This report summarizes mutations in 178 squamous carcinomas; squamous carcinoma seems a different animal.

First, *EGFR* and *ALK* mutations are very rare in this cohort of squamous carcinoma, underscoring again the importance of correct morphologic typing before testing non-small-cell lung carcinomas. Also genetically correlated are 4 gene expression subtype signatures designated as classical, basal, secretory, and primitive in squamous cell carcinoma. The descriptors have not fallen into common use, at least where I work, but can be roughly characterized by a higher frequency of common mutations, in particular, in the classical subtype.

A few interesting findings from this very dense data include (1) almost every squamous cell carcinoma carried a somatic mutation in *TP53*; (2) There was a high rate of inactivating mutations in the *HLA-A* gene, suggesting some role in avoidance of immune destruction and a potential path for immunological therapies; (3) squamous cell carcinoma of the lung bears genetic similarity to head and neck carcinomas; (4) there are frequent alterations in these pathways: *CDKN2A/RB1*, *NFE2L2/KEAP1/CUL3*, *PI3K/AKT*, and *SOX2/TP63/NOTCH1*; (5) *KRAS* mutations, common in pulmonary adenocarcinomas, are very uncommon in squamous carcinomas.

These data are more ammunition in the search for a magic bullet to use for targeted therapy of squamous carcinoma.

A. McCullough, MD

RAS Mutations in Cutaneous Squamous-Cell Carcinomas in Patients Treated with BRAF Inhibitors

Su F, Viros A, Milagre C, et al (Hoffmann—La Roche, Nutley, NJ; Inst of Cancer Res, London, UK; et al)
N Engl J Med 366:207-215, 2012

Background.—Cutaneous squamous-cell carcinomas and keratoacanthomas are common findings in patients treated with BRAF inhibitors.

Methods.—We performed a molecular analysis to identify oncogenic mutations (*HRAS, KRAS, NRAS, CDKN2A,* and *TP53*) in the lesions from patients treated with the BRAF inhibitor vemurafenib. An analysis of an independent validation set and functional studies with BRAF inhibitors in the presence of the prevalent *RAS* mutation was also performed.

Results.—Among 21 tumor samples, 13 had *RAS* mutations (12 in *HRAS*). In a validation set of 14 samples, 8 had *RAS* mutations (4 in *HRAS*). Thus,

60% (21 of 35) of the specimens harbored *RAS* mutations, the most prevalent being *HRAS Q61L*. Increased proliferation of *HRAS Q61L*—mutant cell lines exposed to vemurafenib was associated with mitogen-activated protein kinase (MAPK)—pathway signaling and activation of ERK-mediated transcription. In a mouse model of *HRAS Q61L*—mediated skin carcinogenesis, the vemurafenib analogue PLX4720 was not an initiator or a promoter of carcinogenesis but accelerated growth of the lesions harboring *HRAS* mutations, and this growth was blocked by concomitant treatment with a MEK inhibitor.

Conclusions.—Mutations in *RAS*, particularly *HRAS*, are frequent in cutaneous squamous-cell carcinomas and keratoacanthomas that develop in patients treated with vemurafenib. The molecular mechanism is consistent with the paradoxical activation of MAPK signaling and leads to accelerated growth of these lesions. (Funded by Hoffmann—La Roche and others; ClinicalTrials.gov numbers, NCT00405587, NCT00949702, NCT01001299, and NCT01006980.)

▶ New drugs for the treatment of melanoma have prompted testing of melanomas for the BRAF V600E mutation. Type I BRAF inhibitors (vemurafenib and dabrafenib) have shown antitumor activity more promising than standard chemotherapy.[1]

A fascinating side effect of this new molecular therapy is the development of cutaneous squamous cell carcinomas soon after BRAF inhibitor treatment, with the earliest lesion in this report appearing as soon as 3 weeks posttherapy. This report describes the molecular analysis of these squamous carcinomas developing in BRAF inhibitor—treated patients. The major findings in these squamous carcinomas were mutations in RAS, mostly in HRAS. The apparent mechanism for the development of squamous carcinomas is BRAF inhibitor hyperactivation of the mitogen-activated protein kinase pathway.

So a specific side effect of one targeted therapy is secondary tumor development; no advance comes for free. Aside from revealing another group of people predisposed to squamous carcinomas, these findings suggest increased testing requirements in the future for patients who may be receiving BRAF inhibitors. The accompanying editorial suggests persons planning on receiving BRAF inhibitor therapy should be tested for the presence of RAS mutations. Whether the RAS mutations occur de novo or this therapy causes emergence of previously existing RAS mutations is not completely clear; this study and the putative mechanism in the development of squamous carcinoma suggest RAS mutations antedate BRAF inhibitor therapy.

A. McCullough, MD

Reference

1. Weeraratna AT. RAF around the edges—the paradox of BRAF inhibitors. *N Engl J Med.* 2012;366:271-273.

IgG4-Related Disease

Stone JH, Zen Y, Deshpande V (Massachusetts General Hosp, Boston; King's College Hosp, London, UK)
N Engl J Med 366:539-551, 2012

Background.—IgG4-related disease is a recently recognized fibroinflammatory condition characterized by tumefactive lesions, a dense lymphoplasmacytic infiltrate rich in IgG4-positive plasma cells, storiform fibrosis, and sometimes elevated serum IgG4 concentrations. It can affect virtually all organ systems, with histopathologic features that bear striking similarities regardless of the disease site. Much remains unknown about the behavior of IgG4 in vivo, but the current knowledge regarding the features of IgG4-related disease, potential disease mechanisms, and treatment was reviewed.

Disease Features and Mechanisms.—IgG4 accounts for less than 5% of the total IgG in healthy persons. Although levels vary widely between persons, they tend to be stable within an individual. In theory IgG4 does not activate the classical complement pathway effectively so its role in immune activation has been considered minimal. IgG4 has a unique characteristic: a half-antibody exchange reaction, called the fragment antigen-binding (Fab)-n-arm exchange. As a result, about half of the IgG4 molecules consist of heavy chains linked weakly through noncovalent forces and the remainder have intact disulfide bonds between heavy chains in vivo. IgG4's anti-inflammatory function may be related to rheumatoid factor activity and binding to the Fc portion of IgG antibodies. IgG4 production is mediated by type 2 helper T (Th2) cells.

Misdiagnoses are common. Key morphologic findings are a dense lymphoplasmacytic infiltrate organized in a storiform pattern, obliterative phlebitis, and mild to moderate eosinophil infiltrate. The inflammatory lesion can form a tumefactive mass that destroys involved organs. Diagnosis requires immunohistochemical confirmation with IgG4 immunostaining. Semi-quantitative analysis distinguishes IgG4-related disease from other conditions, such as lymphomas.

Several immune-mediated mechanisms contribute to the fibroinflammatory process of IgG4-related disease. Potential initiating mechanisms are genetic risk factors, bacterial infections and molecular mimicry, and autoimmunity. Specific disease pathways can involve Th2 cells and regulatory immune reaction and IgG4 antibodies.

The epidemiology of IgG4-related disease is poorly described, but most patients are men older than age 50 years. The major clinical manifestations are subacute, so cases are often identified incidentally through radiologic findings or pathologic specimens. One or multiple organs may be involved. A few patients improve spontaneously. Tumefactive lesions and allergic disease are common findings. Major tissue damage and organ failure can occur, but these usually develop subacutely. Untreated IgG4-related cholangitis can produce hepatic failure within months; IgG4-related aortitis can lead to aneurysms and aortic dissections, possibly causing 10% to 50% of inflammatory aortitis cases. Most organs have less aggressive lesions.

Imaging results vary widely, especially in the lung and kidney. Although most patients with IgG4-related disease have elevated serum IgG4 concentrations, the range is wide. Most become lower with glucocorticoid treatment but remain above normal values. The disease may remain in remission or relapse, but insufficient follow-up has been done to predict disease relapse.

Treatment.—Aggressive treatment is undertaken if major organs are involved because IgG4-related disease can lead to serious dysfunction and organ failure. Watchful waiting can be the prudent course in other cases. The correlation between extent of disease and need for treatment is imperfect at best. Treatment with glucocorticoids is typically the first approach, often involving prednisolone 0.6 mg/kg of body weight per day for 2 to 4 weeks initially. Prednisolone can be tapered over 3 to 6 months to 5.0 mg/day, then continued at a dose of 2.5 to 5.0 mg/day for up to 3 years. Some approaches discontinue glucocorticoids completely within 3 months. Disease flares are common. Other agents used as glucocorticoid-sparing agents or remission-maintenance drugs after glucocorticoid-induced remission include azathioprine, mycophenolate mofetil, and methotrexate, but clinical trials supporting their efficacy are lacking. B-cell depletion with rituximab may be useful in patients with recurrent or refractory disease, sometimes producing swift clinical responses and clinical improvement in weeks. A major determinant of treatment responsiveness is the extent of fibrosis in the affected organs. Untreated, IgG4-related disease often progresses from lymphoplasmacytic inflammation to extensive fibrosis. Glucocorticoids and rituximab may be less effective in patients with advanced fibrosis, but some patients respond even with widespread fibrosis.

Conclusions.—IgG4-related disease has pathologic features consistent across many organ systems. Several medical disorders previously thought to be confined to a single organ system may be part of this disease. Greater understanding of the IgG4 molecule, the diverse facets of IgG4-related disease, and treatment responses may reveal more about immune function and other possibly related conditions.

▶ Tumefactive sclerosing fibro inflammatory lesions with lymphoplasmacytic infiltrates, including so-called pseudotumors in various organs of the body, have long been a diagnostic conundrum for surgical pathologists. This review describes the common features of the unifying theme of immunoglobulin G4 (IgG4)—related disease.

Diagnosis of IgG4-related disease is based on a constellation of clinical, radiologic, and serologic findings in the presence of characteristic histopathologic findings. This review is a concise summary of all these features with a discussion of the pathologic findings common to multiple organ sites. The description of accepted immunohistochemical ratios of semiquantitated IgG4 immunostaining is helpful and includes caveats about IgG4 expression in other situations.

Interesting components of this article include proposed roles of autoimmunity, T-cell activation, and cytokine influence as mechanisms of disease causing the ultimately fibrotic state. As a corollary to such a proposed mechanism, there could be abundant opportunities for research concerning the components of this quasi-autoimmune and quasi-allergic phenomenon, including the role and levels of various interleukins, the function and number of type 2 helper and regulatory T cells, and the potential initiating triggers. There is more involved here than plasma cells and IgG4; whether the unique features of the IgG4 molecule are etiologic or a marker of sequelae of more complex etiologic immune mechanisms remains unclear. This review gives a nice summary for a busy pathologist charged with recognizing the characteristic histopathologic milieu and plenty to think about in potential clinical testing requests.

A supplementary appendix (Table 1 in the original article) reproduced electronically, neatly summarizes the clinical conditions of IgG4-related disease throughout the body.

A. McCullough, MD

Comprehensive molecular characterization of human colon and rectal cancer

The Cancer Genome Atlas Network (Baylor College of Medicine, Houston, TX; et al)
Nature 487:330-337, 2012

To characterize somatic alterations in colorectal carcinoma, we conducted a genome-scale analysis of 276 samples, analysing exome sequence, DNA copy number, promoter methylation and messenger RNA and microRNA expression. A subset of these samples (97) underwent low-depth-of-coverage whole-genome sequencing. In total, 16% of colorectal carcinomas were found to be hypermutated: three-quarters of these had the expected high microsatellite instability, usually with hypermethylation and *MLH1* silencing, and one-quarter had somatic mismatch-repair gene and polymerase ε (*POLE*) mutations. Excluding the hypermutated cancers, colon and rectum cancers were found to have considerably similar patterns of genomic alteration. Twenty-four genes were significantly mutated, and in addition to the expected *APC, TP53, SMAD4, PIK3CA* and *KRAS* mutations, we found frequent mutations in *ARID1A, SOX9* and *FAM123B*. Recurrent copy-number alterations include potentially drug-targetable amplifications of *ERBB2* and newly discovered amplification of *IGF2*. Recurrent chromosomal translocations include the fusion of *NAV2* and WNT pathway member *TCF7L1*. Integrative analyses suggest new markers for aggressive colorectal carcinoma and an important role for *MYC*-directed transcriptional activation and repression.

▶ This article is another summary of extensive data from The Cancer Genome Atlas Network, similar to those described in this chapter for breast carcinoma and pulmonary squamous cell carcinoma, but this time for colon and rectal cancer.

The article amplifies and summarizes many of the known genetic abnormalities of colon cancer by a summary of 224 prospectively gathered carcinomas from throughout the colon.

What are some takeaway points for the practicing pathologist? The genetic data in here support the following observations. (1) There is little genetic difference between rectal and colon cancers, and although we distinguish them in our surgery or treatments, this anatomic distinction is not where oncological differences in colon cancers lie. (2) Some colon cancers have relatively few mutations, and some are hypermutated; the authors divide their cohort into these 2 main groups based on mutation rates. Similar to other colon cancer studies, this cohort showed hypermutated cancers predominantly from the right colon; such cancers were predominantly diploid and generally hypermethylated and often showed microsatellite instability. Nonhypermutated tumors showed similarities despite their anatomic site in the colon. (3) Both hypermutated and nonhypermutated cancers showed abnormalities in the WNT signaling pathway; the WNT pathway family embraces the previously studied frequent *APC* mutations. (4) Other commonly abnormal pathways in colon cancer include the transforming growth factor (TGF)-β, PI3K, and RTK-RAS signaling pathways. Several pathways seem to lead back to a critical role of *MYC*. (5) The cohort describes new recurrent mutations in *FAM123B*, *ARDI1A*, and *SOX9* and overexpression of the WNT ligand receptor gene *FZD10*. SOX9 protein facilitates β-catenin degradation, and the authors state this finding represents a novel mutation for any human cancer.

This catalog of mutations supports activation of the WNT signaling pathway, inactivation of TGF-β signaling, and increased activity of *MYC* as common in most colon cancers. After the large diversity seen in the breast and squamous carcinoma genetic descriptions, it's heartening to see some commonality in this report. Sometimes one wonders if all this genomic data will produce so many abnormalities as to split cancer research and drug development off into myriad directions. Suggested drug targets for colon cancer of WNT-signaling inhibitors and small-molecule β-catenin inhibitors seem reasonable based on the common mutations seen here and these new findings.

A. McCullough, MD

Prognostic Relevance of Integrated Genetic Profiling in Acute Myeloid Leukemia
Patel JP, Gönen M, Figueroa ME, et al (Memorial Sloan-Kettering Cancer Ctr, NY; Weill Cornell Med College, NY; et al)
N Engl J Med 366:1079-1089, 2012

Background.—Acute myeloid leukemia (AML) is a heterogeneous disease with respect to presentation and clinical outcome. The prognostic value of recently identified somatic mutations has not been systematically evaluated in a phase 3 trial of treatment for AML.

Methods.—We performed a mutational analysis of 18 genes in 398 patients younger than 60 years of age who had AML and who were randomly assigned to receive induction therapy with high-dose or standard-dose daunorubicin. We validated our prognostic findings in an independent set of 104 patients.

Results.—We identified at least one somatic alteration in 97.3% of the patients. We found that internal tandem duplication in *FLT3* (*FLT3*-ITD), partial tandem duplication in *MLL* (*MLL*-PTD), and mutations in *ASXL1* and *PHF6* were associated with reduced overall survival ($P = 0.001$ for *FLT3*-ITD, $P = 0.009$ for *MLL*-PTD, $P = 0.05$ for *ASXL1*, and $P = 0.006$ for *PHF6*); *CEBPA* and *IDH2* mutations were associated with improved overall survival ($P = 0.05$ for *CEBPA* and $P = 0.01$ for *IDH2*). The favorable effect of *NPM1* mutations was restricted to patients with co-occurring *NPM1* and *IDH1* or *IDH2* mutations. We identified genetic predictors of outcome that improved risk stratification among patients with AML, independently of age, white-cell count, induction dose, and post-remission therapy, and validated the significance of these predictors in an independent cohort. High-dose daunorubicin, as compared with standard-dose daunorubicin, improved the rate of survival among patients with *DNMT3A* or *NPM1* mutations or *MLL* translocations ($P = 0.001$) but not among patients with wild-type *DNMT3A*, *NPM1*, and *MLL* ($P = 0.67$).

Conclusions.—We found that *DNMT3A* and *NPM1* mutations and *MLL* translocations predicted an improved outcome with high-dose induction chemotherapy in patients with AML. These findings suggest that mutational profiling could potentially be used for risk stratification and to inform prognostic and therapeutic decisions regarding patients with AML. (Funded by the National Cancer Institute and others.)

▶ Karyotyping, fluorescent in situ hybridization analysis, and genetic analysis are standard practices in diagnosis and prognostication of acute myeloid leukemia (AML). This article reports on use of a mutational analysis of 18 genes in 398 patients with AML enrolled in clinical trial E1900. The analysis is based on sequencing of a limited number of genes, some associated with improved and some with diminished overall survival. It suggests a model based on this retrospective analysis of stored specimens that could be used to stratify risk, in particular those with intermediate risk, prior to induction. As support for this plan, the authors report data showing that in the accompanying trial those with DNMT3A or NPM1 mutations and those with *MLL* rearrangements had better survival with higher-dose therapy.

In an adjacent article in the same issue of *New England Journal of Medicine*, Walter et al[1] describe a much more comprehensive analysis of 7 cases of secondary AML arising in myelodysplastic syndrome, hundreds of acquired mutations, the emergence of a dominant leukemic subclone, and the description of 11 genes that mutated recurrently, 4 of which (UMODL1, CDH23, SMC3, and ZSWIM4) were not previously known to be significant.

The complexities of the prognostic interaction of these abnormalities and the division of AML into various different prognostic and potentially therapeutic subgroups I leave to hematologists. The juxtaposition of these articles leaves one asking some basic questions about how to approach the explosion of molecular data. Are more data better? If we find more and more abnormalities because of our increasingly finer genomic resolution, how will we find the wheat in all the chaff?

The accompanying editorial[2] brings up the question of how such analyses would be used clinically. Because I seem to have preferentially diagnosed AML late on Friday afternoons, I wonder what the practical implications are of using a panel for genetic mutational abnormalities to obtain data to guide therapy. As we analyze more widely and deeply for the molecular alterations of acute leukemia, we will have to find some new scoring or integrated system to grade the relative weight of significant mutations, and the addition of new testing for newly significant mutations, if we can even get them all analyzed in sufficient time to guide treatment.

A. McCullough, MD

References

1. Walter MJ, Shen D, Ding L, et al. Clonal architecture of secondary acute myeloid leukemia. *N Engl J Med*. 2012;366:1090-1098.
2. Godley LA. Profiles in leukemia. *N Engl J Med*. 2012;366:1152-1153.

Fibulin-3 as a Blood and Effusion Biomarker for Pleural Mesothelioma
Pass HI, Levin SM, Harbut MR, et al (New York Univ Langone Med Ctr; Mount Sinai School of Medicine, NY; Karmanos Cancer Inst, Detroit, MI; et al)
N Engl J Med 367:1417-1427, 2012

Background.—New biomarkers are needed to detect pleural mesothelioma at an earlier stage and to individualize treatment strategies. We investigated whether fibulin-3 in plasma and pleural effusions could meet sensitivity and specificity criteria for a robust biomarker.

Methods.—We measured fibulin-3 levels in plasma (from 92 patients with mesothelioma, 136 asbestos-exposed persons without cancer, 93 patients with effusions not due to mesothelioma, and 43 healthy controls), effusions (from 74 patients with mesothelioma, 39 with benign effusions, and 54 with malignant effusions not due to mesothelioma), or both. A blinded validation was subsequently performed. Tumor tissue was examined for fibulin-3 by immunohistochemical analysis, and levels of fibulin-3 in plasma and effusions were measured with an enzyme-linked immunosorbent assay.

Results.—Plasma fibulin-3 levels did not vary according to age, sex, duration of asbestos exposure, or degree of radiographic changes and were significantly higher in patients with pleural mesothelioma (105 ± 7 ng per milliliter in the Detroit cohort and 113 ± 8 ng per milliliter in the New York cohort) than in asbestos-exposed persons without mesothelioma (14 ± 1 ng per milliliter and 24 ± 1 ng per milliliter, respectively; $P < 0.001$). Effusion fibulin-3 levels were significantly higher in patients with pleural mesothelioma (694 ± 37 ng per milliliter in the Detroit cohort and 636 ± 92 ng per milliliter in the New York cohort) than in patients with effusions not due to mesothelioma (212 ± 25 and 151 ± 23 ng per milliliter, respectively; $P < 0.001$). Fibulin-3 preferentially stained tumor cells in 26 of

26 samples. In an overall comparison of patients with and those without mesothelioma, the receiver-operating-characteristic curve for plasma fibulin-3 levels had a sensitivity of 96.7% and a specificity of 95.5% at a cutoff value of 52.8 ng of fibulin-3 per milliliter. In a comparison of patients with early-stage mesothelioma with asbestos-exposed persons, the sensitivity was 100% and the specificity was 94.1% at a cutoff value of 46.0 ng of fibulin-3 per milliliter. Blinded validation revealed an area under the curve of 0.87 for plasma specimens from 96 asbestos-exposed persons as compared with 48 patients with mesothelioma.

Conclusions.—Plasma fibulin-3 levels can distinguish healthy persons with exposure to asbestos from patients with mesothelioma. In conjunction with effusion fibulin-3 levels, plasma fibulin-3 levels can further differentiate mesothelioma effusions from other malignant and benign effusions. (Funded by the Early Detection Research Network, National Institutes of Health, and others.)

▶ The hunt for worthy individual tumor markers continues in the age of molecular arrays; this report describes a potentially valuable marker for mesothelioma.

Fibulin-3 is a glycoprotein encoded by the gene epidermal growth factor-containing fibulin-like extracellular matrix protein 1 (EFEMP1), expressed in condensing mesenchyme and little expressed in most normal tissues. The authors analyzed archived normal plasma, plasma from persons with pleural mesothelioma and other effusion-causing malignancies, pleural effusions resulting from mesothelioma and other malignancies, and benign pleural effusions in asbestos-exposed persons to demonstrate significantly increased plasma and effusion fibulin-3 levels in persons with malignant mesothelioma. In distinguishing asbestos-exposed persons with benign effusions from those with early mesothelioma, the plasma assay demonstrated sensitivity of 100% and specificity of 94%.

This marker may not be ready for diagnostic prime time yet because of the relatively small numbers, but it seems a promising start. The results are bolstered by the fact that similar results were obtained independently in three separate cohorts at 3 separate centers. Plasma levels of fibulin-3 were significantly elevated in patients with mesothelioma, approximately 2 to 4 times higher than those from other causes. Elevations in fibulin-3 levels in effusions resulting from mesothelioma were also elevated with typically 3 times difference between fibulin-3 levels from mesothelioma and effusions from other causes, including other malignant effusions. A small (n = 26) group of tissues from these mesotheliomas, examined in a tumoral microarray, all showed either nuclear or cytoplasmic expression of fibulin-3 using a Santa Cruz antibody immunohistochemical method (detailed in the supplementary appendix).

We have all been disappointed by tests for novel markers that when more widely used showed disappointing performance compared to the original report. We'll have to wait for more data about how this method performs in larger cohorts prospectively, but this article makes me want to cautiously try these methods out in tissues, effusions, and plasma. I find pleural mesothelial proliferations diagnostically challenging and welcome the chance to vet any protein that seems this strikingly elevated in the presence of malignant mesothelioma.

A. McCullough, MD

Intratumor Heterogeneity and Branched Evolution Revealed by Multiregion Sequencing
Gerlinger M, Rowan AJ, Horswell S, et al (Cancer Res UK London Res Inst; et al)
N Engl J Med 366:883-892, 2012

Background.—Intratumor heterogeneity may foster tumor evolution and adaptation and hinder personalized-medicine strategies that depend on results from single tumor-biopsy samples.

Methods.—To examine intratumor heterogeneity, we performed exome sequencing, chromosome aberration analysis, and ploidy profiling on multiple spatially separated samples obtained from primary renal carcinomas and associated metastatic sites. We characterized the consequences of intratumor heterogeneity using immunohistochemical analysis, mutation functional analysis, and profiling of messenger RNA expression.

Results.—Phylogenetic reconstruction revealed branched evolutionary tumor growth, with 63 to 69% of all somatic mutations not detectable across every tumor region. Intratumor heterogeneity was observed for a mutation within an autoinhibitory domain of the mammalian target of rapamycin (mTOR) kinase, correlating with S6 and 4EBP phosphorylation in vivo and constitutive activation of mTOR kinase activity in vitro. Mutational intratumor heterogeneity was seen for multiple tumor-suppressor genes converging on loss of function; *SETD2*, *PTEN*, and *KDM5C* underwent multiple distinct and spatially separated inactivating mutations within a single tumor, suggesting convergent phenotypic evolution. Gene-expression signatures of good and poor prognosis were detected in different regions of the same tumor. Allelic composition and ploidy profiling analysis revealed extensive intratumor heterogeneity, with 26 of 30 tumor samples from four tumors harboring divergent allelic-imbalance profiles and with ploidy heterogeneity in two of four tumors.

Conclusions.—Intratumor heterogeneity can lead to underestimation of the tumor genomics landscape portrayed from single tumor-biopsy samples and may present major challenges to personalized-medicine and biomarker development. Intratumor heterogeneity, associated with heterogeneous protein function, may foster tumor adaptation and therapeutic failure through Darwinian selection. (Funded by the Medical Research Council and others.)

▶ What pathologist has not seen single malignant tumors with wide variation in histological patterns or malignant tumors where minor primary patterns became the dominant histology in the subsequent metastasis? The assumption that molecular characteristics are similar throughout one tumor seems at odds with much experience in morphology, particularly in solid tumors. Yet for many new molecular tests, it is standard practice to analyze a single sample or a single block, and sometimes quite a small sample from biopsy material. This practice is based on the premise that the result represents the majority of abnormalities in the tumor or the particular target is evenly present, presumably because of some degree of homogeneity in the tumor.

But what of tumoral heterogeneity—words one hears invoked to explain discordant results in simple immunohistochemical discordance and something we know exists because of knowledge of different malignant clones? If such heterogeneity is common, what are the implications for molecular testing?

A snapshot of the possible implications of tumoral heterogeneity in one type of carcinoma is considered in this article, analyzing 4 primary renal cell carcinomas and some of their metastases. Each of the 4 carcinomas was subjected to extensive analysis of multiple samples from multiple areas within a single carcinoma and the results collated. There was extensive intratumoral heterogeneity within a single tumor with 63% to 69% of somatic mutations not detectable in every tumor sample within a single carcinoma. In 1 carcinoma, a prognostic gene expression profile was applied to 1 tumor sampled in multiple areas and gave results suggesting both good and poor outcomes in the same carcinoma, depending on where the sample was taken. The article gives no real information about whether the samples appeared similar histologically, other than being clear cell carcinomas.

Additional heterogeneity between primary tumors and their metastases and heterogeneous mutations within even 1 abnormal gene in a single carcinoma seem to suggest a complexity of unique genetic heterogeneity per tumor that would confound personalized therapy.[1]

On a practical level, will findings such as this one cause a change in testing procedure? Should you send a bigger sample to be genotyped or to search for a specific target? Should you sample several small sites and combine them to reflect a more accurate sample of a whole tumor? How much heterogeneity is present in different families or types of malignancies? Can divergent histological patterns within a single tumor predict such molecular heterogeneity? Should samples be combined and homogenized as is common in microbiology laboratories to increase diagnostic yield? There are no recommendations here except suggestions in the article and accompanying editorial that 1 sample may not be enough. There are implications for searching for specific molecular targets, suggesting that limited sampling in a genetically heterogeneous tumor would significantly underestimate the potential target.

A. McCullough, MD

Reference

1. Longo DL. Tumor heterogeneity and personalized medicine. *N Engl J Med.* 2012; 366:956-957.

Noninvasive Whole-Genome Sequencing of a Human Fetus

Kitzman JO, Snyder MW, Ventura M, et al (Univ of Washington, Seattle; et al)
Sci Transl Med 4:137ra76, 2012

Analysis of cell-free fetal DNA in maternal plasma holds promise for the development of noninvasive prenatal genetic diagnostics. Previous studies have been restricted to detection of fetal trisomies, to specific paternally inherited mutations, or to genotyping common polymorphisms using material obtained invasively, for example, through chorionic villus sampling. Here, we combine genome sequencing of two parents, genome-wide maternal haplotyping, and deep sequencing of maternal plasma DNA to noninvasively determine the genome sequence of a human fetus at 18.5 weeks of gestation. Inheritance was predicted at 2.8×10^6 parental heterozygous sites with 98.1% accuracy. Furthermore, 39 of 44 de novo point mutations in the fetal genome were detected, albeit with limited specificity. Subsampling these data and analyzing a second family trio by the same approach indicate that parental haplotype blocks of ~300 kilo—base pairs combined with shallow sequencing of maternal plasma DNA is sufficient to substantially determine the inherited complement of a fetal genome. However, ultradeep sequencing of maternal plasma DNA is necessary for the practical detection of fetal de novo mutations genome-wide. Although technical and analytical challenges remain, we anticipate that noninvasive analysis of inherited variation and de novo mutations in fetal genomes will facilitate prenatal diagnosis of both recessive and dominant Mendelian disorders.

▶ Did you know that approximately 10% of noncellular DNA in a pregnant woman's plasma derives from the fetus? The discovery of cell-free fetal DNA (cffDNA) in maternal plasma was the basis for noninvasive prenatal diagnosis (NIPD). These small fetal oligonucleotides can be detected early in pregnancy at 8 to 10 weeks postconception. Several companies have been marketing this technology for detection of specific trisomies in the prenatal period. Most of these companies are currently mired in litigation over the method patents. The noninvasive nature of such testing will be changing how we use amniocentesis and chorionic villous sampling when sufficient clinical experience is gained and the legal dust settles.

This report describes an extensive approach to nearly whole-genome sequencing of an 18.5-week fetus (and less complete sequencing of an 8.2-week fetus) from cffDNA obtained from the mother's peripheral blood. The method is complicated and involves family trios (mother, father, and fetus), genome sequencing of both parents, genome-wide maternal haplotyping, and deep sequencing of maternal plasma.

The medical, ethical, and legal implications of a technology that could predict inheritance of most known and some de novo mutations in early pregnancy are huge. Parents, practitioners, managed care companies, and ethicists are only beginning to try to comprehend what extensive genomic data may mean in the antenatal period, especially early in pregnancy when termination of pregnancy may be accomplished with a medication rather than a procedure. Although this report does not describe a method that is ready yet for clinical applications, as NIPD testing matures and is refined, testing for a small set of specific mutations, such as trisomies, may well be replaced by such an extensive approach, possibly in the first trimester. The authors of this article struck a cautionary note, a theme in whole genomic reports, when they concluded, "A final point is that as in other areas of clinical genetics, our capacity to generate data is outstripping our ability to interpret it in ways that are useful to physicians and patients." Physicians, keep your genetic counselor close if you have one.

A. McCullough, MD

PART II

LABORATORY MEDICINE

16 Laboratory Management and Outcomes

The Brain-to-Brain Loop Concept for Laboratory Testing 40 Years After Its Introduction
Plebani M, Laposata M, Lundberg GD (Univ of Padova, Italy; Vanderbilt Univ School of Medicine, Nashville, TN; Stanford Univ, Palo Alto, CA)
Am J Clin Pathol 136:829-833, 2011

Forty years ago, Lundberg introduced the concept of the brain-to-brain loop for laboratory testing. In this concept, in the brain of the physician caring for the patient, the first step involves the selection of laboratory tests and the final step is the transmission of the test result to the ordering physician. There are many intermediary steps, some of which are preanalytic, ie, before performance of the test; some are analytic and relate to the actual performance of the test; and others are postanalytic and involve transmission of test results into the medical record. The introduction of this concept led to a system to identify and classify errors associated with laboratory test performance. Errors have since been considered as preanalytic, analytic, and postanalytic. During the past 4 decades, changes in medical practice have significantly altered the brain-to-brain loop for laboratory testing. This review describes the changes and their implications for analysis of errors associated with laboratory testing (Fig 1).

▶ According to the concept of the "brain-to-brain turnaround time loop" (Fig 1), the generation of any laboratory test result consists of 9 steps, including ordering, collection, identification (at several stages), transportation, separation (or preparation), analysis, reporting, interpretation, and action. The current landscape of medicine has greatly impacted the brain-to-brain loop. In the case of medical laboratories, the challenges are significant for several reasons. Traditionally, laboratory tests have been thought to have merely corroborative or exclusionary value, thus supporting the view of clinical laboratories as an ancillary service and, even more dangerously, laboratory diagnostics as a commodity. The availability of laboratory results derived from testing at home and point-of-care testing

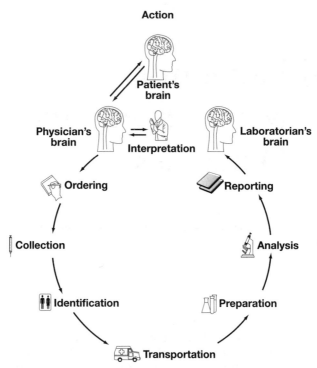

FIGURE 1.—The brain-to-brain loop for laboratory testing 40 years later. (Reprinted from Plebani M, Laposata M, Lundberg GD. The brain-to-brain loop concept for laboratory testing 40 years after its introduction. *Am J Clin Pathol.* 2011;136:829-833, with permission from American Society for Clinical Pathology.)

and the excessive confidence in the value of laboratory results that are generated by all testing devices have led to decontextualizing laboratory diagnostics from the clinical setting to extrapolating test results from all other clinical information. This, in turn, has led to reorganizing laboratory services into "focused factories" actively competing for the business of increasingly savvy customers. Recent technological advances and the new generation of laboratory diagnostics, namely, genetic tests, have occurred despite the relatively low importance given by most stakeholders, including clinicians and policymakers, to the ultimate impact of laboratory information. Major threats and challenges to the brain-to-brain loop mainly originate from 5 factors: the nature of errors in the total testing process, testing and delivery of test results directly to patients, alternative testing sites, increasing difficulties at the laboratory-clinical interface, and a decreased number of trainees in laboratory medicine.

M. G. Bissell, MD, PhD, MPH

Staffing Benchmarks for Clinical Laboratories: A College of American Pathologists Q-Probes Study of Laboratory Staffing at 98 Institutions
Jones BA, Darcy T, Souers RJ, et al (Henry Ford Hosp, Detroit, MI; Univ of Wisconsin School of Medicine and Public Health, Madison; College of American Pathologists, Northfield, IL; et al)
Arch Pathol Lab Med 136:140-147, 2012

Context.—Publicly available information concerning laboratory staffing benchmarks is scarce. One of the few publications on this topic summarized the findings of a Q-Probes study performed in 2004. This publication reports a similar survey with data collected in 2010.

Objective.—To assess the relationship between staffing levels in specified laboratory sections and test volumes in these sections and quantify management span of control.

Design.—The study defined 4 laboratory sections: anatomic pathology (including cytology), chemistry/hematology/immunology, microbiology, and transfusion medicine. It divided staff into 3 categories: management, nonmanagement (operational or bench staff), and doctoral (MD, PhD) supervisory staff. People in these categories were tabulated as full-time equivalents and exclusions specified. Tests were counted in uniform formats, specified for each laboratory section, according to Medicare rules for the bundling and unbundling of tests.

Results.—Ninety-eight participating institutions provided data that showed significant associations between test volumes and staffing for all 4 sections. There was wide variation in productivity based on volume. There was no relationship between testing volume per laboratory section and management span of control. Higher productivity in chemistry/hematology/immunology was associated with a higher fraction of tests coming from nonacute care patients. In both the 2004 and 2010 studies, productivity was inseparably linked to test volume.

Conclusions.—Higher test volume was associated with higher productivity ratios in chemistry/hematology/immunology and transfusion medicine sections. The impact of various testing services on productivity is section-specific.

▶ Despite employee pay and benefits representing more than half of laboratory direct costs, publicly available information on staffing benchmarks is hard to find. A 2004 College of American Pathologists (CAP) Q-Probes study of clinical laboratory staffing in 151 institutions divided the laboratory into 4 sections: anatomic pathology (with histology and cytology separately evaluated), microbiology, transfusion medicine (blood bank), and a section that combined chemistry, immunology, and hematology. The study assessed labor productivity and management span of control within the laboratory sections in relation to laboratory test volumes and institutional characteristics. From a similar survey done in the altered circumstances of 2010, the authors report on a study to compare and contrast with the 2004 results. The latter study benefits from experience accrued in the CAP Laboratory Management Improvement Program (LMIP), which collected information on laboratories' economic characteristics and developed practical definitions of comparable laboratory testing within sections that are key to developing comparable information about various staff positions (line, management, technical, and professional). The LMIP also worked out practical, yet highly reproducible, definitions of tests themselves that could be applied across different institutions. On this basis, staff and the tests that they perform could be counted in a remarkably uniform way to ensure comparability of results.

M. G. Bissell, MD, PhD, MPH

A Decision-Tree Approach to Cost Comparison of Newborn Screening Strategies for Cystic Fibrosis
Wells J, Rosenberg M, Hoffman G, et al (Univ of Wisconsin School of Medicine and Public Health, Madison; Univ of Wisconsin, Madison; Wisconsin State Laboratory of Hygiene, Madison; et al)
Pediatrics 129:e339-e347, 2012

Objectives.—Because cystic fibrosis can be difficult to diagnose and treat early, newborn screening programs have rapidly developed nation-wide but methods vary widely. We therefore investigated the costs and consequences or specific outcomes of the 2 most commonly used methods.

Methods.—With available data on screening and follow-up, we used a simulation approach with decision trees to compare immunoreactive tryp-sinogen (IRT) screening followed by a second IRT test against an IRT/DNA analysis. By using a Monte Carlo simulation program, variation in the model parameters for counts at various nodes of the decision trees, as well as for costs, are included and applied to fictional cohorts of 100 000 newborns. The outcome measures included the numbers of newborns given a diagnosis of cystic fibrosis and costs of screening strategy at each branch and cost per newborn.

Results.—Simulations revealed a substantial number of potential missed diagnoses for the IRT/IRT system versus IRT/DNA. Although the IRT/IRT strategy with commonly used cutoff values offers an average overall cost savings of $2.30 per newborn, a breakdown of costs by societal segments demonstrated higher out-of-pocket costs for families. Two potential system failures causing delayed diagnoses were identified relating to the screening protocols and the follow-up system.

Conclusions.—The IRT/IRT screening algorithm reduces the costs to laboratories and insurance companies but has more system failures. IRT/DNA offers other advantages, including fewer delayed diagnoses and lower out-of-pocket costs to families.

▶ Cystic fibrosis (CF) is a relatively common, life-threatening, autosomal recessive disease that can now be diagnosed routinely through newborn screening (NBS) by using immunoreactive trypsinogen (IRT) as the primary analyte or first tier. After both the Centers for Disease Control and Prevention and CF Foundation endorsed universal adoption of CF screening, it was included in the list of

29 core disorders recommended by the Health Resources and Services Administration for all state NBS programs. Thus, by 2010, all states plus the District of Columbia were screening for CF. With nationwide CF NBS underway, the research climate shifted from one focused on identifying the benefits of screening to one focused on identifying the best screening methodology. Although wide variations in screening methods and cutoff values currently exist throughout the United States and across the world, almost all algorithms begin by evaluating IRT1 levels by using a dried blood specimen collected between 1 and 5 days of age with the second tier being either a second IRT or DNA analysis for CF transmembrane conductance regulator mutations. Further testing and referrals are then made based on the particular screening method in use by the state. This study contributes to the current research by offering a comparison of the costs and consequences, or outcomes, associated with the 2 most popular screening methodologies in the United States by using a decision tree framework that allows for variation in the model parameters. A decision tree visually shows the process of the path a newborn may follow under a screening program. Average assumptions, in terms of rates, are shown for moving along a path, and costs at each point of the process are determined. These results can then be summarized to evaluate the effectiveness of a screening program.

M. G. Bissell, MD, PhD, MPH

A cost-effectiveness model of genetic testing for the evaluation of families with hypertrophic cardiomyopathy
Ingles J, McGaughran J, Scuffham PA, et al (Centenary Inst, Sydney, Australia; Royal Brisbane and Women's Hosp, Australia; Griffith Univ, Brisbane, Australia; et al)
Heart 98:625-630, 2012

Background.—Traditional management of families with hypertrophic cardiomyopathy (HCM) involves periodic lifetime clinical screening of family members, an approach that does not identify all gene carriers owing to incomplete penetrance and significant clinical heterogeneity. Limitations in availability and cost have meant genetic testing is not part of routine clinical management for many HCM families.

Objective.—To determine the cost-effectiveness of the addition of genetic testing to HCM family management, compared with clinical screening alone.

Methods.—A probabilistic Markov decision model was used to determine cost per quality-adjusted life-year and cost for each life-year gained when genetic testing is included in the management of Australian families with HCM, compared with the conventional approach of periodic clinical screening alone.

Results.—The incremental cost-effectiveness ratio (ICER) was $A785 (£510 or €587) per quality-adjusted life-year gained, and $A12 720 (£8261 or €9509) per additional life-year gained making genetic testing a very costeffective strategy. Sensitivity analyses showed that the cost of proband genetic testing was an important variable. As the cost of proband genetic testing decreased, the ICER decreased and was cost saving when the cost fell below $A248 (£161 or €185). In addition, the mutation identification rate was also important in reducing the overall ICER, although even at the upper limits, the ICER still fell well within accepted willingness to pay bounds.

Conclusions.—The addition of genetic testing to the management of HCM families is cost-effective in comparison with the conventional approach of regular clinical screening. This has important implications for the evaluation of families with HCM, and suggests that all should have access to specialised cardiac genetic clinics that can offer genetic testing.

▶ Hypertrophic cardiomyopathy (HCM) is a primary genetic disorder of the myocardium characterized by hypertrophy, usually of the left ventricle, in the absence of other loading conditions such as hypertension. HCM affects 1 in 500 (0.2%) of the general population and importantly remains the most common structural cause of sudden cardiac death (SCD) in people aged less than 35 years. HCM shows marked clinical heterogeneity, which includes individuals with incomplete penetrance, making clinical diagnosis of family members problematic. To date, at least 13 causative genes have been identified in HCM, and genetic testing of the 10 most common genes yields a genetic diagnosis in about 60% of families. In the absence of a genetic diagnosis, first-degree relatives of an affected person are resigned to a lifetime of clinical surveillance based on current guidelines. The efficacy of predictive HCM genetic testing in family members at risk of HCM has been shown, and no negative impact on psychological well-being or health-related quality of life (HR-QoL) has been reported. In fact, genetic testing may impose better HR-QoL and lower anxiety and depression than found in the general population. Genetic testing of inherited heart diseases in Australia is offered through clinical genetics departments or specialized cardiac genetic clinics, which adopt a multidisciplinary approach, including genetic counseling. Despite its clear benefits, genetic testing is not part of routine clinical management for the majority of families. This study sought to identify the incremental costs and effects and the incremental cost-effectiveness ratio of a clinical surveillance strategy, including genetic testing, compared with the traditional method of clinical screening alone in HCM.

M. G. Bissell, MD, PhD, MPH

College of American Pathologists Proposal for the Oversight of Laboratory-Developed Tests
Vance GH (Indiana Univ Med Ctr, Indianapolis)
Arch Pathol Lab Med 135:1432-1435, 2011

Context.—The US Food and Drug Administration (FDA) announced it will exercise authority over laboratory-developed tests (LDTs). Laboratory-developed tests have traditionally been developed and offered in laboratories as a service to patients and regulated under the Clinical

Laboratory Improvement Amendments of 1988 (Clinical Laboratory Improvements Act). Laboratories now face potential dual regulatory oversight from both the Centers for Medicare and Medicaid Services (CMS) and the FDA. The College of American Pathologists (CAP) constructed a proposal to minimize redundancy of agency oversight and burden to laboratories. Modifications to the proposal continue while the laboratory community awaits release of the guidance documents that will stipulate FDA requirements.

Objective.—To describe the historical context framing the entry of FDA into the oversight of LDTs and outline the CAP LDT Proposal in its current form.

Data Sources.—PubMed review of published literature; United States Constitution; and online information resources from the National Institutes of Health, FDA, and US Government.

Conclusion.—The College of American Pathologists is a leader in laboratory quality and has unique insights into the benefits and risks to patients presented by LDTs. Continued dialog with officials from the FDA and CMS will promote public and private collaborative efforts to assure innovation of diagnostic testing, public information, and patient safety for clinical diagnostic testing.

▶ On July 19, 2010, Jeffrey Shuren, MD, JD, director of the Centers for Devices and Radiological Health, announced during a public forum held in Maryland that the US Food and Drug Administration (FDA) would begin exercising oversight of laboratory-developed tests (LDTs). LDTs have traditionally been developed and offered in laboratories as a service to patients and regulated under the Clinical Laboratory Improvement Amendments of 1988 (Clinical Laboratory Improvements Act). Laboratories now face potential dual regulatory oversight from both the Centers for Medicare and Medicaid Services (CMS) and the FDA. The College of American Pathologists constructed a proposal to minimize redundancy of agency oversight and burden to laboratories. Modifications to the proposal continue while the laboratory community awaits release of the guidance documents that will stipulate FDA requirements. Continued dialogue with officials from the FDA and CMS will promote public and private collaborative efforts to assure innovation of diagnostic testing, public information, and patient safety for clinical diagnostic testing.

M. G. Bissell, MD, PhD, MPH

Challenges and Opportunities in the Application Process for Fellowship Training in Pathology: An Independent Survey of Residents and Fellows Demonstrates Limited Interest in an NRMP-Style Matching Program
Bernacki KD, McKenna BJ, Myers JL (Univ of Michigan Med School, Ann Arbor)
Am J Clin Pathol 137:543-552, 2012

A survey completed by 366 pathology residents and fellows examined preferences for 3 fellowship application systems: keeping the current system, a National Resident Matching Program (NRMP)—style match, and a unified time line. All groups showed a strong preference for a time line, accounting for 62.1% of first choices vs the current system (17.3%) or a match (20.6%). When asked for a second choice after time line was ranked first, 60.5% of respondents whose fellowship of choice was available at their residency institution and 63.5% who had accepted fellowship positions at their residency institution preferred the current system; 51.4% whose fellowship of choice was not available at their residency institution and 50.6% of those who had accepted fellowship positions elsewhere preferred a match. Location and family/personal reasons were more important than subspecialty competitiveness and program prestige when accepting fellowship positions. Pressure to choose and apply early for fellowship persists and is greatest for anatomic pathology-only and clinical pathology-only residents.

▶ The Council of the Association of Pathology Chairs (APC) has proposed a pathology subspecialty matching program for applicants matriculating in July 2013. The proposal is driven by a perception that the current system is inequitable and fails to consistently meet the needs of participating residents and programs. Others, including the Council of the Association of Directors of Anatomic and Surgical Pathology, have suggested that a nationally administered match may not be an effective countermeasure for the problems identified and instead misses more important causes of perceived inadequacies in the current process. Proponents of a fellowship match in pathology have focused on the desire among fellowship candidates and program directors for an enforceable and standardized timeline for the application process. The current process is essentially a free market system in which institutions have varying schedules and methods of advertising and recruiting for open fellowship positions. Much of the currently available survey data being used to inform the national debate regarding this contentious issue focuses on the perceptions of residents and residency directors rather than fellows and fellowship directors. Previous surveys that included elements relevant to the current pathology fellowship application system have solicited input primarily from residents, residency program directors, and department chairs. The American Society for Clinical Pathology—sponsored fellowship and job market surveys administered in conjunction with the required annual resident in-service examinations capture responses from all participating pathology residents and a subset of fellows. An additional ad hoc survey of pathology residents was reported on behalf of the APC Council. While these surveys provide important and useful information, they fail to get at some of the key issues underlying not only the problems in need of solutions but also perceptions about a broader range of proposed alternatives. The authors report the results of a survey conducted to learn more about pathology residents' and fellows' experiences with the current fellowship process, their preferences for the fellowship application process, and some of the differences between respondents that might account for the variation in perceptions.

M. G. Bissell, MD, PhD, MPH

Electronic health record donations by laboratories: Is legal necessarily ethical?
Bercovitch L, Grant-Kels JM, Kels BD (Warren Alpert Med School of Brown Univ, Providence, RI; Univ of Connecticut Health Center, Farmington)
J Am Acad Dermatol 66:474-478, 2012

Background.—Federal and state laws govern how hospital and laboratories deal with referring physicians. The Stark law prohibits physicians from referring Medicare or Medicaid patients for certain health services to any entity with which they have a financial arrangement, with a few exceptions. The Antikickback Statute (SKA) makes it illegal to willfully or knowingly accept payment in return for referrals involving federal health care program recipients. Health care providers cannot offer or provide anything of value to induce either a referral of business covered by federal health care programs or the use of federal health care benefits. Exceptions and safe harbors to the AKS permit the donation of health information technology (HIT) services and software to improve e-prescribing and electronic health record (EHR) use. To qualify for the exemption, the HIT training and software must be primarily to create, transmit, receive, and store EHRs. These exceptions are supposed to advance good public policy to encourage the adoption of EHRs, e-prescribing, and better patient care and safety. Although these activities are legal, the question arises as to whether they are ethical practices.

Ethical Considerations.—Ethical issues differ depending on the point of view. Patients want to know that the physician is honoring the fiduciary obligation to place their interests ahead of self-interest. Practitioners are obligated first and foremost to serving in a beneficent manner and doing no harm to their patients. A commercial laboratory that has offered HIT or software has a primary obligation to its owners or shareholders. Therefore its ethical obligations are between those of a business and those of a professional organization. An academic laboratory might feel that it is at a significant economic disadvantage, having to compete with commercial entities yet provide service, education, and training for future practitioners as well as research to advance knowledge in the chosen field. Academic laboratories could become extinct through consolidation or insolvency as a result of this competition from commercial entities. EHR vendors see their mission as maximizing profits and outperforming competitors. They focus on offering the best product within their business capabilities. If steering clients to laboratories that offer their products is good business, that is what they will do. The vendor's ethical obligations consist of dealing honestly with customers, advertising truthfully, and acting legally. The public policy viewpoint would argue the need for HIT and EHRs to improve the efficiency of the health care system, to protect patient safety, to reduce prescribing errors, to control costs, and to facilitate vertical integration of the health care system central to achieving health care reform. Making tools more widely available is a "win-win" situation. The utilitarian viewpoint sees the most ethical decision as that which provides the most beneficent outcome for the most stakeholders.

Results.—The exceptions and safe harbors under the Stark legislation and AKS are based on the premise that anything that advances the adoption of EHRs is good public policy. But using these measures to allow for-profit commercial laboratories to purchase valuable EHRs for clients does not serve any legitimate public good. Rather, it is an inducement to send business to the laboratories.

Conclusions.—How should a medical practice respond if offered an EHR system at a reduced cost by a laboratory in return for its business? Even if the offer is legal, it does not seem ethical to accept a large inducement of this type from a laboratory with which they do business in return for being a client. Interestingly, in 2011, the American Academy of Dermatology Board of Directors formally asked that the federal government eliminate the safe harbor and exceptions for EHR donations by clinical laboratories.

▶ The business practice in which laboratories and hospitals donate up to 85% of the cost of electronic health record (EHR) software, training, and network connectivity interfaces has arisen as a result of a federally mandated exception to the Stark laws on self-referral and a safe-harbor provision in the federal Anti-kickback Statutes (AKS). As the ethical case here illustrates, this has become particularly relevant to dermatologists as commercial dermatopathology laboratories have made such offers to existing and potential clients, and EHR vendors have directed clients to laboratories making such offers. There are federal and state laws that govern how hospitals and laboratories deal with referring physicians. The Stark laws prohibit physicians from referring Medicare or Medicaid patients for certain health services to any entity where the physician has a financial arrangement unless certain exceptions apply. The AKS states that it is illegal to willfully or knowingly accept remuneration in return for referrals involving federal health care program recipients. Under the AKS, it is illegal for health care providers to offer or provide anything of value as an inducement to refer business covered by federal health care programs or to induce in this manner the use of federal health care benefits. In 2006, the Center for Medicare and Medicaid Services (CMS) and the Office of the Inspector General issued 2 new exceptions to the Stark laws and 2 new safe harbors to the AKS to permit donation of health information technology services and software to improve e-prescribing and EHR capabilities. The changes were ostensibly in the interests of good public policy to encourage adoption of EHRs and e-prescribing and to improve quality of care and patient safety. In 2008, the CMS ruled that laboratories could pay for interfaces under the same rules that already allowed them to provide fax machines and dedicated printers for the reporting of test results. These exceptions will automatically sunset on December 31, 2013.

M. G. Bissell, MD, PhD, MPH

The Long and Winding Regulatory Road for Laboratory-Developed Tests

Weiss RL (Univ of Utah School of Medicine, Salt Lake City)
Am J Clin Pathol 138:20-26, 2012

"High complexity" clinical laboratories are approved under the Clinical Laboratory Improvement Amendments to develop, validate, and offer a laboratory-developed test (LDT) for clinical use. The Food and Drug Administration considers LDTs to be medical devices under their regulatory jurisdiction, and that at least certain LDTs should be subject to greater regulatory scrutiny. This review describes the current regulatory framework for LDTs and suggests ways in which to appropriately enhance this framework.

▶ In his 2005 article "Health Care in the 21st Century" in the *New England Journal of Medicine*, William H. Frist, MD, then the majority leader of the US Senate, wrote: "During the next decade, the practice of medicine will change dramatically through genetically based diagnostic tests and personalized, targeted pharmacologic treatments that will enable a move beyond prevention to preemptive strategies. A whole new frontier of medicine will open, with a focus on delaying the onset of many diseases such as cancer, cardiovascular disease, and Alzheimer's disease." Five years later, Margaret A. Hamburg, MO, and Francis S. Collins, MD, PhD, the Commissioner of the Food and Drug Administration, and the Director of the National Institutes of Health, respectively, wrote in their article "The Path to Personalized Medicine:" "Researchers have discovered hundreds of genes that harbor variations contributing to human illness, identified genetic variability in patients' responses to dozens of treatments, and begun to target the molecular causes of some diseases. In addition, scientists are developing and using diagnostic tests based on genetics or other molecular mechanisms to better predict patients' responses to targeted therapy," and "We [the federal government] are now building a national highway system for personalized medicine, with substantial investments in infrastructure and standards. We look forward to doctors and patients navigating these roads to better outcomes and better health." There is a strong belief that personalized medicine tools, such as genetic tests, will continue the momentum toward more precise medical care and dramatic changes in how health care is delivered. As we venture down this personalized medicine superhighway, part of the necessary infrastructure will potentially be a new regulatory framework for oversight of these patient management tests. The challenge will be in creating a framework that ensures safe travels without impeding necessary or desirable progress—that is, ensuring patient protection and innovation, without costly inertia. In designing such a system, it is critical for policy makers and medical professionals alike to fully understand how the current regulatory structure came about. This might lend important clues about how we should proceed from this point on. This article describes a superhighway that has become a long and winding road.

M. G. Bissell, MD, PhD, MPH

Bridging the Chasm: Effect of Health Information Exchange on Volume of Laboratory Testing

Hebel E, Middleton B, Shubina M, et al (Harvard Med School and Clinical Informatics Res and Development, Boston, MA; Brigham and Women's Hosp, Boston, MA)

Arch Intern Med 172:517-519, 2012

Background.—Health information exchanges (HIEs) have been proposed as a way to improve the quality and efficiency of the health care system in the United States. However, few studies document the potential benefits of HIEs, which might have slowed down the acceptance of these exchanges. Provider surveys show that reducing duplicate testing is one of the expected benefits of HIEs. Data from two academic medical centers were assessed to determine if having an HIE was associated with fewer laboratory tests.

Method.—This retrospective study evaluated whether the availability of laboratory test results from a nonencounter hospital reduced the number of subsequent laboratory tests at the encounter hospital. A total of 117,606 patients were included, having received outpatient consultations at two affiliated academic hospitals. The index encounter was the unit of analysis. The number of laboratory tests done until the end of the day of the index encounter was the primary outcome variable. The primary predictor variables were presence of laboratory tests performed during the 7 days before the index encounter and whether the encounter occurred before (1999) or after (2001-2004) the HIE rollout in 2000.

Results.—Patients with recent off-site tests had a mean of 22.07 tests before the index encounter. Patients without recent off-site tests had a mean of 1.62 tests before the index encounter. Most encounters without off-site tests did not include any tests in the preceding week.

Univariate analysis indicated the number of laboratory tests performed after encounters that included off-site laboratory tests decreased by 49% after the HIE was introduced. Multivariate analysis showed that the number of tests for patients with previous off-site tests decreased by 52.6% after HIE integration.

The number of postencounter tests increased by 2.5% for each point increase in the Charlson Comorbidity Index and rose to 51.7% with every subsequent year. The number of tests fell by 0.84% for each $10,000 increase in the patient's median household income. It was also 9.06% lower for patients with Medicaid insurance compared to those having private health insurance.

Conclusions.—The introduction of an internal HIE was related to a significant decrease in the number of laboratory tests ordered for new patients who had undergone recent laboratory tests at another institution. This reduction was as high as 50%, which could produce significant savings when patients often receive care at more than one institution. Thus having access to the patients' laboratory test results through the

HIE alters the decision-making process and should produce financial savings–one of the benefits claimed for the institution of HIEs.

▶ Sharing of patient information between health care providers, including through health information exchanges (HIEs), has been proposed as one of the essential changes to improve the quality and efficiency of the health care system in the United States. It has been estimated that HIEs could decrease health care costs across the country by approximately $78 billion annually. Despite numerous potential advantages of HIEs, there are few studies documenting their benefits. This lack of objective information might have slowed down their acceptance. Studies that show tangible evidence of benefits provided by HIEs are urgently needed. Provider surveys show that reduction in duplicate testing is one of the most commonly expected benefits. The authors, therefore, investigated whether the introduction of an HIE between 2 academic medical centers was associated with a reduction in volume of laboratory testing. They conducted a retrospective study to investigate whether the availability of laboratory test results from a non-encounter hospital reduced the number of subsequent laboratory tests at the encounter hospital (Fig in the original article).

M. G. Bissell, MD, PhD, MPH

A Consensus Curriculum for Laboratory Management Training for Pathology Residents
Weiss RL, Work Group Members (Univ of Utah, Salt Lake City; et al)
Am J Clin Pathol 136:671-678, 2011

Through the combined efforts of the American Pathology Foundation (APF), the American Society for Clinical Pathology (ASCP), and the Program Directors Section (PRODS) of the Association of Pathology Chairs (APC), a needs assessment was performed via a survey on the PRODS listserv, workshops at the APC/PRODS annual meetings in 2009 and 2010, and a Work Group of representatives of APF, ASCP, and PRODS. Residency program needs and resource constraints common to training pathology residents in practice and laboratory management were identified. In addition, a consensus curriculum for management training was created to serve as a resource for residency training program directors and others. The curriculum was converted into a "wiki" design tool for use by program directors, residents, and faculty.

▶ In 1995, the Graylyn Conference Report, "Recommendations for Reform of Clinical Pathology Training," was issued. Subsequently, the Association of Directors of Anatomic and Surgical Pathology and the Academy of Clinical Laboratory Physicians and Scientists each published "curriculum content and evaluation" proposals for resident competency in anatomic and clinical pathology, respectively. Both included specific knowledge and skill sets in laboratory management. Several training programs have also published descriptions of their curricula in laboratory management. Early in 2009, the authors were invited to conduct a workshop on resident laboratory management training for the program directors group at the Association of Pathology Chairs/Program Directors Section (PRODS) Annual Meeting in Seattle, WA, on July 15, 2009. In preparation for that workshop, a survey was developed for distribution to the PRODS listserv. This report describes that survey, summarizes the discussion and action items agreed to during the workshop, and describes a year-long curriculum design process and the development and deployment of this laboratory management curriculum resource to a "wiki" site.

M. G. Bissell, MD, PhD, MPH

17 Clinical Chemistry

Closing the Gaps in Pediatric Laboratory Reference Intervals: A CALIPER Database of 40 Biochemical Markers in a Healthy and Multiethnic Population of Children
Colantonio DA, Kyriakopoulou L, Chan MK, et al (The Hosp for Sick Children, Toronto, Ontario, Canada; et al)
Clin Chem 58:854-868, 2012

Background.—Pediatric healthcare is critically dependent on the availability of accurate and precise laboratory biomarkers of pediatric disease, and on the availability of reference intervals to allow appropriate clinical interpretation. The development and growth of children profoundly influence normal circulating concentrations of biochemical markers and thus the respective reference intervals. There are currently substantial gaps in our knowledge of the influences of age, sex, and ethnicity on reference intervals. We report a comprehensive covariate-stratified reference interval database established from a healthy, nonhospitalized, and multiethnic pediatric population.

Methods.—Healthy children and adolescents (n = 2188, newborn to 18 years of age) were recruited from a multiethnic population with informed parental consent and were assessed from completed questionnaires and according to defined exclusion criteria. Whole-blood samples were collected for establishing age- and sex-stratified reference intervals for 40 serum biochemical markers (serum chemistry, enzymes, lipids, proteins) on the Abbott ARCHITECT c8000 analyzer.

Results.—Reference intervals were generated according to CLSI C28-A3 statistical guidelines. Caucasians, East Asians, and South Asian participants were evaluated with respect to the influence of ethnicity, and statistically significant differences were observed for 7 specific biomarkers.

Conclusions.—The establishment of a new comprehensive database of pediatric reference intervals is part of the Canadian Laboratory Initiative in Pediatric Reference Intervals (CALIPER). It should assist laboratorians and pediatricians in interpreting test results more accurately and thereby lead to improved diagnosis of childhood diseases and reduced patient risk. The database will also be of global benefit once reference intervals are validated in transference studies with other analytical platforms and local populations, as recommended by the CLSI.

▶ Despite this recognized need, pediatric-specific reference intervals remain inadequate or unavailable for many analytes. Many of the reference intervals in current use have been derived from the analysis of a small number of healthy or hospitalized individuals or are focused on a limited age interval with restricted partitions. Because of the challenges with recruiting study participants, only a small number of analytes have been studied. Larger national initiatives have begun to work toward establishing new pediatric reference intervals, but the results remain predominantly unpublished. The Canadian Laboratory Initiative in Pediatric Reference Intervals Project is a collaborative study among pediatric centers across Canada that is addressing critical gaps in pediatric reference intervals by determining the influence of key covariates, such as age, sex, and ethnicity, on pediatric reference intervals. The present report presents age- and sex-specific reference intervals for 40 biochemical markers (serum chemistry, enzyme, lipid, and protein analytes). This new database clearly demonstrates that child age and sex profoundly influence circulating concentrations of these biomarkers, with considerable variation occurring from analyte to analyte.

M. G. Bissell, MD, PhD, MPH

Should I Repeat My 1:2s QC Rejection?

Parvin CA, Kuchipudi L, Yundt-Pacheco JC (Quality Systems Division, Plano, TX)
Clin Chem 58:925-929, 2012

Background.—Repeating a QC that is outside 2SD from the mean (1:2s rule) appears to be a common practice. Although this form of repeat sampling is frowned on by many, the comparative power of the approach has not been formally evaluated.

Methods.—We computed power functions mathematically and by computer simulation for 4 different 1:2s repeat-sampling strategies, as well as the 1:2s rule, the 1:3s rule, and 2 common QC multirules.

Results.—The false-rejection rates for the repeatsampling strategies were similarly low to those of the 1:3s QC rule. The error detection rates for the repeatsampling strategies approached those of the 1:2s QC rule for moderate to large out-of-control error conditions. In most cases, the power of the repeat-sampling strategies was superior to the power of the QC multirules we evaluated. The increase in QC utilization rate ranged from 4% to 13% for the repeat-sampling strategies investigated.

Conclusions.—The repeat-sampling strategies provide an effective tactic to take advantage of the desirable properties of both the 1:2s and 1:3s QC rules. Additionally, the power of the repeat-sampling strategies compares favorably with the power of 2 common QC multirules. These improvements come with a modest increase in the average number of controls tested.

▶ It is considered good laboratory practice to design quality control (QC) strategies—number of QC examinations, QC rules, and frequency of QC evaluations—to ensure that patient results meet the quality required for their intended use. Many laboratories, however, continue to use a 1:2s QC rule for all analytes, without considering the relationship of analytical performance to quality requirements. A 1:2s QC rule rejects results when any QC examination is either 2 standard deviation (SDs) higher or lower than the QC target concentration. One of the undesirable characteristics of the 1:2s QC rule is its high false-rejection rate (4.6% for 1 QC examination, 8.9% for 2 QC examinations, 13.0% for 3 QC examinations). A laboratory that examines 2 QC samples for 20 different analytes and applies a 1:2s QC rule should expect 1 or more analytes to give a QC rule rejection at every QC evaluation. To deal with this unacceptable frequency of false rejections, a common practice is to repeat the QC examination for any failing analytes and again apply the 1:2s rule. Clearly the continued repetition of QC testing until the desired result is achieved is a misguided practice, but what about a single planned repeat evaluation for a failing 1:2s QC rule? The QC performance characteristics of this practice have not been formally investigated. Therefore, the authors considered a number of alternative 1:2s repeat sampling strategies and objectively compared their performance characteristics.

M. G. Bissell, MD, PhD, MPH

A Review of the Methods, Interpretation, and Limitations of the Urine Drug Screen

Markway EC, Baker SN (Univ of Kentucky HealthCare, Lexington)
Orthopedics 34:877-881, 2011

Toxicology screens are used to detect the presence of prescription, nonprescription, or illicit substances. These tests are used in emergency situations to detect intentional or accidental overdose, to monitor drug dependency, and to screen for medical or legal purposes. An initial immunoassay reports qualitative results based on established cut-off concentrations. As a screening test, the initial immunoassay is less sensitive and

TABLE 2.—Selected False Positives Reported in UDS[2,3,6]

Substance	False Positives
Alcohol	Isopropyl alcohol
Amphetamine/ methamphetamine	Amantadine, brompheniramine, bupropion, chlorpromazine, desipramine, dextroamphetamine, ephedrine, isometheptene, labetalol, methylene dioxymethamphetamine, methylphenidate, phentermine, phenylephrine, phenylpropanolamine, promethazine, pseudoephedrine, ranitidine, selegiline, thioridazine, trazodone, trimethobenzamide, trimipramine
Barbiturates	Fenoprofen, ibuprofen, naproxen
Benzodiazepines	Oxaprozin, sertraline
Cannabinoids	Dronabinol, efavirenz, fenoprofen, ibuprofen, naproxen, pantoprazole
Opiates	Dextromethorphan, diphenhydramine, gatifloxacin, ofloxacin, rifampin, verapamil
Methadone	Clomipramine, chlorpromazine, diphenhydramine, doxylamine, quetiapine, thioridazine, verapamil
Phencyclidine	Dextromethorphan, diphenhydraminee, doxylamine, ibuprofen, imipramine, ketamine, meperidine, mesoridazine, thioridazine, tramadol, venlafaxine

Abbreviation: UDS, urine drug screen.
Editor's Note: Please refer to original journal article for full references.

therefore must be interpreted in the context of confounding variables such as the testing method, the substance being screened, and patient-specific characteristics. Either gas chromatography or high-performance liquid chromatography can be used to confirm positive results (Table 2).

▶ Toxicology screens are commonly used in various health care settings. These screening tests can be broadly defined as an examination of a biological specimen to detect the presence of a specific chemical substance or its metabolites. Specimens such as urine, hair, saliva, sweat, and blood may be tested. This article discusses the urine toxicology screen or urine drug screen (UDS) because this is the most frequently used screen in clinical practice. Toxicology screening may provide useful, objective information to clinicians to more effectively treat patients. However, the limitations of these screening methods, especially UDSs, should be recognized for appropriate analysis of results. Positive immunoassay results in the UDS should be confirmed through a more sensitive confirmatory method. Furthermore, it is essential to consider confounding variables such as the potential for false positives (Table 2), substance-specific pharmacokinetic parameters, and patient demographics when interpreting UDS results. There is clinical use to the UDS, but to be effectively used, the results must be analyzed in the context of its limitations.

M. G. Bissell, MD, PhD, MPH

Colonoscopy versus Fecal Immunochemical Testing in Colorectal-Cancer Screening

Quintero E, for the COLONPREV Study Investigators (Hospital Universitario de Canarias, Tenerife, Spain; et al)

N Engl J Med 366:697-706, 2012

Background.—Colonoscopy and fecal immunochemical testing (FIT) are accepted strategies for colorectal-cancer screening in the average-risk population.

Methods.—In this randomized, controlled trial involving asymptomatic adults 50 to 69 years of age, we compared one-time colonoscopy in 26,703 subjects with FIT every 2 years in 26,599 subjects. The primary outcome was the rate of death from colorectal cancer at 10 years. This interim report describes rates of participation, diagnostic findings, and occurrence of major complications at completion of the baseline screening. Study outcomes were analyzed in both intention-to-screen and as-screened populations.

Results.—The rate of participation was higher in the FIT group than in the colonoscopy group (34.2% vs. 24.6%, $P < 0.001$). Colorectal cancer was found in 30 subjects (0.1%) in the colonoscopy group and 33 subjects (0.1%) in the FIT group (odds ratio, 0.99; 95% confidence interval [CI], 0.61 to 1.64; $P = 0.99$). Advanced adenomas were detected in 514 subjects (1.9%) in the colonoscopy group and 231 subjects (0.9%) in the FIT group (odds ratio, 2.30; 95% CI, 1.97 to 2.69; $P < 0.001$), and nonadvanced adenomas were detected in 1109 subjects (4.2%) in the colonoscopy group and 119 subjects (0.4%) in the FIT group (odds ratio, 9.80; 95% CI, 8.10 to 11.85; $P < 0.001$).

Conclusions.—Subjects in the FIT group were more likely to participate in screening than were those in the colonoscopy group. On the baseline screening examination, the numbers of subjects in whom colorectal cancer was detected were similar in the two study groups, but more adenomas were identified in the colonoscopy group. (Funded by Instituto de Salud Carlos III and others; ClinicalTrials.gov number, NCT00906997.)

▶ Colorectal cancer is the third most common cancer worldwide and the second leading cause of cancer-related deaths. Several studies have found that colorectal cancer screening is effective and cost effective in the average-risk population. Recommended strategies for colorectal cancer screening fall into 2 broad categories: stool tests (occult blood and exfoliated DNA tests) and structural examinations (flexible sigmoidoscopy, colonoscopy, and computed tomographic colonography). Stool tests primarily detect cancer, and structural examinations detect both cancer and premalignant lesions. Stool tests for occult blood (guaiac testing and fecal immunochemical testing [FIT]) are predominantly used in Europe and Australia, whereas colonoscopy is the predominant screening method in the United States. The authors conducted a randomized, controlled trial to compare semiquantitative FIT with colonoscopy. They hypothesized that FIT screening every 2 years would be noninferior to one-time colonoscopy with respect to a reduction in mortality related to colorectal cancer among average-risk subjects. This interim report describes rates of participation, diagnostic findings, and the occurrence of major complications at the completion of the baseline screening.

M. G. Bissell, MD, PhD, MPH

A comparison of plasma-free metanephrines with plasma catecholamines in the investigation of suspected pheochromocytoma
Lee GR, Johnston PC, Atkinson AB, et al (Royal Victoria Hosp, Belfast, UK)
J Hypertens 29:2422-2428, 2011

Objective.—To compare the diagnostic performance of plasma metanephrines by ELISA and plasma catecholamine measurements by HPLC in patients selected for clonidine suppression testing.

Methods.—Plasma catecholamines adrenaline (ADR) and noradrenaline (NOR) were measured by HPLC and metanephrine with normetanephrine (NMN) by ELISA ($n = 67$). The diagnostic performance of metanephrines was determined by receiver operating characteristic (ROC) curve analysis.

Results.—Phaeochromocytoma was confirmed by histological analysis in 14 patients and excluded in 53 patients by a negative clonidine suppression test (CST), abdominal computerized tomography scan and clinical follow-up (median 2.5 years). A sensitivity and specificity of 100 and 96%, respectively, was obtained by using our current CST diagnostic criteria for ADR and NOR values. ROC curve analysis revealed optimum sensitivity and specificity for plasma-free metanephrines using a threshold of 784 pmol/l at baseline and 663 pmol/l at 180 min. Baseline measurements of metanephrine with NMN showed 100% sensitivity and 98% specificity, as assessed by ROC curve analysis-derived criteria or when evaluated against published decision thresholds. A sensitivity and specificity of 100% was obtained for the combined measurements of metanephrine with NMN at 180 min.

Conclusion.—Plasma metanephrines (metanephrine with NMN) were equally effective as plasma catecholamines during CST. This study supports the use of measuring plasma metanephrines by ELISA as a less labour-intensive and equally effective biochemical test for phaeochromocytoma in patients with a high clinical suspicion. There was still overlap between groups with and without phaeochromocytoma at baseline under controlled conditions and clinically some patients still need to undergo clonidine suppression testing.

▶ Pheochromocytoma is a rare but important cause of hypertension. Its clinical presentation can be varied with nonspecific signs and symptoms. Secretion of catecholamines can be episodic or biochemically silent and, therefore, can present difficulty in diagnosis. Failure to diagnose can have potentially fatal cardiovascular consequences so it is, therefore, important to consider the diagnosis in all hypertensive patients and then to have accurate biochemical assays for diagnosis in those in whom testing is considered necessary. In the initial biochemical investigation, a superior diagnostic sensitivity of measuring fractionated metanephrines (metanephrine and normetanephrine [NMN] measured separately), in urine or plasma, has been reported in comparison with the widely used measurement of urinary catecholamines. For patients with a high clinical suspicion and equivocal results after initial biochemical testing, clonidine suppression testing, based on the principle that clonidine suppresses catecholamine release from sympathetic nerves but does not affect autonomous tumor production, is helpful in differentiating patients with essential hypertension who have borderline increases in catecholamines and some suggestive symptoms from those who actually have a pheochromocytoma. The authors' practice has been to continue with dynamic testing incorporating plasma catecholamines measured by high-performance liquid chromatography (HPLC) and to proceed directly to the clonidine suppression test (CST) for the sake of patient convenience. In equivocal cases, their experience in the use of clonidine suppression testing has been excellent over many years. Immunoassays have emerged recently as an alternative method to HPLC for measuring metanephrines in plasma, offering an attractive alternative to the more labor-intensive measurement of catecholamines by HPLC. Against this background, the aim of this study was to compare measurement of the plasma catecholamine metabolites, metanephrine and normetanephrine, with plasma catecholamines during CSTs in R/O pheochromocytoma patients.

M. G. Bissell, MD, PhD, MPH

Evaluation of the Test-mate ChE (Cholinesterase) Field Kit in Acute Organophosphorus Poisoning

Rajapakse BN, Thiermann H, Eyer P, et al (South Asian Clinical Toxicology Res Collaboration, Peradeniya, Sri Lanka; Bundeswehr Inst of Pharmacology and Toxicology, Munich, Germany; Ludwig-Maximilians Univ, Munich, Germany; et al)

Ann Emerg Med 58:559-564, 2011

Study Objective.—Measurement of acetylcholinesterase (AChE) is recommended in the management of organophosphorus poisoning, which results in 200,000 deaths worldwide annually. The Test-mate ChE 400 is a portable field kit designed for detecting occupational organophosphorus exposure that measures RBC AChE and plasma cholinesterase (PChE) within 4 minutes. We evaluate Test-mate against a reference laboratory test in patients with acute organophosphorus self-poisoning.

Methods.—This was a cross-sectional comparison study of 14 patients with acute organophosphorus poisoning between May 2007 and June 2008. RBC AChE and PChE were measured in 96 and 91 samples, respectively, with the Test-mate ChE field kit and compared with a reference laboratory, using the limits of agreement method (Bland and Altman), κ statistics, and Spearman's correlation coefficients.

Results.—There was good agreement between the Test-mate ChE and the reference laboratory for RBC AChE. The mean difference (Test-mate—reference) was −0.62 U/g hemoglobin, 95% limits of agreement −10.84 to 9.59 U/g hemoglobin. Good agreement was also observed between the categories of mild, moderate, and severe RBC AChE inhibition (weighted κ 0.85; 95% confidence interval [CI] 0.83 to 0.87). Measurement of PChE also showed good agreement, with a mean difference (Test-mate—reference) of +0.06 U/mL blood, 95% limits of agreement −0.41 to 0.53 U/mL blood. Spearman's correlation coefficients were 0.87 (95% CI 0.81 to 0.91) for RBC AChE and 0.76 (95% CI 0.66 to 0.84) for PChE. Analysis for within-subject correlation of subjects did not change the limits of agreement.

Conclusion.—The Test-mate ChE field kit reliably provides rapid measurement of RBC AChE in acute organophosphorus poisoning.

▶ Organophosphorus pesticide self-poisoning is a serious public health problem, resulting in approximately 200 000 deaths annually worldwide. The case fatality is as high as 15% to 30%, depending on the type and amount of organophosphorus agent consumed and the delay in initiation of treatment. Poisoning is due to the inhibition of acetylcholinesterase (AChE; EC 3.1.1.7). The measurement of AChE in red blood cells (RBCs) and plasma cholinesterase (PChE; EC 3.1.1.8) is recommended in managing organophosphorus poisoning. AChE levels can be used to confirm the diagnosis and grade severity of poisoning and may also have a role in guiding oxime therapy and facilitating early discharge of patients with mild poisoning. A major challenge in performing RBC AChE assays is the need for special measures during blood collection, such as immediate dilution and cooling of samples to prevent ex vivo reactions occurring over time in cases of acute poisoning. This is particularly important for patients who are receiving oxime antidote therapy, because results may be inaccurate when such precautions are omitted. Despite the benefits of AChE monitoring, this test is not available in most parts of the developing world in which there is a high caseload of organo-phosphorus poisoning. Even in the developed world, a rapid and accurate system of AChE testing is not available for acute organophosphorus poisoning. Improved methods to rapidly monitor severe organophosphorus poisoning may also be rele-vant to chemical warfare attacks.

M. G. Bissell, MD, PhD, MPH

An Examination of the Usefulness of Repeat Testing Practices in a Large Hospital Clinical Chemistry Laboratory

Deetz CO, Nolan DK, Scott MG (Washington Univ School of Medicine, St Louis, MO; Barnes-Jewish Hosp, St Louis, MO)
Am J Clin Pathol 137:20-25, 2012

A long-standing practice in clinical laboratories has been to automatically repeat laboratory tests when values trigger automated "repeat rules" in the laboratory information system such as a critical test result. We examined 25,553 repeated laboratory values for 30 common chemistry tests from December 1, 2010, to February 28, 2011, to determine whether this practice is necessary and whether it may be possible to reduce repeat testing to improve efficiency and turnaround time for reporting critical values. An "error" was defined to occur when the difference between the initial and verified values exceeded the College of American Pathologists/Clinical Laboratory Improvement Amendments allowable error limit. The initial values from 2.6% of all repeated tests (668) were errors. Of these 668 errors, only 102 occurred for values within the analytic measurement range. Median delays in reporting critical values owing to repeated testing ranged from 5 (blood gases) to 17 (glucose) minutes.

▶ Since the early 1970s, laboratory medicine specialists have used computer tech-nology and automation to identify and confirm critical laboratory values. The historic practice in clinical laboratories has been to automatically repeat laboratory tests when values are greater than or less than a critical threshold or when they trigger other automated "repeat rules," such as a delta check. These practices were established when laboratory instruments were far less reliable than today, yet they persist in many laboratories (including the authors'). In fact, recent studies show that analytic issues account for only 8% to 15% of clinical laboratory—related errors, with preanalytic and postanalytic errors representing 85% to 92% of all errors. Contemporary laboratory instruments use numerous safeguards in their hardware and software to improve the accuracy and reliability of results. A recent summary of data from a College of American Pathologists Q-Probes survey suggests 61% of laboratories still repeat testing for critical chemistry values. The survey also suggests that laboratory test repeat practices have the potential to delay reporting by 10 to 14 minutes and waste resources without significantly preventing analytic errors. These observations led the authors to question whether automated repeated testing is necessary in their laboratory. They examined 25 553 repeat laboratory values from a total of 855 009 results during a 3-month period to determine whether it may be possible to reduce repeat testing and improve efficiency and turnaround time for reporting laboratory values.

M. G. Bissell, MD, PhD, MPH

Accuracy of 6 Routine 25-Hydroxyvitamin D Assays: Influence of Vitamin D Binding Protein Concentration
Heijboer AC, Blankenstein MA, Kema IP, et al (VU Univ Med Ctr, Amsterdam, the Netherlands; Univ Med Ctr, Groningen, the Netherlands; et al)
Clin Chem 58:543-548, 2012

Background.—Recent recognition of its broad pathophysiological importance has triggered an increased interest in 25-hydroxyvitamin D [25(OH)D]. By consequence, throughput in 25(OH)D testing has become an issue for clinical laboratories, and several automated assays for measurement of 25(OH)D are now available. The aim of this study was to test the accuracy and robustness of these assays by comparing their results to those of an isotope dilution/online solid-phase extraction liquid chromatography/tandem mass spectrometry (ID-XLC-MS/MS) method. We put specific focus on the influence of vitamin D—binding protein (DBP) by using samples with various concentrations of DBP.

Methods.—We used 5 automated assays (Architect, Centaur, iSYS, Liaison, and Elecsys), 1 RIA (Diasorin) preceded by extraction, and an ID-XLC-MS/MS method to measure 25(OH)D concentrations in plasma samples of 51 healthy individuals, 52 pregnant women, 50 hemodialysis patients, and 50 intensive care patients. Using ELISA, we also measured DBP concentrations in these samples.

Results.—Most of the examined 25(OH)D assays showed significant deviations in 25(OH)D concentrations from those of the ID-XLC-MS/MS method. As expected, DBP concentrations were higher in samples of pregnant women and lower in samples of IC patients compared to healthy controls. In 4 of the 5 fully automated 25(OH)D assays, we observed an inverse relationship between DBP concentrations and deviations from the ID-XLC-MS/MS results.

Conclusions.—25(OH)D measurements performed with most immunoassays suffer from inaccuracies that are DBP concentration dependent. Therefore, when interpreting results of 25(OH)D measurements, careful consideration of the measurement method is necessary.

▶ Vitamin D sufficiency plays an important role not only in the prevention of osteoporosis or osteomalacia but also, as suggested recently, in the prevention of other diseases such as cancer and autoimmune diseases. Consequently, clinical laboratories receive numerous requests for measuring 25-hydroxyvitamin D (25[OH]D) concentrations. Traditionally, assays for 25(OH)D have involved extraction with organic solvents, reconstitution of the specimen in a suitable matrix, and quantification by immunoassay. Alternative methods include high-performance liquid chromatography. Because such methods are rather laborious, automation of 25(OH)D measurements is desirable, and many automated methods have been developed recently. A major challenge in measuring 25(OH)D is the displacement of 25(OH)D from vitamin D—binding protein (DBP). The organic solvents used to release 25(OH)D from its binding protein are not compatible with most immunoassays or protein-binding assays. Alternative methods for displacement have been devised, but it remains unclear whether the automated methods are sufficiently effective in liberating 25(OH)D from DBP. The aim of this study was to test the accuracy of the currently available 25(OH)D assays by comparing 6 available routine vitamin D assays with an isotope dilution/online solid-phase extraction liquid chromatography/tandem mass spectrometry method, using plasma not only from healthy individuals, but also from patients with a broad range of DBP concentrations, to assess the sensitivity of the various assays to differences in circulating DBP concentrations (Fig 3 in the original article).

M. G. Bissell, MD, PhD, MPH

Comparison of Serum Creatinine and Cystatin C for Early Diagnosis of Contrast-Induced Nephropathy after Coronary Angiography and Interventions

Ribichini F, Gambaro G, Graziani MS, et al (Univ of Verona, Italy; Catholic Univ, Rome, Italy; Ospedale Civile Maggiore, Verona, Italy)
Clin Chem 58:458-464, 2012

Background.—The diagnostic accuracy of serum creatinine and cystatin C (Cys) as early predictors of contrast-induced nephropathy (CIN) has been debated. We investigated the diagnostic sensitivities, diagnostic specificities, and variations from baseline for serum creatinine and Cys in CIN.

Methods.—We prospectively evaluated 166 patients at risk for CIN at baseline, and at 12, 24, and 48 h after exposure to contrast media. CIN occurred in 30 patients (18%). Changes (Δ) compared to baseline in serum creatinine and Cys were evaluated at the predefined time points. ROC curve analysis was performed for the Δ 12-h basal serum creatinine and Cys.

Results.—The Δ serum creatinine at 12 h from baseline was the earliest predictor of CIN [area under the ROC curve (AUC) = 0.80; $P < 0.001$]. The Δ serum creatinine 15% variation [0.15 mg/dL (13.2 μmol/L)] yielded 43% diagnostic sensitivity and 93% diagnostic specificity. The ΔCys at 12 h from baseline performed significantly worse than serum creatinine (AUC = 0.48; $P = 0.74$).

Conclusions.—Variations from the serum creatinine baseline offer better diagnostic accuracy for predicting CIN at an earlier stage than similar variations in Cys. An additional diagnostic value of Cys over the determination of serum creatinine in the setting of CIN was not observed.

▶ Acute kidney injury (AKI) is a well-recognized complication following angiographic examinations. AKI prolongs hospitalization, may cause renal failure, and substantially increases morbidity and mortality. The most common form of AKI after cardiovascular invasive procedures with administration of iodine contrast media is contrast-induced nephropathy (CIN), conventionally defined as an acute impairment of renal function, expressed as a relative increase in serum creatinine concentration of at least 25% or an absolute increase in serum creatinine from 0.3 mg/dL or up to 0.5 mg/dL within 48 hours in the absence of other related causes. CIN is diagnosed on the basis of the dynamic changes in serum creatinine after exposure to iodine contrast media. However, because serum creatinine is not a perfect glomerular filtration rate (GFR) biomarker owing to its tubular secretion and variable production rate, the perception is that serum creatinine is insensitive to early changes in GFR. Cystatin C (Cys) is a cationic low-molecular-weight cysteine protease that is produced at a constant rate by all nucleated cells, is not metabolized in the serum, and is freely filtered by the glomeruli. Cys has been proposed as an alternative to serum creatinine to evaluate GFR, owing to the absence of variations related to age, sex, and muscle mass. In the study reported here, the authors compared the diagnostic sensitivity and diagnostic specificity of serum creatinine and Cys for early CIN prediction in a population of patients undergoing coronary angiography and interventions who were at risk for AKI (Fig 1 in the original article).

M. G. Bissell, MD, PhD, MPH

Long-Term Biological Variation of Serum Protein Electrophoresis M-Spike, Urine M-Spike, and Monoclonal Serum Free Light Chain Quantification: Implications for Monitoring Monoclonal Gammopathies

Katzmann JA, Snyder MR, Rajkumar SV, et al (Mayo Clinic, Rochester, MN)
Clin Chem 57:1687-1692, 2011

Background.—We analyzed serial data in patients with clinically stable monoclonal gammopathy to determine the total variation of serum M-spikes [measured with serum protein electrophoresis (SPEP)], urine M-spikes [measured with urine protein electrophoresis (UPEP)], and monoclonal serum free light chain (FLC) concentrations measured with immunoassay.

Methods.—Patients to be studied were identified by (*a*) no treatment during the study interval, (*b*) no change in diagnosis and <5 g/L change in

TABLE 4.—Total, Analytical, and Biological CVs[a]

	Measurable Serum M-Spike[b]	Urine M-Spike (≥200 mg/24 h)	Measurable Serum iFLC[c]	Serum IgG
Total CV	8.1	35.8	28.4	13
Analytical CV	2.1	4.5	5.8	4.2
Biological CV	7.8	35.5	27.8	12.3

[a]Total CVs are from Table 2, analytical CVs are from laboratory validation studies, and biological CVs are derived from the relationship of the biological CV being equal to the square root of the difference of the square of the total CV minus the square of the analytical CV.
[b]Values >10 g/L.
[c]Values >100 mg/L.

serum M-spike over the course of observation; (c) performance of all 3 tests (SPEP, UPEP, FLC immunoassay) in at least 3 serial samples that were obtained 9 months to 5 years apart; (d) serum M-spike ≥10 g/L, urine M-spike ≥200 mg/24 h, or clonal FLC ≥100 mg/L. The total CV was calculated for each method.

Results.—Among the cohort of 158 patients, 90 had measurable serum M-spikes, 25 had urine M-spikes, and 52 had measurable serum FLC abnormalities. The CVs were calculated for serial SPEP M-spikes (8.1%), UPEP M-spikes (35.8%), and serum FLC concentrations (28.4%). Combining these CVs and the interassay analytical CVs, we calculated the biological CV for the serum M-spike (7.8%), urine M-spike (35.5%), and serum FLC concentration (27.8%).

Conclusions.—The variations in urine M-spike and serum FLC measurements during patient monitoring are similar and are larger than those for serum M-spikes. In addition, in this group of stable patients, a measurable serum FLC concentration was available twice as often as a measurable urine M-spike (Table 4).

▶ The authors analyzed serial data in patients with clinically stable monoclonal gammopathy to determine the total variation of serum M-spikes, urine M-spikes, and monoclonal serum free light chain (FLC) concentrations measured with immunoassay (Table 4). There is a large body of work regarding within-person variation and the meaning of differences between sequential laboratory results. These studies have recognized the variation to be the sum of preanalytic and analytical variability as well as intra-individual biological variability. Traditionally, these studies have focused on healthy individuals with results within the working range of an assay. Serum immunoglobulins can be quantified in patients with monoclonal immunoglobulins and variations can be compared with reference intervals for serum immunoglobulins, but there are no normal counterparts to serum and urine M -spikes. The authors have analyzed serial samples in clinically stable patients to assess the total variability (analytical plus biological) of these monitoring tests. Intrinsic to this approach is that the biological variability also may contain disease variability despite restricting the patient cohort to clinically defined stable patients. The authors have undertaken these studies to evaluate disease-monitoring recommendations, with particular emphasis on the recommendations for serum FLC.

M. G. Bissell, MD, PhD, MPH

Investigating Interferences of a Whole-Blood Point-of-Care Creatinine Analyzer: Comparison to Plasma Enzymatic and Definitive Creatinine Methods in an Acute-Care Setting

Straseski JA, Lyon ME, Clarke W, et al (Univ of Utah Health Sciences Ctr, Salt Lake City; Univ of Calgary, Alberta, Canada; Johns Hopkins Med Institutions, Baltimore, MD; et al)
Clin Chem 57:1566-1573, 2011

Background.—Although measurement of whole-blood creatinine at the point of care offers rapid assessment of renal function, agreement of point-of-care (POC) results with central laboratory methods continues to be a concern. We assessed the influence of several potential interferents on POC whole-blood creatinine measurements.

Methods.—We compared POC creatinine (Nova Stat Sensor) measurements with plasma enzymatic (Roche Modular) and isotope dilution mass spectrometry (IDMS) assays in 119 hospital inpatients. We assessed assay interference by hematocrit, pH, pO_2, total and direct bilirubin, creatine, prescribed drugs, diagnosis, red blood cell water fraction, and plasma water fraction.

Results.—CVs for POC creatinine were 1.5- to 6-fold greater than those for plasma methods, in part due to meter-to-meter variation. Regression comparison of POC creatinine to IDMS results gave a standard error $(S_{y|x})$ of 0.61 mg/dL (54 μmol/L), whereas regression of plasma enzymatic creatinine to IDMS was $S_{y|x}$ 0.16 mg/dL (14 μmol/L). By univariate analysis, bilirubin, creatine, drugs, pO_2, pH, plasma water fraction, and hematocrit were not found to contribute to method differences. However, multivariate analysis revealed that IDMS creatinine, red blood cell and plasma water fractions, and hematocrit explained 91.8% of variance in POC creatinine results.

Conclusions.—These data suggest that whole-blood POC creatinine measurements should be used with caution. Negative interferences observed with these measurements could erroneously suggest adequate renal function near the decision threshold, particularly if estimated glomerular filtration rate is determined. Disparity between whole-blood and plasma matrices partially explains the discordance between whole-blood and plasma creatinine methods.

▶ Patients with limited renal filtration are susceptible to contrast-induced nephropathy (CIN) after contrast computed tomography (CT) or magnetic resonance imaging (MRI) studies. Monitoring whole-blood creatinine at the point of care has gained favor as an immediate assessment of renal impairment to avoid CIN. Direct biosensors for point-of-care (POC) measuring of analytes such as creatinine, glucose, or lactate detect chemical bioactivity as a function of analyte molality (amount of analyte per unit of water mass, eg, mmol/kg). However, most meters report results in units of molarity (amount of analyte per volume of sample, eg, mmol/L). Conversion between blood creatinine molality detected and plasma creatinine molarity reported is affected by device calibration that typically assumes healthy mean values for plasma water mass, red blood cell water mass, and hematocrit. In the past, comparisons of novel whole-blood creatinine methods with plasma enzymatic creatinine reference methods were susceptible to systematic bias because of the lack of creatinine standardization. To address these concerns and reduce the risk of reference assay interference, the authors compared POC results with an isotope-dilution mass spectrometry (IDMS) creatinine assay. The goal of this study was to assess the performance of the Nova StatSensor POC whole-blood creatinine analyzer by comparing its performance with the Roche Diagnostics plasma enzymatic creatinine method (Fig 1 in the original article) and an IDMS plasma creatinine method (Fig 3 in the original article). The authors investigated possible causes of observed discrepancies, including whole-blood matrix components.

M. G. Bissell, MD, PhD, MPH

18 Clinical Microbiology

Visual Detection of High-Risk Human Papillomavirus Genotypes 16, 18, 45, 52, and 58 by Loop-Mediated Isothermal Amplification with Hydroxynaphthol Blue Dye

Luo L, Nie K, Yang M-J, et al (Chinese Ctr for Disease Control and Prevention, Beijing, China)

J Clin Microbiol 49:3545-3550, 2011

A simple, rapid, sensitive, qualitative, colorimetric loop-mediated isothermal amplification (LAMP) with hydroxynaphthol blue dye (HNB) was established to detect high-risk human papillomavirus (HPV) genotypes 16, 18, 45, 52, and 58. All initial validation studies with the control DNA proved to be type specific. The colorimetric type-specific LAMP assay could achieve a sensitivity of 10 to 100 copies at 63°C for 65 min, comparable to that of real-time PCR. In order to evaluate the reliability of HPV type-specific LAMP, the assay was further evaluated with HPV DNAs from a panel of 294 clinical specimens whose HPV status was previously determined with a novel one-step typing method with multiplex PCR. The tested panel comprised 108 HPV DNA-negative samples and 186 HPV-DNA-positive samples of 14 genotypes. The results showed that the sensitivity of HPV type-specific LAMP for HPV types 16, 18, 45, 52, and 58 was 100%, 100%, 100%, 100%, and 100%, respectively, and the specificity was 100%, 98.5%, 100%, 98.8%, and 99.2%, respectively, compared with a novel one-step typing method with multiplex PCR. No cross-reactivity with other HPV genotypes was observed. In conclusion, this qualitative and colorimetric LAMP assay has potential usefulness for the rapid screening of HPV genotype 16, 18, 45, 52, and 58 infections, especially in resource-limited hospitals or rural clinics of provincial and municipal regions in China (Fig 3).

▶ So far, at least 14 high-risk human papillomavirus (HPV) genotypes have been shown to cause cervical cancer. Technologies available for HPV genotyping vary by method and platform and may offer type-specific characterization for a multitude of different high- and low-risk HPV types. However, these methods might not be suitable in primary clinical settings in developing countries or for field use, because of the sophisticated instrumentation required, elaborate and complicated assay procedures, and expensive reagents. There is therefore a growing demand for simple and economical molecular tests. Loop-mediated isothermal amplification (LAMP) is a nucleic acid amplification method that has emerged as a powerful gene amplification tool because of its

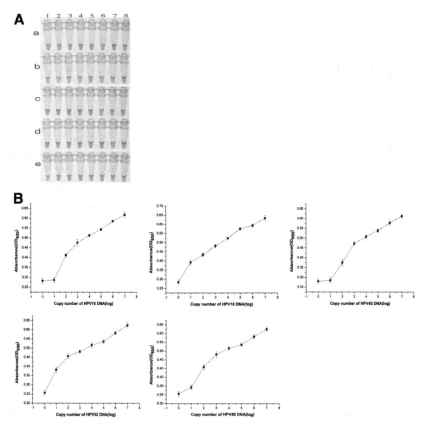

FIGURE 3.—Sensitivity analysis of colorimetric type-specific LAMP assay using serial dilutions of a cloned pMD18-T plasmid containing HPV16, HPV18, HPV45, HPV52, or HPV58 DNA, respectively. (A) Tubes contained HPV16 (a), HPV18 (b), HPV45 (c), HPV52 (d), and HPV58 (e). Dilutions were 10^7 copies (tube 1), 10^6 copies (tube 2), 10^5 copies (tube 3), 10^4 copies (tube 4), 10^3 copies (tube 5), 10^2 copies (tube 6), 10^1 copies (tube 7), and 10^0 copies (tube 8). (B) The average result for each concentration of HPV DNA was determined from three independent colorimetric tests and is represented as the means ± 2 times the standard deviation. The absorbance (OD_{650}) cutoff value (0.3) is calculated by adding two standard deviations to the mean of the negative reaction. When the absorbance (OD_{650}) value is over 0.3, it is defined as a positive reaction. (Reprinted from Luo L, Nie K, Yang M-J, et al. Visual detection of high-risk human papillomavirus genotypes 16, 18, 45, 52, and 58 by loop-mediated isothermal amplification with hydroxynaphthol blue dye. *J Clin Microbiol.* 2011;49:3545-3550, with permission from American Society for Microbiology.)

simplicity, speed, specificity, and cost-effectiveness. The use of this technique with hydroxynaphthol blue (HNB) dye was first developed in the authors' laboratory and is being used increasingly for rapid and visual detection and typing of emerging viruses. In this study, a simple and visual type-specific LAMP assay for the detection of high-risk HPV genotypes 16, 18, 45, 52, and 58 is described, in which the reaction was carried out in a single tube by mixing primers and DNA polymerase with the tested samples at 63°C for 65 min. The LAMP assay was further evaluated with HPV DNAs from 294 clinical cervical scrape samples; the results demonstrate that this assay is sensitive and specific. One of the most attractive features of this LAMP assay is that the results can be observed and determined by HNB dye-mediated visualization using the naked eye and without opening the tubes after amplification (Fig 3).

M. G. Bissell, MD, PhD, MPH

Rapid Identification of *Staphylococcus aureus* and Methicillin Resistance by Flow Cytometry Using a Peptide Nucleic Acid Probe

Shrestha NK, Scalera NM, Wilson DA, et al (Cleveland Clinic, OH; et al)
J Clin Microbiol 49:3383-3385, 2011

A total of 56 *Staphylococcus aureus* isolates incubated for 2 h in the presence or absence of oxacillin were analyzed by flow cytometry after labeling with an *S. aureus*-specific peptide nucleic acid (PNA) probe. Two defined

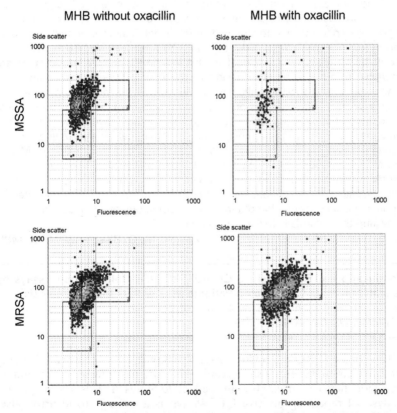

MHB without oxacillin   MHB with oxacillin

FIGURE 1.—Representative dot plots of MRSA and MSSA strains on flow cytometry after incubation in the presence or absence of oxacillin for 2 h, with gate 1 (red) and gate 2 (blue) shown, highlighting differences in signal events. For interpretation of the references to color in this figure legend, the reader is referred to web version of this article. (Reprinted from Shrestha NK, Scalera NM, Wilson DA, et al. Rapid identification of *Staphylococcus aureus* and methicillin resistance by flow cytometry using a peptide nucleic acid probe. *J Clin Microbiol.* 2011;49:3383-3385, with permission from American Society for Microbiology.)

ratios, the paired signal count ratio (PSCR) and the gate signal count ratio (GSCR), differentiated methicillin-resistant *S. aureus* (MRSA) and methicillin- susceptible *S. aureus* (MSSA) with sensitivities of 100% each and specificities of 96% and 100%, respectively (Fig 1).

▶ The authors have demonstrated that methicillin-resistant *Staphylococcus aureus* (MRSA) and methicillin-susceptible *S. aureus* (MSSA) isolates can be accurately and rapidly differentiated by flow cytometry based on fluorescence intensity and side scatter differences after brief exposure to oxacillin using a nonspecific fluorescent nucleic acid dye (Fig 1). Flow cytometry to differentiate MRSA from MSSA would be even more useful if the method could incorporate *S. aureus*-specific probe labeling instead of using a nonspecific dye. *S. aureus* and other microorganisms can be accurately identified by labeling with specific peptide nucleic acid-fluorescence in situ hybridization (PNAFISH) probes. Such probes are currently being used in clinical microbiology laboratories to rapidly identify *S. aureus* in blood culture bottles found to be growing gram-positive cocci in clusters. This study demonstrates the potential to use flow cytometry to go one step further and to rapidly determine methicillin susceptibility in addition to identifying *S. aureus*. The total time to run a batch of 10 samples was about 3.5 h, including the 2 h of incubation time. Many of these steps are amenable to automation. The design of the flow cytometer instrument used and the nature of the test also allow for random access testing, another advantage for an assay for clinical application. The cost per sample of the flow cytometry test using this method is estimated to be about $24, compared with about $45 for the same identification using a commercially available real-time polymerase chain reaction assay. Rapid identification of *S. aureus* and differentiation of MRSA and MSSA can be accomplished by real-time polymerase chain reaction also, but the potential advantages of whole-cell analysis via flow cytometry include simplified sample preparation, the ability for random access testing, the potential for direct visual confirmation of target cell morphology by fluorescence microscopy, and the potentially lower cost per test.

M. G. Bissell, MD, PhD, MPH

Identification of False-Positive QuantiFERON-TB Gold In-Tube Assays by Repeat Testing in HIV-Infected Patients at Low Risk for Tuberculosis
Gray J, Reves R, Johnson S, et al (Univ of Colorado, Aurora)
Clin Infect Dis 54:e20-e23, 2012

The QuantiFERON-TB Gold In-Tube assay (QFT) is increasingly being used for latent tuberculosis screening in patients infected with human immunodeficiency virus (HIV) in the United States. This is a retrospective analysis of repeating positive QFT assays as a strategy to identify false-positive results in HIV-infected patients at low risk for tuberculosis.

▶ The incidence of tuberculosis and the proportion of individuals co-infected with human immunodeficiency virus (HIV) in the United States is falling.

HIV-infected patients remain an important group to target for latent tuberculosis infection (LTBI) testing and treatment because of their increased risk of progression to active tuberculosis. Preventive isoniazid therapy in HIV-infected people has proven beneficial if given to patients with positive tuberculin skin tests (TSTs), but has the risk of toxicity without proven benefit in patients who are TST-negative. The commercially available interferon-γ release assays (IGRAs)—QuantiFERON-TB Gold In-Tube (QFT; Cellestis) and T-Spot. TB (Oxford Immunotec)—are alternatives to TST for screening HIV-infected patients. IGRAs are increasingly used because of their higher specificity and requirement of 1 patient visit. As with TSTs, IGRAs rely on functioning cell-mediated immunity and therefore have higher rates of failed tests in HIV-infected patients. There are no data on the predictive value of IGRAs in HIV-infected patients in the United States, and poor concordance between the TST and IGRAs has been reported. Because of poor rates of LTBI screening using TST, the HIV clinics at Denver Health and University of Colorado switched to QFT in 2009. Rates of testing increased, but unexpected positive QFTs were observed in patients with low risk for tuberculosis exposure, such as US-born Coloradans among whom the tuberculosis incidence in 2010 was 0.6 per 100 000. To assess the validity of the QFT results, both clinics began repeating unexpected positive QFTs prior to recommending LTBI therapy.

M. G. Bissell, MD, PhD, MPH

A Critical Appraisal of the Role of the Clinical Microbiology Laboratory in the Diagnosis of Bloodstream Infections

Weinstein MP, Doern GV (Robert Wood Johnson Med School, New Brunswick, NJ; Univ of Iowa Carver College of Medicine, Iowa City)
J Clin Microbiol 49:S26-S29, 2011

The detection of bloodstream infections is one of the most important functions of clinical microbiology laboratories. Despite advances in blood culture technology and clinical studies that have focused on the detection of bacteremia and fungemia, perfection has not been achieved and uncertainties persist. This review provides perspectives on a number of areas, including the recommended number of blood cultures, duration of incubation of blood cultures, use of anaerobic, in addition to aerobic, blood culture media, value of the lysis-centrifugation method, processing and reporting of probable blood culture contaminants, and limitations of current blood culture methods and systems. We also address the handling of blood cultures in point-of-care locations that lack full microbiology capabilities.

▶ The detection of bacteremia and fungemia is arguably one of the most important functions of the clinical microbiology laboratory. Although much has been learned in recent decades and guidelines for blood cultures have been published, absolute certainties remain elusive. There are many questions still without clear answers. For example, why are there so many negative blood cultures? Only 10% to 15% of all blood cultures show growth, and approximately half of these grow contaminants, raising questions about whether current methods are not sufficiently sensitive and whether clinicians use the wrong clinical triggers to initiate orders for blood cultures. What is the optimal number of blood cultures that should be obtained when sepsis is suspected? Can the duration of the routine incubation of routine blood cultures be reduced to fewer than 5 days? Should a routine blood culture set combine aerobic and anaerobic culture vials or should a culture set use only aerobic culture vials, with anaerobic vials included selectively for patients with a high probability of anaerobic bacteremia? Does the lysis-centrifugation blood culture method have any value? How should blood culture contaminants be assessed? How can the number of negative blood cultures be reduced? Should blood cultures be done in a stat lab or point-of-care location? What microorganisms are missed consistently with conventional blood culture approaches?

M. G. Bissell, MD, PhD, MPH

Accuracy of microscopic urine analysis and chest radiography in patients with severe sepsis and septic shock
Capp R, Chang Y, Brown DFM (Massachusetts General Hosp, Boston)
J Emerg Med 42:52-57, 2012

Background.—Diagnosis of source of infection in patients with septic shock and severe sepsis needs to be done rapidly and accurately to guide appropriate antibiotic therapy.

Objective.—The purpose of this study is to evaluate the accuracy of two diagnostic studies used in the emergency department (ED) to guide diagnosis of source of infection in this patient population.

Methods.—This was a retrospective review of ED patients admitted to an intensive care unit with the diagnosis of severe sepsis or septic shock over a 12-month period. We evaluated accuracy of initial microscopic urine analysis testing and chest radiography in the diagnosis of urinary tract infections and pneumonia, respectively.

Results.—Of the 1400 patients admitted to intensive care units, 170 patients met criteria for severe sepsis and septic shock. There were a total of 47 patients diagnosed with urinary tract infection, and their initial microscopic urine analysis with counts >10 white blood cells were 80% sensitive (95% confidence interval [CI] .66—.90) and 66% specific (95% CI .52—.77) for the positive final urine culture result. There were 85 patients with final diagnosis of pneumonia. The sensitivity and specificity of initial chest radiography were, respectively, 58% (95% CI .46—.68) and 91% (95% CI .81—.95) for the diagnosis of pneumonia.

Conclusion.—In patients with severe sepsis and septic shock, the chest radiograph has low sensitivity of 58%, whereas urine analysis has a low specificity of 66%. Given the importance of appropriate antibiotic selection and optimal but not perfect test characteristics, this population may benefit from broad-spectrum antibiotics, rather than antibiotics tailored toward a particular source of infection.

▶ Septic shock and severe sepsis carry high mortality rates, and septic shock has been identified as the most common cause of death in noncoronary intensive care units (ICUs). Recently, 2 studies have found that early effective antibiotic treatment is highly associated with lower mortality rates and that inappropriate antibiotic treatment in patients with septic shock has a 5-fold increased mortality rate compared with patients who received effective antibiotic treatment. To date, effective antibiotic treatment is selected based on identification of source of infection. Emergency physicians use the history and physical examination, as well as laboratory studies and radiology testing, to diagnose sources of infection. Microscopic urine analysis and chest x-ray study are widely utilized tests in the emergency department to help diagnose 2 common causes of severe sepsis and septic shock: pneumonia and urinary tract infections. No studies to date have looked at overall sensitivities and specificities of these 2 tests in the adult population with severe sepsis and septic shock. In this study, the accuracy of these 2 commonly used diagnostic tests in patients with severe sepsis and septic shock is reviewed.

M. G. Bissell, MD, PhD, MPH

Trends and Characteristics of Culture-Confirmed *Staphylococcus aureus* Infections in a Large U.S. Integrated Health Care Organization
Ray GT, Suaya JA, Baxter R (Northern California Region, Oakland, CA; North America Vaccine Development, Philadelphia, PA; Kaiser Permanente Vaccine Study Ctr and The Permanente Med Group, Oakland, CA)
J Clin Microbiol 50:1950-1957, 2012

Infections due to *Staphylococcus aureus* present a significant health problem in the United States. Between 1990 and 2005, there was a dramatic increase in community-associated methicillin-resistant *S. aureus* (MRSA), but recent reports suggest that MRSA may be declining. We retrospectively identified *S. aureus* isolates (n = 133,450) that were obtained from patients in a large integrated health plan between 1 January 1998 and 31 December 2009. Trends over time in MRSA were analyzed, and demographic risk factors for MRSA versus methicillin-susceptible *S. aureus* (MSSA) were identified. The percentage of *S. aureus* isolates that were MRSA increased from 9% to 20% between 1998 and 2001 and from 25% to 49% between 2002 and 2005 and decreased from 49% to 43% between 2006 and 2009. The increase in MRSA was seen in blood and in other bacteriological specimens and occurred in all age and race/ethnicity groups, though it was most pronounced in persons aged 18 to < 50 years and African-Americans. Hospital onset infections were the most likely to be MRSA (odds ratio [OR], 1.58; confidence interval [CI], 1.46 to 1.70, compared to community-associated cases), but the largest increase in MRSA was in community-associated infections. Isolates from African-Americans (OR, 1.73; CI, 1.64 to 1.82) and Hispanics (OR, 1.11; CI, 1.06 to 1.16) were more likely to be MRSA than those from whites. After substantial increases between 1998 and 2005 in the proportion of *S. aureus* isolates that were MRSA, the proportion decreased between 2006 and 2009. Hospital onset *S. aureus* infections are disproportionately MRSA, as are those among African-Americans.

▶ Infections due to *Staphylococcus aureus* present a substantial health problem in the United States. *S. aureus* is a major cause of hospital-acquired pneumonia and lower respiratory tract infections and the primary cause of surgical site infections and skin and soft tissue infections (SSTIs) and is now likely the leading cause of invasive bacterial disease. Throughout the 1990s, *S. aureus* infections in hospitalized patients were increasingly caused by methicillin-resistant *S. aureus* (MRSA), making treatment of these infections more difficult. Moreover, between 1990 and 2005, there was an even more dramatic increase in community-associated MRSA (CAMRSA) infections. However, there are indications that MRSA may be on the decline. A recent US study found that the incidence of health care–associated invasive MRSA declined from 2005 to 2008, and an analysis of *S. aureus* isolates from outpatient pediatric patients with SSTIs found the percentage of isolates that were MRSA was lower in 2008 and 2009 than in 2005 to 2007. In general, surveillance activity for MRSA has been limited to bloodstream or invasive infections and to health care–associated and hospital-onset disease, and there have been few population-based studies. As the epidemiology of *S. aureus* disease changes, inclusion of community-associated, community-onset, and noninvasive disease is important for assessing the magnitude of the burden of disease in the population, for setting priorities for prevention and control, and for creating guidelines for empirical antibiotic treatment. In this retrospective study covering 12 years, the authors describe laboratory-confirmed *S. aureus* infections in a large cohort of persons of all ages, using isolates from sterile and nonsterile sites in both ambulatory and inpatient settings. They describe trends in methicillin resistance of laboratory-confirmed *S. aureus* isolates and trends in the incidence of *S. aureus* bloodstream infections, and they explore the relationship of patient demographics and infection onset type to the likelihood of *S. aureus* infections being methicillin resistant.

M. G. Bissell, MD, PhD, MPH

Invasive Mycoses: Diagnostic Challenges
Ostrosky-Zeichner L (Univ of Texas Health Med School, Houston)
Am J Med 125:S14-S24, 2012

Despite the availability of newer antifungal drugs, outcomes for patients with invasive fungal infections (IFIs) continue to be poor, in large part due to delayed diagnosis and initiation of appropriate antifungal therapy. Standard histopathologic diagnostic techniques are often untenable in at-risk patients, and culture-based diagnostics typically are too insensitive or nonspecific, or provide results after too long a delay for optimal IFI management. Newer surrogate markers of IFIs with improved sensitivity and specificity are needed to enable earlier diagnosis and, ideally, to provide prognostic information and/or permit therapeutic monitoring. Surrogate assays should also be accessible and easy to implement in the hospital. Several nonculture-based assays of newer surrogates are making their way into the medical setting or are currently under investigation. These new or up-and-coming surrogates include antigens/antibodies (mannan and antimannan antibodies) or fungal metabolites (D-arabinitol) for detection of invasive candidiasis, the *Aspergillus* cell wall component galactomannan used to detect invasive aspergillosis, or the fungal cell wall component and panfungal marker β-glucan. In addition, progress continues with use of polymerase chain reaction— or other nucleic acid— or molecular-based assays for diagnosis of either specific or generic IFIs, although the various methods must be better standardized before any of these approaches can be more fully implemented into the medical setting. Investigators are also beginning to explore the possibility of combining newer surrogate markers with each other or with more standard diagnostic approaches to improve sensitivity, specificity, and capacity for earlier diagnosis, at a time when fungal burden is still relatively low and more responsive to antifungal therapy.

▶ The incidence of invasive fungal infections (IFIs) is on the rise, largely due to an increasing pool of immunocompromised or severely ill patients at elevated risk for IFIs. IFIs are associated with significant morbidity and mortality, and are increasingly caused by fungal pathogens or subspecies with diminished susceptibility or resistance to many standard antifungal agents. Poor outcome in patients with IFIs can often be related to delayed treatment with an effective antifungal agent or combination of agents due to limitations of standard diagnostic techniques. Diagnosis of IFIs is extremely challenging, because current diagnostic methods are not sufficiently sensitive or specific, and results are often available too late to be clinically useful. Newer diagnostic markers and techniques are available and continue to evolve, but many clinicians are unfamiliar with these approaches. Early diagnosis and/or treatment have been shown to improve patient outcomes. Hence, there is a clear need to educate clinicians about different techniques available to diagnose and manage patients with IFIs. This article provides a general overview of the importance of early diagnosis, the need for surrogates in medical mycology, and the relative advantages and disadvantages of standard histopathologic and culture-based approaches to IFI diagnosis and newer nonculture-based diagnostic techniques.

M. G. Bissell, MD, PhD, MPH

A Highly Efficient Ziehl-Neelsen stain: Identifying *De Novo* Intracellular *Mycobacterium tuberculosis* and Improving Detection of Extracellular *M. tuberculosis* in Cerebrospinal Fluid

Chen P, Shi M, Feng G-D, et al (Fourth Military Med Univ, Xi'an, Shaanxi, China)
J Clin Microbiol 50:1166-1170, 2012

Tuberculous meningitis leads to a devastating outcome, and early diagnosis and rapid chemotherapy are vital to reduce morbidity and mortality. Since *Mycobacterium tuberculosis* is a kind of cytozoic pathogen and its numbers are very few in cerebrospinal fluid, detecting M. *tuberculosis* in cerebrospinal fluid from tuberculous meningitis patients is still a challenge for clinicians. Ziehl-Neelsen stain, the current feasible microbiological method for the diagnosis of tuberculosis, often needs a large amount of cerebrospinal fluid specimen but shows a low detection rate of M. *tuberculosis*. Here, we developed a modified Ziehl-Neelsen stain, involving cytospin slides with Triton processing, in which only 0.5 ml of cerebrospinal fluid specimens was required. This method not only improved the detection rate of extracellular M. *tuberculosis* significantly but also identified intracellular M. *tuberculosis* in the neutrophils, monocytes, and lymphocytes clearly. Thus, our modified method is more effective and sensitive than the conventional Ziehl-Neelsen stain, providing clinicians a convenient yet powerful tool for rapidly diagnosing tuberculous meningitis.

▶ Tuberculous meningitis (TBM) is the most severe form of tuberculosis and causes substantial morbidity and mortality. The early diagnosis of and prompt initiation of chemotherapy for TBM are crucial to a successful outcome. However, the early and accurate detection of mycobacteria in tuberculosis in the cerebrospinal fluid (CSF) of TBM patients still remains a challenge for clinicians, mainly because of the lack of rapid, efficient, and practical detection methods. Currently, mycobacterial culture is the gold standard for detecting *Mycobacterium tuberculosis*, but it is time consuming and requires specialized safety procedures in laboratories. Serologic methods are convenient but lack sensitivity and specificity. Although the polymerase chain reaction technique is rapid, it is costly for routine use in developing countries where most tuberculosis cases occur. Conventional smear microscopy with the Ziehl-Neelsen (ZN) stain is a rapid and practical method for detecting acid-fast bacilli, especially in low-income countries, because of its rapidity, low cost, and high positive predictive value for tuberculosis. However, the ZN method is severely handicapped by its low detection rate, ranging from 0% to 20% for CSF specimens. To reveal the presence of intracellular M. *tuberculosis* and improve the detection of extracellular M. *tuberculosis* from a small volume of CSF specimens, the authors developed a highly efficient ZN stain involving the use of only 0.5-ml CSF specimens from TBM cases.

M. G. Bissell, MD, PhD, MPH

A Sample Extraction Method for Faster, More Sensitive PCR-Based Detection of Pathogens in Blood Culture

Regan JF, Furtado MR, Brevnov MG, et al (Life Technologies, Foster City, CA; et al)
J Mol Diagn 14:120-129, 2012

Three mechanistically different sample extraction methodologies, namely, silica spin columns, phenol-chloroform, and an automated magnetic capture of polymer-complexed DNA (via an Automate Express instrument), were compared for their abilities to purify nucleic acids from blood culture fluids for use in TaqMan assays for detection of *Staphylococcus aureus*. The extracts from silica columns required 100- to 1000-fold dilutions to sufficiently reduce the powerful PCR inhibitory effects of the anticoagulant sodium polyanetholsulfonate, a common additive in blood culture media. In contrast, samples extracted by either phenol-chloroform or the Automate Express instrument required little or no dilution, respectively, allowing for an approximate 100-fold improvement in assay sensitivity. Analysis of 60 blood culture bottles indicated that these latter two methodologies could be used to detect lower numbers of pathogens and that a growing *S. aureus* culture could be detected 2 hours earlier than when using silica columns. Of the three tested methodologies, the Automate Express instrument had the shortest time to result, requiring only approximately 80 minutes to process 12 samples. These findings highlight the importance of considering the mechanism when selecting a DNA extraction methodology, given that certain PCR inhibitors act in a similar fashion to DNA in certain chemical environments, resulting in copurification, whereas other methodologies use different chemistries that have advantages during the DNA purification of certain types of samples.

▶ Molecular analysis of blood cultures is increasingly being used to identify bloodborne pathogens. Although it is considered the gold standard, culturing blood can generate false-negative results up to 31% of the time and false-positive results up to 10% of the time, making confirmation by polymerase chain reaction (PCR) desirable. Achieving accurate PCR results from blood culture samples is difficult, however, because of the presence of powerful PCR inhibitor additives. These inhibitors must be sufficiently removed from a blood culture sample to minimize the potential for false-negative PCR results. High-molecular-weight polysaccharide-based purification has proven to be particularly useful in forensics applications, where PCR inhibitors are commonly encountered, but this newer technology has not yet been tested on routine blood cultures. After several analytical experiments designed to examine the utility of these extraction methodologies in removing inhibitors found in culture media, 3 methodologies were compared for their ability to purify DNA from 60 blood cultures for accurate TaqMan analysis and to determine whether any of the methodologies offers an advantage in reducing time to result. The target organisms for the present study were methicillin-resistant *Staphylococcus aureus* and methicillin-sensitive *S. aureus*. These pathogens are responsible for approximately 756 000 hospitalizations and > 18 650 deaths per year, at a cost of approximately $26.8 billion to the US health care system. Improving the accuracy and speed of detecting these pathogens is extremely important, given that an improper or delayed diagnosis can result in increased morbidity and mortality for infected individuals.

M. G. Bissell, MD, PhD, MPH

Bacteriuria Screening by Automated Whole-Field-Image-Based Microscopy Reduces the Number of Necessary Urine Cultures
Falbo R, Sala MR, Signorelli S, et al (Hosp of Desio, Italy)
J Clin Microbiol 50:1427-1429, 2012

We evaluated a new automated urine sediment analyzer that provides whole-field images for the screening of urine samples prior to bacterial culture. Sterile urine samples from 1,011 male and female outpatients and inpatients (mean age 54.7) with a urinary tract infection prevalence of 18.3% were studied. Screening rapidly provides negative results.

▶ Urinary tract infection is one of the most common diseases diagnosed in the clinical microbiology laboratory through bacterial count per volume of urine. Approximately 80% of routine cultures are negative, and screening urine samples with significant bacteriuria from those without will anticipate negative results and reduce labor. In this study, the authors used a new automated urine sediment analyzer that provides whole-field images of the sediment for the screening of urine samples without significant bacteriuria. A total of 1011 consecutive midstream clean catch and catheter urine specimens were collected in sterile containers from 213 inpatients and 798 outpatients of all age groups (range, 0 to 95 years; mean, 54.7 years) and both genders, from November 2009 to January 2010, which were examined within 3 hours of receipt in the laboratory. Assessment of screening performance by the imaging technique was done by calculating sensitivity, specificity, positive predictive value, negative predictive value, efficiency, false-negative rate, and false-positive rate according to Clinical and Laboratory Standards Institute document EP12-A and was compared to that by automated strip analysis.

M. G. Bissell, MD, PhD, MPH

A Critical Appraisal of the Role of the Clinical Microbiology Laboratory in the Diagnosis of Urinary Tract Infections
Burd EM, Kehl KS (Emory Univ School of Medicine, Atlanta, GA; Med College of Wisconsin, Milwaukee)
J Clin Microbiol 49:S34-S38, 2011

Background.—Urinary tract infections (UTI) are common in outpatient and inpatient settings, so urine cultures are a large part of the workload for many clinical microbiology laboratories. Urine cultures should be used only when appropriate, and laboratories should provide meaningful results to obtain optimal care for patients.

Use of Urine Cultures.—The existing guidelines suggest that urine cultures are no longer recommended as part of the routine workup for young women suffering their first episode of acute uncomplicated cystitis. In most cases, culture and susceptibility testing add little to either diagnosing the condition or choosing an antibiotic for treatment. Laboratories could help to ensure that only appropriate specimens are submitted for culture by educating ordering physicians about these guidelines. Publishing data showing the reduction in laboratory costs associated with treating first-episode cystitis based on symptoms alone may help to persuade providers to restrict their use of urine cultures. Microbiologists should develop comprehensive practice guidelines for diagnosing UTIs that parallel those already in place but include methods for obtaining susceptibility data to guide empirical therapy for acute, uncomplicated UTIs when cultures are not done.

Pyuria Screening.—The sensitivity and specificity data for dipstick leukocyte esterase tests for pyuria are poor, so these tests should probably not be used. Newer automated systems are better choices, but studies that correlate results with UTI do not yet support their routine use.

Bacteruria.—Few published studies support the practice of urinalysis with reflex to culture only if the urinalysis is positive. Outcome studies based on current culture criteria, with an exclusion for women with first-episode cystitis, are lacking. Guidelines for how to manage complex patient populations are also needed. Current guidelines state that a colony count of $\geq 10^3$ colony-forming units (CFU)/ml of a single bacterial species is indicative of UTI in patients with indwelling catheters, whether urethral or suprapubic. However, indwelling catheter cultures with more than three bacterial species should not be worked up, since these catheters tend to be readily colonized by organisms not found in the bladder. New recommendations for children should also be developed. Recommendations for how to handle yeast in urine and its correlation to UTI are also needed.

Antimicrobial Susceptibility Testing.—Current guidelines recommend doing susceptibility testing for all cultures, but the relevance of these tests for urinary tract isolates is unclear. It would be helpful to have well-designed studies to determine their relevance and generate urine-specific breakpoints.

Conclusions.—Changes are needed concerning the role of clinical microbiology laboratories in diagnosing UTIs. New clinical studies are needed in some areas, as well as cooperative new recommendations.

▶ Urinary tract infection (UTI) is a common health problem in both outpatient and inpatient settings, and urine cultures occupy much of the workload in many clinical microbiology laboratories. Appropriate utilization of urine cultures by health care providers and generation of meaningful results by the laboratory are important for optimal care of patients as well as efficient operation of laboratories. The discussion in this article focuses on some potential opportunities for generation of meaningful test results and improving laboratory utilization. These include limiting utilization of urine cultures in first-time uncomplicated acute cystitis; developing comprehensive practice guidelines for the laboratory diagnosis of UTI in all situations; advocating evidence-based practice as the basis for reimbursement; discontinuing the use of dipstick leukocyte esterase tests as a screening method; revisiting antibiotic susceptibility patterns for urinary tract isolates; and conducting cost and outcomes studies of recurrent cystitis in both typical and more complex patient populations, such as catheterized and immunosuppressed patients.

M. G. Bissell, MD, PhD, MPH

19 Hematology and Immunology

Using the Antinuclear Antibody Test to Diagnose Rheumatic Diseases: When Does a Positive Test Warrant Further Investigation?
Volkmann ER, Taylor M, Ben-Artzi A (Univ of California-Los Angeles)
South Med J 105:100-104, 2012

The anti-nuclear antibody (ANA) test is ordered commonly as a screening test for rheumatic diseases. Although ANA positivity is highly sensitive for certain rheumatic diseases, the presence of ANA is nonspecific and can be associated with numerous nonrheumatic factors, including environmental exposures, malignancies, drugs, and infections. This article describes a practical approach for physicians when evaluating patients using a positive ANA test. In the absence of connective tissue disease symptoms, the ANA test has minimal clinical significance in diagnosing rheumatic diseases. Understanding how to use ANA test results appropriately may reduce unnecessary referrals and costly workups.

▶ For more than 50 years, detection of antinuclear antibody (ANA) in human sera has been associated with the presence of autoimmune disease. For conditions such as systemic lupus erythematosus (SLE), the sensitivity of the ANA test approaches 100%; however, a positive ANA test in the setting of nonspecific complaints often poses a clinical dilemma for physicians. In light of myriad nonrheumatic conditions associated with a positive ANA test, interpretation of the test results can be challenging. This review proposes a novel paradigm that may be used when evaluating patients with a positive ANA test. After describing the process of detecting ANA, the authors examine both nonrheumatic and rheumatic causes of a positive ANA test and review clinical signs and symptoms that may increase the specificity of a positive ANA test for particular rheumatic diseases. There are 2 considerations that would make the ANA assay more specific for detecting rheumatic diseases: raising the threshold for a positive test or coupling the test with more specific signs and symptoms of a particular rheumatic disease.

M. G. Bissell, MD, PhD, MPH

349

Expression of Hemoglobin Variant Migration by Capillary Electrophoresis Relative to Hemoglobin A₂ Improves Precision

Keren DF, Shalhoub R, Gulbranson R, et al (The Univ of Michigan, Ann Arbor;
Warde Med Laboratory, Ann Arbor, MI)
Am J Clin Pathol 137:660-664, 2012

We report the precision of the mean migration position of hemoglobin (Hb)S, HbC, HbG (Philadelphia), and HbD (Los Angeles) in 193 samples of whole blood assayed by capillary electrophoresis (CE) and high–performance liquid chromatography (HPLC). By expressing the migration of Hb variants by CE relative to that of HbA_2 in the same sample, there was a significant improvement in the coefficient of variation for each variant studied. The potential usefulness of expressing Hb variants relative to that of HbA_2 was evaluated by comparing the separation of 2 closely migrating Hbs. When expressed by their initial migrations on CE, 25 of the 43 cases of HbG and HbD overlapped. However, when the migrations of these variants were expressed relative to the HbA_2 in the same sample, the 24 cases of HbG separated completely from the 19 cases of HbD. These findings suggest that expressing Hb variants relative to an internal standard, such as HbA_2, may be of value for establishing a library of variant Hbs evaluated by CE.

▶ Identification of structural hemoglobin (Hb) variants and thalassemias traditionally has relied on alkaline and acid gel electrophoresis and, more recently, high-performance liquid chromatography (HPLC). These methods detect structural variants by electrophoretic migration or elution patterns. Precision of measurement of HbA is needed to detect thalassemia and can be helpful in cases of thalassemia and iron deficiencies. Capillary electrophoresis (CE) has been shown to be a reliable alternative to HPLC and is one that provides a more user-friendly interpretive format. All 3 methods readily separate the most common variants such as HbS, HbC, and HbE. However, some variants, such as HbG and HbD, are more difficult to separate from each other because they have identical migration on gels, overlapping elution times by HPLC, and similar migration by CE. Although HbG and HbD are readily distinguished because of their alpha and beta variants, respectively, the ability to separate such closely eluting or migrating proteins can be used as a test of the precision of each method. In this article, the authors describe their findings for the precision of the migration position for common Hb variants evaluated by CE. They have demonstrated that expressing the migration position relative to HbA improves the ability of CE to distinguish between 2 closely migrating variant Hbs (HbG and HbD).

M. G. Bissell, MD, PhD, MPH

Is the Blood Basophil Count Sufficiently Precise, Accurate, and Specific?: Three Automated Hematology Instruments and Flow Cytometry Compared

Amundsen EK, Henriksson CE, Holthe MR, et al (Oslo Univ Hosp, Ullevaal, Norway)

Am J Clin Pathol 137:86-92, 2012

We compared the performance of the basophil count of 3 hematology instruments with a flow cytometric method (FCM) in which CD123 and CD193 were used as basophil markers. By analyzing 112 patient samples, we found the ADVIA 120 (Siemens Healthcare Diagnostics, Deerfield, IL) and CELL-DYN Sapphire (Abbott Diagnostics, Santa Clara, CA) to underestimate the number of basophils by approximately 50% and the Sysmex XE-2100 (Sysmex, Kobe, Japan) and ADVIA to overestimate the basophil count in some samples with pathologic leukocytes. All 3 instruments had large (25%-50%) analytic within-run coefficients of variation. Compared with the FCM, we found a relatively good correlation for the CELL-DYN basophil count ($r = 0.81$), an intermediate correlation for the Sysmex ($r = 0.64$), and a poor correlation for the ADVIA ($r = 0.24$). When excluding the 52 samples flagged for the presence of pathologic leukocytes, these correlations were found to be 0.84, 0.90, and 0.57, respectively. The basophil count of the 3 instruments is, at least presently, of unsatisfactory quality.

▶ Basophils are granulocytes present at low concentrations in human peripheral blood that have important functions in the immune system. Through the 5-part differential leukocyte count, they have been counted in blood for decades, yet the importance of the count remains uncertain. One reason might be that basophils usually constitute less than 1% of the total leukocyte count and may, therefore, be difficult to count. The reference method for the basophil count is by microscopic slide examination as described in the H20-A2 standard from the Clinical and Laboratory Standards Institute (CLSI). But when counting the recommended 400 leukocytes, one might expect to find only 0 to 4 basophils, which leads to poor precision. This problem is also recognized by the CLSI, which states that the manual count is not suitable as a reference method for cells less frequent than 5% of the total leukocyte count. Hematology instruments count some thousand leukocytes and, therefore, may potentially offer more reliable estimates of the basophil count. However, many studies show a low correlation between the basophil count of different instruments and between instruments and the reference method. In part, this discrepancy may be caused by nonspecificity, that is, cells other than basophils being counted as basophils. The aim of this study was to evaluate the performance of the basophil count of 3 commonly used hematology instruments with a modified form of a previously published flow cytometric method (FCM) using monoclonal antibodies against CD193 (CCR3) and CD123 (IL-3R). The specificity of the FCM was confirmed by morphologic examination of flow cytometrically sorted cells. The performance of the basophil count of the hematology instruments was evaluated with focus on specificity, imprecision, and accuracy.

M. G. Bissell, MD, PhD, MPH

Low activated leukocyte cell adhesion molecule expression is associated with advanced tumor stage and early prostate-specific antigen relapse in prostate cancer

Minner S, Kraetzig F, Tachezy M, et al (Univ Med Ctr Hamburg-Eppendorf, Germany)

Hum Pathol 42:1946-1952, 2011

Activated leukocyte cell adhesion molecule (CD166) is a member of the immunoglobulin superfamily and is aberrantly expressed in different tumors, including prostate cancer. To learn more on the prevalence and clinical significance of activated leukocyte cell adhesion molecule expression in prostate cancer, a tissue microarray containing 3261 primary prostate cancers treated by radical prostatectomy was used. A total of 2390 different prostate cancers were analyzed by immunohistochemistry in a tissue microarray format. Activated leukocyte cell adhesion molecule immunostaining in cancers was compared with clinical follow-up, which was available for 1746 patients. Membranous activated leukocyte cell adhesion molecule immunostaining was recorded in 1663 (69.6%) of cases. High activated leukocyte cell adhesion molecule expression levels were significantly associated with favorable tumor features (pT: $P = .0015$; pN: $P = .0008$; preoperative prostate-specific antigen: $P = .0057$) and a lower risk of a biochemical recurrence ($P = .0067$). Cytoplasmatic activated leukocyte cell adhesion molecule staining was usually associated with membranous staining. The small number of cancers with pure cytoplasmatic staining did not reveal any particularities with respect to clinical outcome or tumor phenotype. It is concluded that activated leukocyte cell adhesion molecule protein is almost always expressed in prostate cancer and that decreased levels of activated leukocyte cell adhesion molecule expression may lead to an aggressive behavior of tumor cells. The abundant presence of activated leukocyte cell adhesion molecule and its membranous localization in prostate cancer epithelium make activated leukocyte cell adhesion molecule a potentially attractive structure for targeted therapy.

▶ Activated leukocyte cell adhesion molecule (ALCAM; CD166) is a member of the immunoglobulin superfamily. ALCAM is a cell adhesion molecule expressed by epithelial cells in several organs and is involved in embryogenesis, angiogenesis, hematopoiesis, and immune response. Alterations in expression of ALCAM have been reported in different malignancies, including melanoma, bladder cancer, breast cancer, colorectal cancer, esophageal squamous cell cancer, pancreatic cancer, oral squamous cell cancer, ovarian cancer, neuroblastoma, and prostate cancer. ALCAM expression is increased in some tumors and down-regulated in others. An association between high ALCAM expression and unfavorable prognosis has been shown for colorectal cancer, pancreatic cancer, esophageal squamous cell cancer, and neuroblastoma.

In contrast, several studies on breast cancer suggested that reduced ALCAM expression is associated with poor prognosis. ALCAM expression occurs in normal prostate epithelium. The role of ALCAM in prostate cancer is unclear. An increased

ALCAM expression in low-grade as compared with high-grade prostate cancer was described in a study analyzing 54 cancers by immunohistochemistry. However, the same group found a significant association between high cytoplasmatic ALCAM staining and early biochemical recurrence in a series of 42 patients. In addition to its prognostic role, ALCAM represents a potential future target for therapy. The utility of ALCAM as a drug target structure may be further enhanced by ligand-induced endocytosis. Moreover, in a recently described internalizing single-chain antibody, targeting ALCAM has been suggested for potential intracellular delivery of various therapeutic agents to prostate cancer cells.

The aim of this study was to clarify the prevalence and prognostic role of ALCAM expression in prostate cancer by using a preexisting tissue microarray (TMA), including more than 3000 prostate cancers, mostly with clinical follow-up data. The data show that ALCAM expression is abundant in prostate cancer, and that high-level ALCAM expression is associated with favorable tumor phenotype and good prognosis.

M. G. Bissell, MD, PhD, MPH

Cytogenetic Profile of Patients With Acute Myeloid Leukemia and Central Nervous System Disease
Shihadeh F, Reed V, Faderl S, et al (The Univ of Texas MD Anderson Cancer Ctr, Houston; et al)
Cancer 118:112-117, 2012

Background.—Acute myeloid leukemia (AML) infrequently involves the central nervous system (CNS). This study was undertaken in patients with AML to determine whether cytogenetic findings predict CNS involvement.

Methods.—The medical records of 1354 patients with AML who were treated at The University of Texas MD Anderson Cancer Center between January 2000 and December 2008 were reviewed. Forty patients (3%) had CNS involvement at time of presentation or disease recurrence, of whom 37 had conventional cytogenetics performed on bone marrow aspirate material. Demographics, treatment, and status at last follow-up were collected.

Results.—Eleven patients (30%) had a diploid karyotype, and 14 patients (38%) had complex cytogenetics. Only 5 of the 40 patients had CNS disease at diagnosis, and the remaining patients had CNS disease at relapse. Patients who developed CNS disease were younger $(P = .019)$, had a higher white blood cell (WBC) count at diagnosis $(P = .001)$, had higher lactate dehydrogenase level (LDH) levels $(P < .0001)$, and had higher percentages peripheral blast cells $(P = .024)$ at diagnosis compared with the rest of the population. In addition, patients with CNS disease had higher rates of chromosome 16 inversion $(P < .001)$, chromosome 11 abnormality $(P = .005)$, and trisomy 8 $(P = .02)$ and had a tendency toward complex cytogenetics $(P = .2)$ compared with the control group (patients who had AML with no CNS involvement).

Conclusions.—Patients with AML and CNS disease often had higher LDH levels and WBC counts at diagnosis, and they often presented with chromosome 16 inversion and chromosome 11 abnormalities. The current study indicated that the overall survival of patients with AML who had CNS involvement is poor.

▶ Conventional cytogenetic analysis of acute leukemia is a mainstay of the diagnostic workup. Cytogenetic results have been integrated, in part, into the current World Health Organization classification of both acute myeloid leukemia (AML) and acute lymphoblastic leukemia (ALL). Three important multicenter clinical trials by the Cancer and Leukemia Group B, the United Kingdom Medical Research Council, and the Southwest Oncology Group have demonstrated the importance of an initial cytogenetic assessment on the outcome of patients with AML. Cytogenetic abnormalities commonly are divided into 3 prognostic groups: favorable, intermediate, and unfavorable. Treatment regimens for patients with AML are tailored, in part, on the basis of risk factors, including cytogenetic data. The risk of central nervous system (CNS) involvement in patients with acute leukemia is far greater in patients with ALL than it is in patients with AML. Consequently, cytogenetic data have been correlated with CNS disease in patients with ALL, but there is a paucity of literature on patients with AML. Conversely, clinical presentation and treatment of CNS disease associated with AML have been addressed in the literature. In this study, the objective was to identify patients with AML who had CNS involvement and to review clinicopathologic findings with a particular emphasis on the results of conventional cytogenetic analysis. The authors also compared this group with a large group of patients who presented with AML without CNS involvement.

M. G. Bissell, MD, PhD, MPH

Predictive Parameters for a Diagnostic Bone Marrow Biopsy Specimen in the Work-Up of Fever of Unknown Origin
Ben-Baruch S, Canaani J, Braunstein R, et al (Tel Aviv Sourasky Med Ctr, Israel)
Mayo Clin Proc 87:136-142, 2012

Objective.—To determine the role of bone marrow biopsy (BMBX), performed in association with comprehensive blood and imaging tests, in the evaluation of patients with fever of unknown origin (FUO).

Patients and Methods.—We reviewed the medical records of 475 hospitalized patients who underwent BMBX in our medical center from January 1, 2005, to April 30, 2010. We identified 75 patients who fulfilled the accepted classic Petersdorf criteria for FUO. All patients underwent in-hospital investigation for fever, including chest and abdominal computed tomography.

Results.—In 20 patients (26.7%), BMBX established the final diagnosis. Sixteen patients had hematologic disorders, including 8 patients with non-Hodgkin lymphoma, 2 with acute leukemia, 1 with multiple myeloma, 1 with myelodysplastic syndrome, and 4 with myeloproliferative disorders. The remaining patients with diagnostic BMBX specimens had solid tumors (2 patients), granulomatous disease (1 patient), and hemophagocytic syndrome (1 patient). Multivariate analysis revealed the following as the significant positive predictive parameters for a diagnostic BMBX spec-imen: male sex (odds ratio [OR], 7.35; 95% confidence interval [CI], 1.19-45.45), clinical lymphadenopathy (OR, 21.98; 95% CI, 1.97-245.66), anemia (OR, 2.21; 95% CI, 1.28-3.80), and increased lactate dehydrogenase levels (OR, 1.003; 95% CI, 1.001-1.006).

Conclusion.—Bone marrow biopsy is still a useful ancillary procedure for establishing the diagnosis of FUO, particularly if used in the appropriate clin-ical setting. Clinical and laboratory parameters associated with hematologic disease are predictive of a diagnostic BMBX specimen in patients with FUO.

▶ Even in the current era of widespread use of advanced medical technologies, the investigation of fever of unknown origin (FUO) still remains a major diagnostic challenge for many physicians. The working definition of FUO is: an illness of more than 3 weeks' duration, accompanied by a temperature greater than 38.3°C on several occasions, the cause of which was uncertain after 1 week of in-hospital investigation. Diagnosing FUO is difficult for both patients and physicians because the spectrum of diseases causing FUO is wide and includes numerous conditions entailing many noninvasive and invasive diagnostic procedures. The use of bone marrow biopsy (BMBX) has been traditionally considered a second-line procedure to achieve diagnosis because of the invasive nature of the procedure. Nevertheless, BMBX was shown in earlier studies to be a useful but limited adjunct to the clinical workup of FUO. These reported studies were mostly undertaken in patients with human immunodeficiency virus infection and in those suspected of having mycobacterial disease. A recent study conducted in hospitalized patients identified anemia and thrombocytopenia as positive predictors for a diagnostic BMBX specimen. However, the exact role for BMBX in the evaluation of patients who have already undergone extensive blood tests and computed tomography of the chest and abdomen has not yet been defined. The authors present the diagnostic yield of BMBX in the evaluation of 75 patients with prolonged fever who were admitted to a tertiary medical center. The results identify simple clinical and laboratory parameters as predictive indicators that increase the diagnostic yield of BMBX in the modern investigation of FUO. Implementing these predictive laboratory findings may aid in optimal selection of patients best suited for BMBX as part of the clinical workup of patients with FUO.

M. G. Bissell, MD, PhD, MPH

Early Cytogenetic and Molecular Response During First-Line Treatment of Chronic Myeloid Leukemia in Chronic Phase: Long-Term Implications
Quintás-Cardama A, Cortes JE, Kantarjian HM (The Univ of Texas MD Anderson Cancer Ctr Houston)
Cancer 117:5261-5270, 2011

Chronic myeloid leukemia (CML) depends on the kinase activity of the BCR-ABL1 fusion protein. This dependency has led to the development of BCR-ABL1 inhibitors, such as imatinib, dasatinib, and nilotinib, which have proved to be highly efficacious treatments for CML. The European

LeukemiaNet guidelines have established the importance of achieving a certain depth of response at different time points during imatinib therapy for patients with newly diagnosed CML in chronic phase. Patients who achieve a complete cytogenetic response by 12 months or a major molecular response by 18 months are classified as optimal responders and deemed to have excellent long-term outcomes. Conversely, failing to achieve such milestones is associated with an increased risk of worse long-term outcomes, such as loss of response, disease progression, or death. With ongoing treatment, patients not in complete cytogenetic response face a decreasing probability of ever achieving a complete cytogenetic response or major molecular response and increasing risk of disease progression. Available data therefore support treatment recommendations based on achieving defined levels of response within a specified duration of treatment. Recent data have shown that dasatinib and nilotinib used as frontline CML therapy result in higher response rates that are achieved at earlier time points compared with standard-dose imatinib therapy. Future analyses will need to determine whether these higher rates of deep and fast responses translate into improved long-term survival.

▶ Chronic myeloid leukemia (CML) is a malignant hematologic disorder in which clonal expansion of leukemic stem cells depends on constitutive expression of the BCR-ABL1 oncoprotein. BCR-ABL1 is a fusion protein encoded in most patients by the Philadelphia chromosome, formed by reciprocal translocations between chromosomes 9 and 22. Almost 10 years ago, CML therapy was radically changed by the introduction of imatinib (formerly STI571), a BCR-ABL1—targeting tyrosine kinase inhibitor. Imatinib 400 mg once daily became rapidly established as the preferred first-line therapy for patients with newly diagnosed CML in chronic phase after showing superior efficacy and safety compared with interferon-ex plus cytarabine, the previous standard of care. With ongoing treatment, patients not in complete cytogenetic response face a decreasing probability of ever achieving a complete cytogenetic response or major molecular response and an increasing risk of disease progression. Available data therefore support treatment recommendations based on achieving defined levels of response within a specified duration of treatment. Recent data have shown that dasatinib and nilotinib used as frontline CML therapy result in higher response rates that are achieved at earlier time points compared with standard-dose imatinib therapy. Future analyses will need to determine whether these higher rates of deep and fast responses translate into improved long-term survival.

M. G. Bissell, MD, PhD, MPH

Detection of Leukemic Lymphoblasts in CSF Is Instrument-Dependent
Huppmann AR, Rheingold SR, Bailey LC, et al (The Children's Hosp of Philadelphia, PA)
Am J Clin Pathol 137:795-799, 2012

Staging and monitoring of pediatric acute lymphoblastic leukemia (ALL) includes examination of the cerebrospinal fluid (CSF). At our institution, we noted an increased incidence of low-level leukemic blasts in CSF samples from patients with ALL. This increase coincided with a conversion from the Shandon CytoSpin 4 (Thermo Fisher Scientific, Waltham, MA) to the Wescor Cytopro Rotor AC-060 (Wescor, Logan, UT). This study directly compared these 2 machines using patient samples and known concentrations of cultured leukemia cells. With patient samples, the Wescor Cytopro led to a 5- to 9-fold increase in the number of cells on a slide compared with the Shandon CytoSpin; furthermore, leukemic blasts were detected only with the Wescor Cytopro in 2 cases. Similar findings were observed using cultured leukemia cells. Thus, the detection of blasts in CSF is highly instrument-dependent. The newer, more sensitive cytocentrifuge machines identify blasts that were previously missed by older machines, but the clinical significance remains under investigation (Fig 2).

▶ The 5-year survival rate of pediatric patients with acute lymphoblastic leukemia (ALL) has increased from 54.1% in the 1975–1977 period to 85.1% in the 1999–2005 period because of numerous treatment advances. Despite this progress, approximately 1 in 5 patients will have a recurrence of ALL, including some as isolated central nervous system (CNS) relapses. High cerebrospinal fluid (CSF) blast count at initial diagnosis (CNS 3, cell count > 5 white blood cells [WBCs]/μL with blasts present) is correlated with a poorer prognosis. However, the prognostic significance of a lower blast count in the CSF (CNS 2a, cell count < 5 WBCs/μL, < 10 red blood cells/μL, and blasts identifiable on cytocentrifuged samples) is unclear, with varying implications reported among different studies. In either case, initial successful therapy includes the clearance of blasts from the CSF. In present-day Children's Oncology Group and international

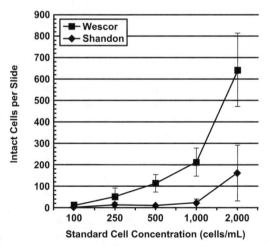

FIGURE 2.—The mean number of cells counted per slide (y-axis) plotted against input number of K562 cells in 1 mL of RPMI (x-axis) for the Wescor Cytopro Rotor AC-060 vs the Shandon CytoSpin 4. Each sample was done in quintuplicate. Error bars indicate the standard deviation. (Reprinted from Huppmann AR, Rheingold SR, Bailey LC, et al. Detection of leukemic lymphoblasts in CSF is instrument-dependent. *Am J Clin Pathol.* 2012;137:795-799, with permission from American Society for Clinical Pathology.)

cooperative trials, the CSF cell count and cytocentrifuge data are obtained with each administration of intrathecal chemotherapy. CSF with CNS 3 findings represent ALL CNS relapse, and patients with these findings are eligible for ALL relapse trials with intensified systemic and focused CNS therapy. Some cooperative groups also define a subset of patients as having an event if there are 2 episodes of CNS 2 findings (ideally blasts are confirmed by immunophenotyping) during a 4-week interval, but patients with these findings are not currently eligible for relapse trials until they have a diagnosis of CNS 3. At The Children's Hospital of Philadelphia, the authors noted an apparent increased incidence of CSF with CNS 2a findings during the last 3 years. This increase coincided with the introduction of a new cytocentrifuge machine in their pathology laboratory (Fig 2). In this report, they describe a causal relationship between the new cytocentrifuge machine and the increased incidence of CNS 2a disease, indicating that the detection of blasts in the CSF is highly instrument dependent.

M. G. Bissell, MD, PhD, MPH

Translational Applications of Flow Cytometry in Clinical Practice
Jaye DL, Bray RA, Gebel HM, et al (Emory Univ, Atlanta, GA)
J Immunol 188:4715-4719, 2012

Flow cytometry has evolved over the past 30 y from a niche laboratory technique to a routine tool used by clinical pathologists and immunologists for diagnosis and monitoring of patients with cancer and immune deficiencies. Identification of novel patterns of expressed Ags has led to the recognition of cancers with unique pathophysiologies and treatment strategies. FACS had permitted the isolation of tumor-free populations of hematopoietic stem cells for cancer patients undergoing stem cell transplantation. Adaptation of flow cytometry to the analysis of multiplex arrays of fluorescent beads that selectively capture proteins and specific DNA sequences has produced highly sensitive and rapid methods for high through-put analysis of cytokines, Abs, and HLA genotypes. Automated data analysis has contributed to the development of a "cytomics" field that integrates cellular physiology, genomics, and proteomics. In this article, we review the impact of the flow cytometer in these areas of medical practice (Fig 2, Table1).

▶ Flow cytometry began as *microfluorimetry* in the 1960s as an analytic technique to measure the properties of individual cells in a fluid stream following illumination with a laser. The basic operation of a flow cytometer involves breaking the fluid stream into a series of small droplets, segregating individual cells into a minority of the formed droplets and quickly interrogating the light properties of individual droplets following laser illumination. Droplets containing single cells could be electrostatically charged and separated from the majority of the cells in the fluid stream by deflecting the droplets into collection tubes during their flight in air using charged deflector plates. The harnessing of

Number of publications per year

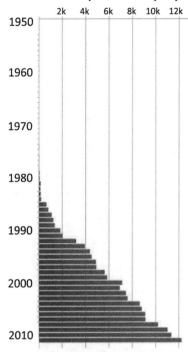

*(1953) The Coulter Principle. Invention of A method of counting cells suspended in A fluid

*(1965) Van Dilla at Los Alamos Labs invents the cell sorter.

*(1969) Gohde develops the first fluorescent flow cytometer; Van Dilla et al use cell microfluorimetry to measure cell properties

*(1972) Herzenberg and his team at Stanford Invent fluorescence activated cell sorting (FACS)

*(1975) Kohler and Millstein produce monoclonal antibodies in hybridomas

*(1979) Reinherz separate subsets of T cells using monoclonal antibodies

*Early 1980's, high speed flow cytometry used to sort chromosomes for the Human Genome Project.

*(1985) The same year the HIV/AIDS pandemic announced, new techniques for assessing cell morphology using two parameters of light scatter were developed by Smart et al.

*(2002) New fluorescent dyes with narrow excitations and emission wavelength bands

FIGURE 2.—Milestones in flow cytometry. Key events in the development of flow cytometry are shown in a vertical timeline (*left panel*), with the number of publications/y identified in http://apps.webofknowledge.com listing "microfluorimetry or flow cytometry" as key words (*right panel*). (Reprinted from Jaye DL, Bray RA, Gebel HM, et al. Translational applications of flow cytometry in clinical practice. *J Immunol.* 2012;188:4715-4719, with permission from The American Association of Immunologists, Inc.)

mAbs that specifically bound to cell surface markers and the discovery of a variety of fluorescent dyes with narrow excitation and emission spectra allowed the application of this technology to basic immunology research, clinical immunology diagnostics, and cell selection for preclinical models and clinical trials of transplanting phenotypically defined cell subsets. The timeline for the technical milestones of flow cytometry is shown in Fig 2, with the introduction of clinical applications of flow cytometry shown in Table 1. This review highlights the emerging clinical applications of flow cytometry and describes the unique bioinformatics issues that must be addressed when large list-mode files containing data on 6 or more parameters from millions of analyzed cells are generated from clinical samples.

M. G. Bissell, MD, PhD, MPH

TABLE 1.—Summary of Clinical Applications of Flow Cytometry

Clinical Situation	Cell/Analyte of Interest	Patient Specimen Types	Period of Clinical Use
Cancer	Diagnosis of hematolymphoid cancers (mostly leukemias/lymphomas)	Cancer cells	Blood, bone marrow, various tissues	Early 1980s
	Determine cell DNA content for prognosis (e.g. childhood lymphoblastic leukemia)	Cancer cells	Blood, bone marrow	Late 1980s
	Monitoring of hematolymphoid cancers after therapy	Residual cancer cells	Blood, bone marrow	Early 1990s
Immunologic diseases	Diagnosis and monitoring of HIV/AIDS	CD4$^+$ andCD8$^+$ T cell subsets	Blood	Early 1980s
	Diagnosis of primary immunodeficiencies	B cells, T cells, and T cell subsets	Blood, lymphoid tissues	Late 1980s
Cell therapy and transplantation	Determine adequacy of hematopoietic stem cell grafts (bone marrow transplantation) to repopulate bone marrow	CD34$^+$ stem cells	Stem cell graft	Early 1990s
	Risk assessment for graft rejection of solid organs and graft-versus-host disease after hematopoietic stem cell transplantation	Abs to HLA proteins HLA genotype genomic DNA	Recipient's serum Donor's blood cells	Early 2000s Middle 2000s

Prognostic Impact of Discordant Results From Cytogenetics and Flow Cytometry in Patients With Acute Myeloid Leukemia Undergoing Hematopoietic Cell Transplantation

Fang M, Storer B, Wood B, et al (Fred Hutchinson Cancer Res Ctr, Seattle, WA; Seattle Cancer Care Alliance, WA)
Cancer 118:2411-2419, 2012

Background.—Cytogenetics and multicolor flow cytometry (MFC) are useful tools for monitoring outcome of treatment in acute myeloid leukemia (AML). However, no data are available regarding the meaning of results when the 2 tests do not agree.

Methods.—The authors of this report analyzed 1464 pairs of concurrent cytogenetics and flow results from 424 patients, before and after hematopoietic cell transplantation, and compared the prognostic impact of discordant and concordant results.

Results.—Informative discordant results were observed in 22% of patients. Compared with patients who had double-negative test results, either positive result had a significant impact on overall survival and relapse-free survival. The hazard ratios with either positive cytogenetic results or positive MFC results pretransplantation were 3.1 ($P = .009$) and 2.5 ($P = .0008$), respectively, for reduced overall survival and 2.7 ($P = .01$) and 4.1 ($P < .0001$), respectively, for decreased recurrence-free survival. Similar findings were obtained post-transplantation. Molecular cytogenetics, ie, fluorescence in situ hybridization (FISH), added value to the evaluation of discordant cases.

Conclusions.—The detection of residual AML by either cytogenetics or flow cytometry in patients who underwent hematopoietic cell transplantation predicted early relapse and shortened survival (Fig 1).

▶ Cytogenetics and immunophenotyping by flow cytometry are part of the standard evaluation of newly diagnosed acute myeloid leukemia (AML), and both techniques are also used to monitor results of therapy. Most of the available information about the utility of these techniques to monitor therapeutic response comes from their application after conventional chemotherapy. In that setting, for patients in morphologic complete remission, abnormal cytogenetics predict significantly shorter disease-free survival (DFS) and overall survival. However, because of limited sensitivity, the estimated false-negative rate for conventional cytogenetics as an indicator of minimal residual disease (MRD) is approximately 50%; in addition, almost 50% of all patients with AML are cytogenetically normal at diagnosis. Molecular cytogenetics with interphase fluorescence in situ hybridization (FISH) has greater sensitivity for the detection of specific chromosome abnormalities, especially for patients with poor chromosome morphology or low or no yield of metaphase cells. Flow cytometric methods for MRD detection rely on the degree of immunophenotypic deviation of abnormal populations from normal hematopoietic maturation and, hence, have a variable. The advent of high-level multicolor flow cytometry analysis (MFC) allows for the routine detection of up to 10 simultaneous fluorochromes and offers theoretical improvements

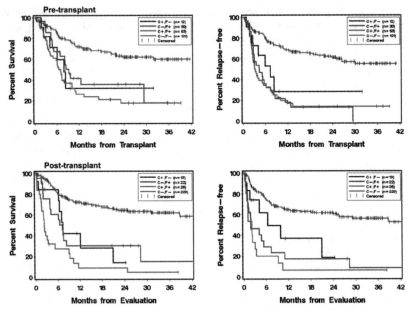

FIGURE 1.—These Kaplan-Meier plots illustrate (*Left*) overall survival and (*Right*) relapse-free survival according to test results obtained (*Top*) pretransplantation and (*Bottom*) post-transplantation. The analysis was based on the last test result for the pretransplantation window (days −60 to −1) and the first test result for the post-transplantation window (Days 1 to 100). C+/F− indicates the patients who had abnormal cytogenetic (C) results (including fluorescence in situ hybridization results) but normal flow cytometry (F) results. C−/F+ indicates the patients who had normal cytogenetic results but abnormal flow cytometry results. C+/F+ indicates those who had both abnormal cytogenetic and flow cytometry results. C−/F− indicates those who had normal cytogenetic results and normal flow cytometry results. (Reprinted from Fang M, Storer B, Wood B, et al. Prognostic impact of discordant results from cytogenetics and flow cytometry in patients with acute myeloid leukemia undergoing hematopoietic cell transplantation. *Cancer.* 2012;118:2411-2419, Copyright 2012 American Cancer Society. This material is reproduced with permission of Wiley-Liss, Inc., a subsidiary of John Wiley & Sons, Inc.)

in both specificity and sensitivity. Because a direct comparison of cytogenetic and MFC results for their prognostic impact in the transplantation setting is not available, especially when the analyses yield discordant results, the authors conducted a comparison of 1464 paired results from 424 patients with AML who underwent allogeneic HCT. In this study, a positive result from either cytogenetic or MFC testing was associated with a poor prognosis of similar degree. FISH analysis provided further prognostic information in both concordant and discordant cases. These data demonstrated that MRD either pre-transplantation or post-transplantation, regardless of how it is measured, predicts outcome.

M. G. Bissell, MD, PhD, MPH

A prospective randomised study of a rotary powered device (OnControl) for bone marrow aspiration and biopsy
Swords RT, Anguita J, Higgins RA, et al (Univ of Texas Health Science Ctr, San Antonio; University Hospital Gregorio Marañón, Madrid, Spain; et al)
J Clin Pathol 64:809-813, 2011

Introduction.—Bone marrow aspiration and biopsy is an invasive procedure associated with morbidity and mortality risk. We compared a powered bone marrow aspiration and biopsy device to the traditional method by relatively assessing pain scores, procedure times, biopsy capture rates, quality of material retrieved, and safety and operator satisfaction.

Methods.—Two large academic medical centres participated in this trial. Patients were randomised to have procedures carried out using the powered system or the manual technique. A visual analogue scale pain score was recorded immediately following skin puncture and once again at the end of the procedure for each patient. Procedure time was measured from skin puncture to core specimen acquisition. Pathologic assessment of 30 randomised samples was carried out. Operator satisfaction with devices was measured on a scale of 0–10, with 10 as the highest rating.

Results.—Five operators from two sites enrolled 50 patients (powered, n = 25; manual, n = 25). Groups were evenly matched, with no significant differences in the means for age, weight and height. The powered system was superior to the manual system with respect to patient perceived pain from needle insertion (2.6 ± 2.0 vs 4.1 ± 2.5, $p = 0.022$) and procedural time (100.0 ± 72.8 s vs 224.1 ± 79.0 s, $p < 0.001$). Overall pain scores at the end of both procedures were comparable (3.2 ± 2.2 vs 3.8 ± 3.0, $p = 0.438$). No complications were observed in either arm of the study. Blinded pathologic analysis of the specimens retrieved revealed that cores obtained using the powered system were longer and wider than those obtained using the manual technique (25.4 ± 12.3 mm^2 vs 11.9 ± 5.6 mm^2, $p = 0.001$). For marrow aspiration, no difference was seen between groups for clot/particle spicules or smear spicules. Operator assessment favoured the use of the powered device.

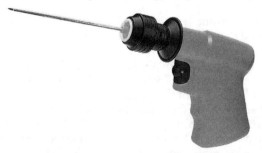

FIGURE 1.—The OnControl bone marrow aspiration and biopsy system (Vidacare Corporation). (Reprinted from Swords RT, Anguita J, Higgins RA, et al. A prospective randomised study of a rotary powered device (OnControl) for bone marrow aspiration and biopsy. *J Clin Pathol.* 2011;64:809-813, with permission from the BMJ Publishing Group Ltd.)

Conclusions.—Results of this trial suggest that the use of a powered bone marrow biopsy device significantly reduces needle insertion pain and procedural time when compared to a manual technique. The superior size and overall quality of core specimens retrieved by the powered device provides more material for pathologic evaluation, thereby increasing diagnostic yield and reducing the need for repeat procedures (Fig 1).

▶ Bone marrow aspiration procedures are valuable for differential cell counts and individual cell morphology evaluation. For the evaluation of marrow cellularity, determination of the number of megakaryocytes, and the detection of lymphoma, granulomas, and metastatic carcinomas, the trephine biopsy procedure is preferred. Percutaneous needle core biopsy has historically been a safe and effective mode for diagnosing bone and soft-tissue lesions. The trend in modern diagnostic medicine is for minimally invasive procedures to be selected for use where possible. Studies have reported duration of needle insertion as the sole predictor of patient pain during the procedure, with needle insertion lasting an average of 7 minutes. A validation study of a new powered aspiration system (Fig 1) showed a substantially faster time for needle insertion into the medullary space of the iliac crest, with a mean insertion time of 5 seconds, but this was limited in that only aspirates and not cores could be obtained. The authors reported both the preclinical and early clinical results of a newer powered device with the ability to obtain both aspirate and core biopsy of good quality. However, that sample size was limited, and no comparison was made to traditional trephine biopsy devices. The purpose of this study was to substantiate the findings from previous studies of the powered aspiration and biopsy system as well as a randomized comparison with the standard nonpowered technique.

M. G. Bissell, MD, PhD, MPH

Mutations of *NOTCH1* are an independent predictor of survival in chronic lymphocytic leukemia

Rossi D, Rasi S, Fabbri G, et al (Amedeo Avogadro Univ of Eastern Piedmont, Novara, Italy; Columbia Univ, NY; et al)
Blood 119:521-529, 2012

Analysis of the chronic lymphocytic leukemia (CLL) coding genome has recently disclosed that the *NOTCH1* proto-oncogene is recurrently mutated at CLL presentation. Here, we assessed the prognostic role of *NOTCH1* mutations in CLL. Two series of newly diagnosed CLL were used as training (n = 309) and validation (n = 230) cohorts. *NOTCH1* mutations occurred in 11.0% and 11.3% CLL of the training and validation series, respectively. In the training series, *NOTCH1* mutations led to a 3.77-fold increase in the hazard of death and to shorter overall survival (OS; $P < .001$). Multivariate analysis selected *NOTCH1* mutations as an independent predictor of OS after controlling for confounding clinical and biologic variables. The independent prognostic value of *NOTCH1* mutations was externally confirmed in the validation series. The poor prognosis conferred by *NOTCH1* mutations was attributable, at least in part, to shorter treatment-free survival and higher risk of Richter transformation. Although *NOTCH1* mutated patients were devoid of *TP53* disruption in more than 90% cases in both training and validation series, the OS predicted by *NOTCH1* mutations was similar to that of *TP53* mutated/deleted CLL. *NOTCH1* mutations are an independent predictor of CLL OS, tend to be mutually exclusive with *TP53* abnormalities, and identify cases with a dismal prognosis.

▶ Chronic lymphocytic leukemia (CLL) is a lymphoproliferative disorder and the most common form of leukemia in the Western world. It is a heterogeneous disease with an extremely variable course ranging from very indolent, with a nearly normal life expectancy, to rapidly progressive, leading to death and occasionally undergoing transformation to aggressive lymphoma, known as *Richter syndrome* (RS). Therefore, treatment can be challenging, and management of CLL has become increasingly personalized for each patient depending on certain clinical and biological features. Several prognostic markers have been discovered, including a disruption in *TP53*, which is identified in a fraction of high-risk CLL patients. However, not all high-risk CLL patients have a *TP53* disruption, and other cancer genes are implicated in the aggressive cases. One of the genes recently discovered in high-risk CLL patients is the *NOTCH1* proto-oncogene. Activating mutations of *NOTCH1* are seen in approximately 10% of CLL patients at the time of diagnosis, and this frequency increases as the disease progresses and may be associated with an unfavorable outcome. However, many of the clinical implications of *NOTCH1* mutations in CLL remain to be evaluated, including the distribution among CLL patients with *TP53* disruption and unmutated immunoglobulin heave variable (IGHV) genes. The authors of this study evaluated for *NOTCH1* mutations in untreated CLL patients and correlated the data with molecular results for *TP53* and *IGHV* mutations. They also looked at prognostic parameters to evaluate if *NOTCH1* predicts overall survival in CLL patients. The results of this study show the robustness and reproducibility of *NOTCH1* as a risk factor. This discovery opens the door for possible targeted therapy for *NOTCH1* inhibitors, which are currently under development in other clinical contexts.

H. Signorelli, DO

Cytogenetic Profile of Patients With Acute Myeloid Leukemia and Central Nervous System Disease

Shihadeh F, Reed V, Faderl S, et al (The Univ of Texas MD Anderson Cancer Ctr, Houston; et al)
Cancer 118:112-117, 2012

Background.—Acute myeloid leukemia (AML) infrequently involves the central nervous system (CNS). This study was undertaken in patients with AML to determine whether cytogenetic findings predict CNS involvement.

Methods.—The medical records of 1354 patients with AML who were treated at The University of Texas MD Anderson Cancer Center between January 2000 and December 2008 were reviewed. Forty patients (3%) had

CNS involvement at time of presentation or disease recurrence, of whom 37 had conventional cytogenetics performed on bone marrow aspirate material. Demographics, treatment, and status at last follow-up were collected.

Results.—Eleven patients (30%) had a diploid karyotype, and 14 patients (38%) had complex cytogenetics. Only 5 of the 40 patients had CNS disease at diagnosis, and the remaining patients had CNS disease at relapse. Patients who developed CNS disease were younger ($P = .019$), had a higher white blood cell (WBC) count at diagnosis ($P = .001$), had higher lactate dehydrogenase level (LDH) levels ($P < .0001$), and had higher percentages peripheral blast cells ($P = .024$) at diagnosis compared with the rest of the population. In addition, patients with CNS disease had higher rates of chromosome 16 inversion ($P < .001$), chromosome 11 abnormality ($P = .005$), and trisomy 8 ($P = .02$) and had a tendency toward complex cytogenetics ($P = .2$) compared with the control group (patients who had AML with no CNS involvement).

Conclusions.—Patients with AML and CNS disease often had higher LDH levels and WBC counts at diagnosis, and they often presented with chromosome 16 inversion and chromosome 11 abnormalities. The current study indicated that the overall survival of patients with AML who had CNS involvement is poor.

▶ Conventional cytogenetic analysis is an important predictive and prognostic factor for many hematologic malignancies including acute myeloid leukemia (AML). Cytogenetic results have been incorporated into the current World Health Organization classification system and are usually divided into 3 prognostic groups: favorable, intermediate, and unfavorable. It is uncommon for patients with AML to have central nervous system (CNS) involvement and therefore there is a paucity of literature correlating cytogenetic data and prognosis for this patient subgroup. The authors of this study reviewed clinicopathologic findings, emphasizing conventional cytogenetic results in AML patients with CNS disease. They also correlated the cytogenetic findings with the risk of CNS disease as well as with overall survival in patients with AML. The results presented in this paper have also been observed by other investigators, such as a higher frequency of chromosome 16 inversion in AML patients with CNS disease as compared with AML patients without CNS disease. However, because of the low number of patients with CNS disease, it is not possible to make therapeutic recommendations based on cytogenetic analysis for this group. Only additional monitoring for CNS disease in patients with high-risk cytogenetics can be recommended at this time. More studies will need to be completed to confirm the findings from this article.

H. Signorelli, DO

Expanding Nilotinib Access in Clinical Trials (ENACT): An Open-Label, Multicenter Study of Oral Nilotinib in Adult Patients With Imatinib-Resistant or Imatinib-Intolerant Philadelphia Chromosome-Positive Chronic Myeloid Leukemia in the Chronic Phase

Nicolini FE, Turkina A, Shen Z-X, et al (Edouard Herriot Hosp, Lyon, France; Hematology Res Ctr, Moscow, Russia; Hematology Dept, Shanghai Ruijin Hosp, China; et al)
Cancer 118:118-126, 2012

Background.—Nilotinib is a selective, potent BCR-ABL inhibitor. Previous studies demonstrated the efficacy and safety of nilotinib in Philadelphia chromosome-positive chronic myeloid leukemia patients in chronic phase (CML-CP) or accelerated phase who failed prior imatinib.

Methods.—This expanded access trial further characterized the safety of nilotinib 400 mg twice daily in patients with CML-CP (N = 1422).

Results.—In this large, heavily pretreated population, nilotinib demonstrated significant efficacy, with complete hematologic response and complete cytogenetic response achieved in 43% and 34% of patients, respectively. Responses were rapid, mostly occurring within 6 months, and were higher in patients with suboptimal response to imatinib, with 75% and 50% achieving major cytogenetic response and complete cytogenetic response, respectively. At 18 months, the progression-free survival rate was 80%. Most patients achieved planned dosing of 400 mg twice daily and maintained the dose >12 months. Nonhematologic adverse events (AEs) were mostly mild to moderate and included rash (28%), headache (25%), and nausea (17%). Grade 3 or 4 thrombocytopenia (22%), neutropenia (14%), and anemia (3%) were low and managed by dose reduction or brief interruption. Grade 3 or 4 elevations in serum bilirubin and lipase occurred in 4% and 7% of patients, respectively. The incidence of newly occurring AEs decreased over time. Of patients who experienced a dose reduction because of AEs and attempted a re-escalation, 87% successfully achieved re-escalation to the full dose.

Conclusions.—This large study confirms that nilotinib was well tolerated and that grade 3 or 4 AEs occurred infrequently and were manageable through transient dose interruptions.

▶ Chronic myeloid leukemia (CML) is a clonal myeloproliferative disorder characterized by the Philadelphia chromosome (Ph), which is formed by a reciprocal translocation1 involving chromosomes 9 and 22 and results in an oncogenic fusion gene encoding the BCR-ABL protein, having a constitutively active tyrosine kinase domain. Imatinib mesylate is a BCR-ABL inhibitor that is currently the standard of care for CML patients. Nilotinib was developed to be a more potent inhibitor of BCR-ABL than imatinib and work against imatinib-resistant mutant forms. Clinical trials have demonstrated that nilotinib is safe and efficacious in patients with imatinib-resistant or imatinib-intolerant CML in chronic phase (CML-CP) and CML in accelerated phase (CML-AP). Nilotinib is generally well-tolerated with infrequent adverse events and has gained approval for imatinib-resistant, imatinib-intolerant, and newly diagnosed CML treatment in many countries including the United States, Japan, and those in the European Union. The authors of this article discuss the findings of the Expanding Nilotinib Access in Clinical Trials (ENACT) multinational trial. The ENACT trial is the largest safety trial of any tyrosine kinase inhibitor in CML to date and evaluated the safety of nilotinib in a large patient population that closely resembles clinical practice. However, the patients in this trial, as in any clinical trial, were typically younger than seen in the real clinical setting, and data in older patients would be necessary. The trial provided efficacy data as well as guidance to physicians on how to manage CML patients on nilotinib.

H. Signorelli, DO

A Double-Blind, Placebo-Controlled Trial of Ruxolitinib for Myelofibrosis
Verstovsek S, Mesa RA, Gotlib J, et al (Univ of Texas MD Anderson Cancer Ctr, Houston; Mayo Clinic, Scottsdale, AZ; Stanford Cancer Inst, CA; et al)
N Engl J Med 366:799-807, 2012

Background.—Ruxolitinib, a selective inhibitor of Janus kinase (JAK) 1 and 2, has clinically significant activity in myelofibrosis.

Methods.—In this double-blind trial, we randomly assigned patients with intermediate-2 or high-risk myelofibrosis to twice-daily oral ruxolitinib (155 patients) or placebo (154 patients). The primary end point was the proportion of patients with a reduction in spleen volume of 35% or more at 24 weeks, assessed by means of magnetic resonance imaging. Secondary end points included the durability of response, changes in symptom burden (assessed by the total symptom score), and overall survival.

Results.—The primary end point was reached in 41.9% of patients in the ruxolitinib group as compared with 0.7% in the placebo group ($P < 0.001$). A reduction in spleen volume was maintained in patients who received ruxolitinib; 67.0% of the patients with a response had the response for 48 weeks or more. There was an improvement of 50% or more in the total symptom score at 24 weeks in 45.9% of patients who received ruxolitinib as compared with 5.3% of patients who received placebo ($P < 0.001$). Thirteen deaths occurred in the ruxolitinib group as compared with 24 deaths in the placebo group (hazard ratio, 0.50; 95% confidence interval, 0.25 to 0.98; $P = 0.04$). The rate of discontinuation of the study drug because of adverse events was 11.0% in the ruxolitinib group and 10.6% in the placebo group. Among patients who received ruxolitinib, anemia and thrombocytopenia were the most common adverse events, but they rarely led to discontinuation of the drug (in one patient for each event). Two patients had transformation to acute myeloid leukemia; both were in the ruxolitinib group.

Conclusions.—Ruxolitinib, as compared with placebo, provided significant clinical benefits in patients with myelofibrosis by reducing spleen size, ameliorating debilitating myelofibrosis-related symptoms, and improving overall survival. These benefits came at the cost of more frequent anemia and thrombocytopenia in the early part of the treatment period. (Funded by Incyte; COMFORT-I ClinicalTrials.gov number, NCT00952289.)

▶ Myelofibrosis is a myeloproliferative disorder characterized by abnormal blood counts, splenomegaly, and debilitating symptoms. Survival ranges from approximately 2 to 11 years, depending on defined prognostic factors. The pathogenesis of the disease is related to activation of the intracellular Janus kinase (JAK)-signal transducer and activator of transcription (STAT) pathway. However, only 50% of patients with primary myelofibrosis have the gain-of-function mutation in the gene encoding JAK2 (JAK2 V617F), but other mechanisms of activation are known to dysregulate this pathway in patients with myelofibrosis. Ruxolitinib has been shown to be a potent inhibitor of JAK1 and JAK2 and has shown promising results in clinical trials in reducing splenomegaly and improving myelofibrosis-related symptoms regardless of their JAK2 V617F mutational status. The authors of this article evaluated the efficacy and safety of ruxolitinib in a randomized, double-blind, placebo-controlled trial in patients with intermediate-2 or high-risk myelofibrosis. The study showed that ruxolitinib therapy was significantly more effective than placebo with a number of significant clinical benefits, including improved overall survival (Fig 3 in the original article). Adverse events that were more common in patients receiving ruxolitinib included anemia and thrombocytopenia, but these events were manageable in this study. Additional findings in this study included a return to baseline symptoms in patients who had interruption of ruxolitinib therapy.

H. Signorelli, DO

CD117 Expression Is a Sensitive but Nonspecific Predictor of *FLT3* Mutation in T Acute Lymphoblastic Leukemia and T/Myeloid Acute Leukemia

Hoehn D, Medeiros LJ, Chen SS, et al (The Univ of Texas MD Anderson Cancer Ctr, Houston)
Am J Clin Pathol 137:213-219, 2012

Others have suggested that CD117, or an immunophenotypic profile including CD117, can serve as surrogate for *FLT3* mutation in T acute lymphoblastic leukemia (ALL), thereby guiding targeted therapy. We report the results of flow cytometry immunophenotypic analysis in 42 cases of T-ALL and T/myeloid acute leukemia also assessed for *FLT3* mutation. CD117 was expressed in 21 (50%), and *FLT3* was mutated in 8 cases (19%; 1 T-ALL and 7 T/myeloid). *FLT3*-mutated cases were terminal deoxynucleotidyl transferase (TdT)+/CD2+ (7/8), cytoplasmic CD3+/CD5+ (5/8), CD7+/CD13+/CD15+(4/6), CD33+ (4/8), CD34+, and CD117+ (bright). Cytochemistry showed myeloperoxidase-positive cells in all T/myeloid acute leukemias (3%-50%). We conclude that *FLT3* mutation is rare in T-ALL, and its presence supports T/myeloid lineage. CD117 expression alone is sensitive but not specific for *FLT3* mutation. The immunophenotypic profile of TdT, CD7, CD13, CD34, and CD117 (bright) is helpful for predicting *FLT3* mutation, with a sensitivity of 100% and specificity of 94%.

▶ The FMS-like tyrosine kinase 3 (FLT3) gene is a class III tyrosine kinase, and its product is expressed in early hematopoietic progenitors. Mutations of FLT3 cause constitutive activation and occur mainly in cases of acute myeloid leukemia (AML) or myelodysplastic syndrome (MDS). It is associated with a high risk for relapse and an overall poor outcome. Acute lymphoblastic leukemia (ALL) cases rarely have FLT3 mutations. The cases of ALL with FLT3 mutations are usually B-cell neoplasms and associated with mixed lineage leukemia (MLL) gene alterations. Targeted therapy against FLIT3 has been developed and is currently being evaluated for clinical use. Mutations of FLT3 in T-ALL cases are uncommon with reports of less than 5% of cases, and therefore testing for FLT3 mutations is low yield. It would be helpful to stratify which T-ALL cases get worked up for FLT3 mutations and reduce unnecessary molecular testing. Prior studies have shown that cases of T-ALL with FLT3 mutations also show CD117 expression. The suggested immunoprofile that predicts the presence FLT3 mutations in T-ALL cases was CD2+/CD7+/CD13+/CD34+/CD62L+/CD117+/surface CD3-/CD4-/CD5-/CD8-. The authors of this study evaluate the usefulness of CD117 expression and this immunophenotype to predict FLT3 mutations in their institutions T-ALL and T/AML cases.

H. Signorelli, DO

Prognostic Value of *MYC* Rearrangement in Cases of B-cell Lymphoma, Unclassifiable, With Features Intermediate Between Diffuse Large B-Cell Lymphoma and Burkitt Lymphoma
Lin P, Dickason TJ, Fayad LE, et al (The Univ of Texas MD Anderson Cancer Ctr, Houston)
Cancer 118:1566-1573, 2012

Background.—B-cell lymphoma, Unclassifiable with features intermediate between diffuse large B-cell lymphoma (DLBCL) and Burkitt lymphoma, for convenience referred to here as unclassifiable B-cell lymphoma, is a category in the 2008 World Health Organization system used for a group of histologically aggressive neoplasms that are difficult to classify definitively. Currently, there is no established standard therapy for these neoplasms.

Methods.—The authors assessed *MYC* status and correlated it with treatment response and outcome in a group of 52 patients with unclassifiable B-cell lymphoma treated with either a standard DLBCL regimen (R-CHOP [rituximab plus cyclophosphamide, doxorubicin, vincristine, and prednisolone-related therapy]) or more intensive regimens, such as R-hyper-CVAD (rituximab plus hyperfractionated cyclophosphamide, vincristine, doxorubicin, and dexamethasone alternating with high-dose methotrexate and cytarabine). The regimens were selected by the treating clinicians based on the overall clinical and pathological findings.

Results.—Thirty (58%) unclassifiable B-cell lymphomas had *MYC* abnormalities (*MYC*⁺) including 27 with rearrangement, 2 with amplification, and 1 with both. The *MYC*⁺ and *MYC*⁻ groups were similar in their age distribution and International Prognostic Index scores. Progression-free survival of patients with *MYC*⁺ unclassifiable B-cell lymphoma treated initially with R-CHOP was significantly worse than patients treated with R-hyper-CVAD (*P* = .0358). In contrast, for the *MYC*⁻ unclassifiable B-cell lymphoma group, some patients responded to R-CHOP, and others were refractory to R-hyper-CVAD.

Conclusions.—*MYC* aberrations are common in unclassifiable B-cell lymphoma. The presence of *MYC* aberrations identifies a patient subset that requires more aggressive therapy than R-CHOP. In contrast, *MYC*⁻ unclassifiable B-cell lymphoma patients responded variably to either R-CHOP or aggressive therapy, and the latter showed no survival advantage.

▶ High-grade B-cell lymphoma is often times difficult to classify as either diffuse large B-cell lymphoma (DLBCL) or Burkitt lymphoma (BL). This is because there are aggressive cases that are considered borderline with overlapping features. The 2008 World Health Organization (WHO) classification recognized this gray zone and proposed the category, "B-cell lymphoma, unclassifiable with features intermediate between diffuse large B-cell lymphoma and Burkitt lymphoma." These unclassifiable B-cell lymphoma cases also show molecular profiles that are intermediate between DLBCL and BL with a subset showing MYC gene rearrangements. MYC gene rearrangements are characteristic of BL and are only found in 5% to 10% of cases of conventional DLBCL. Although this new category in the 2008 WHO classification has been helpful for classifying the neoplasm, it does not address the issue of therapy for the patient which has been difficult to address. The authors of this study looked at cases of lymphomas at their institution that met criteria for unclassifiable B-cell lymphoma and assessed the MYC status to predict therapeutic response and prognosis.

H. Signorelli, DO

Blockade of Lymphocyte Chemotaxis in Visceral Graft-Versus-Host Disease

Reshef R, Luger SM, Hexner EO, et al (Univ of Pennsylvania, Philadelphia)
N Engl J Med 367:135-145, 2012

Background.—Graft-versus-host disease (GVHD) is a major barrier to successful allogeneic hematopoietic stem-cell transplantation (HSCT). The chemokine receptor CCR5 appears to play a role in alloreactivity. We tested whether CCR5 blockade would be safe and limit GVHD in humans.

Methods.—We tested the in vitro effect of the CCR5 antagonist maraviroc on lymphocyte function and chemotaxis. We then enrolled 38 high-risk patients in a single-group phase 1 and 2 study of reduced-intensity allogeneic HSCT that combined maraviroc with standard GVHD prophylaxis.

Results.—Maraviroc inhibited CCR5 internalization and lymphocyte chemotaxis in vitro without impairing T-cell function or formation of hematopoietic-cell colonies. In 35 patients who could be evaluated, the cumulative incidence rate ($\pm$ SE) of grade II to IV acute GVHD was low at 14.7 $\pm$ 6.2% on day 100 and 23.6 $\pm$ 7.4% on day 180. Acute liver and gut GVHD were not observed before day 100 and remained uncommon before day 180, resulting in a low cumulative incidence of grade III or IV GVHD on day 180 (5.9 $\pm$ 4.1%). The 1-year rate of death that was not preceded by disease relapse was 11.7 $\pm$ 5.6% without excessive rates of relapse or infection. Serum from patients receiving maraviroc prevented CCR5 internalization by CCL5 and blocked T-cell chemotaxis in vitro, providing evidence of antichemotactic activity.

Conclusions.—In this study, inhibition of lymphocyte trafficking was a specific and potentially effective new strategy to prevent visceral acute GVHD. (Funded by Pfizer and others; ClinicalTrials.gov number, NCT00948753.)

▶ Acute graft-versus-host disease (GVHD) is a serious complication of hemato-poietic stem cell transplantation with a high morbidity and mortality rate. It occurs in 30% to 50% of patients who receive a human leukocyte antigen—matched transplant from a related donor and 50% to 70% of those who receive a transplant from an unrelated donor. GVHD is most likely caused by the proliferation of viable donor T-lymphocytes that recognize the recipient as foreign, resulting in the damage of host tissue. One of the key steps in the pathogenesis of GVHD involves the T cells interacting with host antigen-presenting cells that lead to the release of cytokines and chemokines, which contribute to the tissue damage. A mediator that is thought to play an important role is chemokine receptor 5 (CCR5) involved in lymphocyte recruitment. Some studies have even shown that certain mutations in the CCR5 region have proved to be protective against GVHD. Maraviroc is one of the first drugs developed that antagonizes the class of CCR5. It works through a noncompetitive and slowly reversible mechanism. Currently, maraviroc is used for antiretroviral therapy in patients with human immunodeficiency virus. The authors in this study proposed that the drug may also have a role on chemo-taxis and alloreactivity and inhibition of GVHD. They analyzed both in vitro and in vivo results of maraviroc on T-cell chemotaxis and on preventing GVHD.

H. Signorelli, DO

Predicting Survival of Patients With Hypocellular Myelodysplastic Syndrome: Development of a Disease-Specific Prognostic Score System
Tong W-G, Quintás-Cardama A, Kadia T, et al (The Univ of Texas MD Anderson Cancer Ctr, Houston)
Cancer 118:4462-4470, 2012

Background.—Although most patients with myelodysplastic syndrome (MDS) exhibit bone marrow hypercellularity, a subset of them present with a hypocellular bone marrow. Specific factors associated with poor prognosis have not been investigated in patients with hypocellular MDS.

Methods.—The authors studied a cohort of 253 patients with hypocellular MDS diagnosed at The University of Texas MD Anderson Cancer Center between 1993 and 2007 and a cohort of 1725 patients with hyper-/normocellular MDS diagnosed during the same time period.

Results.—Patients with hypocellular MDS presented more frequently with thrombocytopenia ($P < .019$), neutropenia ($P < .001$), low serum β-2 microglobulin ($P < .001$), increased transfusion dependency ($P < .001$), and intermediate-2/high-risk disease (57% vs 42%, $P = .02$) compared with patients with hyper-/normocellular MDS. However, no difference in overall survival was observed between the 2 groups ($P = .28$). Multivariate analysis identified poor performance status (Eastern Cooperative Oncology Group ≥ 2), low hemoglobin (<10 g/dL), unfavorable cytogenetics ($-7/7q$ or complex), increased bone marrow blasts ($\geq 5\%$), and high serum lactate dehydrogenase (>600 IU/L) as adverse independent factors for survival.

Conclusions.—A new prognostic model based on these factors was built that segregated patients into 3 distinct risk categories independent of International Prognostic Scoring System (IPSS) score. This model is independent from the IPSS, further refines IPSS-based prognostication, and may be used to develop risk-adapted therapeutic approaches for patients with hypocellular MDS.

▶ Myelodysplastic syndrome (MDS) is a clonal bone marrow disorder characterized by dysplastic changes in hematopoietic progenitors, ineffective hematopoiesis, peripheral blood cytopenias, and an increased risk of transformation to acute myeloid leukemia (AML). MDS patients typically show a hypercellular or normocellular marrow, reflecting excessive bone marrow apoptosis and rapid cellular proliferation. MDS is extremely heterogeneous and therefore multiple prognostic modules are available including: the French-American-British (FAB), World Health Organization, and International Prognostic Scoring System (IPSS) classification system. The IPSS classifies patients based on the percentage of bone marrow blasts, conventional cytogenetics, and number of cytopenias and is the one most often employed in clinical practice today. However, the original IPSS classification system has some limitations because it was designed for patients with newly diagnosed, untreated MDS, and excluded those patients with secondary MDS and chronic myelomonocytic leukemia. The IPSS also fails to identify patients with low-risk MDS with a poor prognosis who may benefit from earlier treatment. Therefore, multiple new prognostic models are currently under review. Although the new models apply to a greater variety of MDS patients and take into account treatment, they do not address patients with hypocellular MDS, which accounts for 10% to 20% and appears to have a different prognosis. Patients with hypocellular MDS have been difficult to differentiate from aplastic anemia and it is not currently recognized as a distinct entity. The authors of this study wanted to get a better understanding of hypocellular MDS by analyzing patients with hypocellular MDS and looking at the associations between disease characteristics and survival. They compared these results with a cohort of patients with hyper-/normocellular MDS. Their results support the notion that hypocellular

MDS and hyper-/normocellular MDS are 2 biologically distinct entities with independent prognostic factors that can be used to devise a new prognostic model. Although this new model proved to be useful in hypocellular MDS patients at this institution, it would need to be validated with a larger cohort of patients to confirm its utility. Other, newer prognostic models that have been proposed were not evaluated in this study.

H. Signorelli, DO

Eltrombopag and Improved Hematopoiesis in Refractory Aplastic Anemia

Olnes MJ, Scheinberg P, Calvo KR, et al (Natl Heart, Lung, and Blood Inst, Bethesda, MD; Mark O. Hatfield Clinical Res Ctr, Bethesda, MD)
N Engl J Med 367:11-19, 2012

Background.—Severe aplastic anemia, which is characterized by immune-mediated bone marrow hypoplasia and pancytopenia, can be treated effectively with immunosuppressive therapy or allogeneic transplantation. One third of patients have disease that is refractory to immunosuppression, with persistent, severe cytopenia and a profound deficit in hematopoietic stem cells and progenitor cells. Thrombopoietin may increase the number of hematopoietic stem cells and progenitor cells.

Methods.—We conducted a phase 2 study involving patients with aplastic anemia that was refractory to immunosuppression to determine whether the oral thrombopoietin mimetic eltrombopag (Promacta) can improve blood counts. Twenty-five patients received eltrombopag at a dose of 50 mg, which could be increased, as needed, to a maximum dose of 150 mg daily, for a total of 12 weeks. Primary end points were clinically significant changes in blood counts or transfusion independence. Patients with a response continued to receive eltrombopag.

Results.—Eleven of 25 patients (44%) had a hematologic response in at least one lineage at 12 weeks, with minimal toxic effects. Nine patients no longer needed platelet transfusions (median increase in platelet count, 44 000 per cubic millimeter). Six patients had improved hemoglobin levels (median increase, 4.4 g per deciliter); 3 of them were previously dependent on red-cell transfusions and no longer needed transfusions. Nine patients had increased neutrophil counts (median increase, 1350 per cubic millimeter). Serial bone marrow biopsies showed normalization of trilineage hematopoiesis in patients who had a response, without increased fibrosis. Monitoring of immune function revealed no consistent changes.

Conclusions.—Treatment with eltrombopag was associated with multilineage clinical responses in some patients with refractory severe aplastic anemia. (Funded by the National Heart, Lung, and Blood Institute; ClinicalTrials.gov number, NCT00922883.)

▶ Aplastic anemia is an acquired bone marrow disease resulting from an autoimmune attack on the bone marrow, which is characterized by trilineage marrow hypoplasia and a paucity of hematopoietic stem and progenitor cells. Standard treatment for aplastic anemia includes immunosuppressive therapy with hematologic responses seen in approximately two-thirds of patients. The patients who fail to respond to immunosuppressive therapy may undergo allogenic hematopoietic stem-cell transplantation if a suitable donor is available. Patients who are refractory to these treatment options are left without other options besides supportive treatment. The c-MPL molecule expressed on megakaryocytes binds with thrombopoietin, which potentiates platelet maturation and release. This molecule is also thought to reside on the surface of hematopoietic stem cells and progenitor cells, suggesting that these cells may be stimulated by thrombopoietin and result in a hematologic response in patients with treatment-refractory aplastic anemia. The authors of this study looked at eltrombopag, an oral thrombopoietin drug that promotes megakaryopoiesis and release of platelets, in patients with aplastic anemia that did not respond to standard immunosuppressive treatment. Patients in this study received increasing doses of eltrombopag and were monitored for hematologic responses and toxic effects. Bone marrow features were also followed.

H. Signorelli, DO

Molecular and Clinicopathologic Characterization of AML With Isolated Trisomy 4
Bains A, Lu G, Yao H, et al (Univ of Texas MD Anderson Cancer Ctr, Houston)
Am J Clin Pathol 137:387-394, 2012

Acute myeloid leukemia (AML) with isolated trisomy 4 is rare. Associations with *KIT* mutations on chromosome 4q12 have been documented. The clinicopathologic features and mutational status of *KIT*, *FLT3*, *NPM1*, *CEBPA*, and *RAS* were assessed in 13 AML cases with isolated trisomy 4. There were 9 men and 4 women with a median age of 54 years. Median blast count was 84% (range, 24%−93%). Morphologic features varied across five 2008 World Health Organization categories. *FLT3* (5/10) and *NPM1* (4/10) mutations were observed at a frequency similar to normal−karyotype AML cases. *KIT* D816V (1/10), *RAS* (1/11; *NRAS*), and *CEBPA* (0/9) mutations were rare or absent. In 11 of 13 cases, complete remission was achieved. In 8 cases, relapse occurred, with median relapse−free survival of 11 months. Median overall survival was 28 months. AML with isolated trisomy 4 is rare and associated with high bone marrow blast counts and an intermediate to poor prognosis. *KIT* mutations are uncommon.

▶ Patients with acute myeloid leukemia (AML) who harbor an isolated trisomy 4 are extremely rare. In a literature review of multiple references between 1986 and 2009, only 83 cases were reported. Therefore, it has been difficult to approximate the frequency of this abnormality among AML patients. The exact pathogenesis of trisomy 4 in AML is unknown, but some studies have shown either an association with KIT gene mutations or propose that the KIT gene is overexpressed because of its location on chromosome 4. The authors of this study looked at the largest reported series of patients to date with AML and isolated trisomy 4. They determined the frequency within their institution along with the clinicopathologic and molecular characteristics. A total of 20 029 cases of AML as the primary diagnosis were reviewed that resulted in 13 different cases of trisomy 4 as the sole cytogenetic abnormality. They also looked at the mutational status of a number of genes that were often mutated in AML, including KIT, FLT3, NPM1, CEBPA, and RAS in these cases. Although this cytogenetic event is extremely rare, most of these patients were shown to have similar characteristics, including a high bone marrow blast count along with an intermediate to poor prognosis. The mutational frequencies analyzed were not shown to be increased in the patients of this series compared with those seen in AML cases with a normal karyotype.

H. Signorelli, DO

The Role of CD19 and CD27 in the Diagnosis of Multiple Myeloma by Flow Cytometry: A New Statistical Model

Cannizzo E, Carulli G, Del Vecchio L, et al (Univ of Pisa, Italy; Federico II Univ, Naples, Italy; et al)
Am J Clin Pathol 137:377-386, 2012

We have developed a new statistical diagnostic model that examines the correlation between immunophenotype and clonality as detected by flow cytometry (FC) and histology, defining the diagnostic role of FC in multiple myeloma (MM). The 192 bone marrow samples from patients and control subjects were studied for routine diagnostic analysis of MM; a minimum of 100 plasma cells (PCs) were analyzed for each patient sample. A direct 7- or 8-color method was applied to study the immunophenotype of PCs, utilizing a FACSCanto II (BD Biosciences, San Jose, CA). Samples were labeled with fluorochrome–conjugated monoclonal antibodies (AmCyan, Pac Blue, fluorescein isothiocyanate, phycoerythrin [PE], PECy7, peridinin-chlorophyll protein, allophycocyanin [APC], and APC-Cy7) to the following antigens: CD138, CD81, CD200, CD221, CD45, CD38, CD28, CD19, CD27, CD117, CD38, CD33, CD20, CD56, CD10, and immunoglobulin κ and λ light chains. Among all antigens tested, CD19 and CD27, when applied to our model, resulted in optimal concordance with histology. This model defines the effective diagnostic role FC could have in MM and in the detection of minimal residual disease.

▶ Multiple myeloma (MM) is a clonal B-cell neoplasm characterized by infiltration of the bone marrow by malignant plasma cells (PCs), often with evidence of lytic lesions, monoclonal protein, and end-organ damage. Currently the diagnosis is based on histologically evaluating the morphologic features, analysis of M-protein, immunophenotyping, cytogenetics, and the labeling-index proliferation of plasma cells. Flow cytometry (FC) has an important role not only in immunophenotyping but also in guiding clinicians with prognosis and treatment. Some of the potential advantages of FC include: the ability to discern between normal and malignant plasma cells, defining the risk of progression from monoclonal gammopathy of unknown significance, detecting prognostic markers, and evaluating for minimal residual disease (MRD). A disadvantage of FC has been in providing quantitative information in MM. However, there are difficulties with the methodology of FC, leading to discrepancies over the exact immunophenotype of plasma cells and the associated clinical significance. This study used 8-color FC analysis to define a new diagnostic approach between the histology and phenotype in MM. Additionally, the study addressed the important role FC may have in detecting MRD in MM, especially when levels of PCs are below 5%.

H. Signorelli, DO

20 Transfusion Medicine and Coagulation

Whole blood gene expression analyses in patients with single versus recurrent venous thromboembolism
Lewis DA, Stashenko GJ, Akay OM, et al (Duke Univ Med Ctr, Durham, NC)
Thromb Res 128:536-540, 2011

Introduction.—Venous thromboembolism may recur in up to 30% of patients with a spontaneous venous thromboembolism after a standard course of anticoagulation. Identification of patients at risk for recurrent venous thromboembolism would facilitate decisions concerning the duration of anticoagulant therapy.

Objectives.—In this exploratory study, we investigated whether whole blood gene expression data could distinguish subjects with single venous thromboembolism from subjects with recurrent venous thromboembolism.

Methods.—40 adults with venous thromboembolism (23 with single event and 17 with recurrent events) on warfarin were recruited. Individuals with antiphospholipid syndrome or cancer were excluded. Plasma and serum samples were collected for biomarker testing, and PAXgene tubes were used to collect whole blood RNA samples.

Results.—D-dimer levels were significantly higher in patients with recurrent venous thromboembolism, but P-selectin and thrombin-antithrombin complex levels were similar in the two groups. Comparison of gene expression data from the two groups provided us with a 50 gene probe model that distinguished these two groups with good receiver operating curve characteristics (AUC 0.75). This model includes genes involved in mRNA splicing and platelet aggregation. Pathway analysis between subjects with single and recurrent venous thromboembolism revealed that the Akt pathway was upregulated in the recurrent venous thromboembolism group compared to the single venous thromboembolism group.

Conclusions.—In this exploratory study, gene expression profiles of whole blood appear to be a useful strategy to distinguish subjects with single venous thromboembolism from those with recurrent venous thromboembolism. Prospective studies with additional patients are needed to validate these results (Fig 1).

▶ Venous thromboembolism (VTE) is a major cause of morbidity and mortality. Each year, approximately 350 000 to 600 000 individuals in the United States will

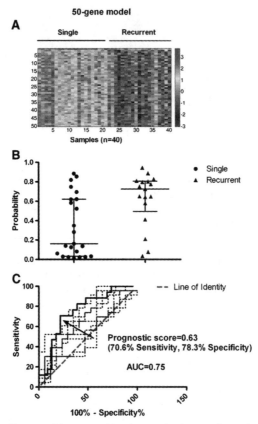

FIGURE 1.—Development of the gene model to distinguish subjects with a single VTE from those with recurrent VTE. (A) The heat map representing the expression of the 50 genes probes used to develop the metagenes model is shown with blue and red representing extremes of expression with visually apparent differences in gene expression. Samples from single VTE subjects are on the left (n = 23), and samples from subjects with recurrent VTE are on the right (n = 17). (B) Leave-one-out cross validation: a comparison of the individual and median (with interquartile range) estimated classification probability of recurrent VTE predicted by the 50 gene model is shown. (C) Leave-one-out cross validation: the ROC curve identifying the probability score of 0.63 as the optimal cut-point to be used to classify samples is shown (black solid line). The area under the curve (AUC) is 0.75. The ROC curves for the 10 random permutations are shown as dotted lines. For interpretation of the references to color in this figure legend, the reader is referred to web version of this article. (Reprinted from Lewis DA, Stashenko GJ, Akay OM, et al. Whole blood gene expression analyses in patients with single versus recurrent venous thromboembolism. *Thromb Res.* 2011;128:536-540, Copyright 2011, with permission from Elsevier.)

develop a VTE and up to 100 000 will die. Recurrent VTE develops within 8 years in as many as 30% of patients after stopping a standard course of anticoagulant therapy. This fact is consistent with a growing body of data suggesting that VTE is a chronic disease with acute exacerbations (manifested as recurrent thromboembolism). Inherited and acquired risk factors contribute to an individual's risk for VTE, but these factors are frequently inadequate at predicting who will develop an initial VTE or recurrent VTE. Current evidence suggests against evaluating most patients with spontaneous VTE for thrombophilia. As a consequence of this increased risk for recurrent VTE, many patients with VTE would benefit from a longer course of anticoagulant therapy. Furthermore, recent studies in subjects with VTE have shown that an extended course of anticoagulation will decrease the risk of recurrence. Determining which patients are at highest risk for recurrence is therefore clearly a vital health concern. D-dimer has been studied extensively for its effectiveness as a biomarker for recurrent VTE. In this exploratory study, the authors used a heterogeneous group of patients with VTE to investigate whether selected biomarkers, including D-dimer, P-selectin, thrombin-antithrombin complex levels, and/or gene expression information could be used distinguish patients with a single VTE event from patients with recurrent VTE (Fig 1).

M. G. Bissell, MD, PhD, MPH

A Diagnosis of Heparin-Induced Thrombocytopenia with Combined Clinical and Laboratory Methods in Cardiothoracic Surgical Intensive Care Unit Patients

Demma LJ, Winkler AM, Levy JH (Emory Univ, Atlanta, GA)
Anesth Analg 113:697-702, 2011

Background.—Diagnosing postoperative heparin-induced thrombocytopenia (HIT) in cardiothoracic surgical patients is complicated because of the profound thrombocytopenia that occurs with cardiopulmonary bypass (CPB). CPB predisposes patients to develop a frequent incidence of antibodies directed against platelet factor 4 (PF4)/heparin complexes and HIT. The sensitivity of readily available antibody immunoassays is high, but specificity is quite low. The use of both a clinical probability score and rapid laboratory immunoassay has been shown to increase specificity, which is of particular importance in the CPB setting. Prompt diagnosis is crucial because cessation of heparin and treatment with alternative anticoagulation can reduce the risk of thromboembolic events.

Methods.—We retrospectively reviewed records from cardiothoracic surgical patients whose serum was tested with both the serotonin release assay (SRA) and the PF4/heparin immunoassay from January 2007 through December 2010. We assigned a high, intermediate, or low clinical "4Ts" probability score that quantifies thrombocytopenia, timing of platelet decrease, and thrombotic complications in each patient. We then compared the clinical score and the PF4/heparin immunoassay against the "gold standard" diagnostic test, the SRA.

Results.—The sensitivity and specificity for PF4/heparin optical density > 0.40 were 100% and 26%, respectively. Sensitivity and specificity for the diagnosis of HIT with a combination of PF4/heparin optical density > 0.40 and high/intermediate 4Ts score were 100% and 70%, respectively. The negative predictive value was 100% for low 4Ts score.

Conclusions.—We demonstrated that the use of the 4Ts clinical score combined with the PF4/heparin immunoassay for HIT diagnosis increases the sensitivity and specificity of HIT testing compared with the PF4/heparin

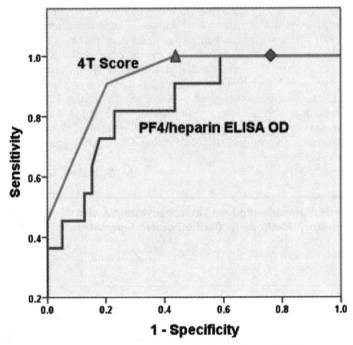

FIGURE 2.—Receiver operating characteristic curve for platelet factor 4 (PF4)/heparin enzyme-linked immunosorbent assay (ELISA), area under the curve = 0.84 (95% confidence interval [CI], 0.71−0.97), and "4Ts" clinical probability score, area under the curve = 0.92 (95% CI, 0.85−1.00). The data point for the PF4/heparin ELISA cutoff value of 0.40 is shown with a diamond (sensitivity 100%, 1 − specificity 74%); data point for 4Ts clinical probability score cutoff value of ≥4 is shown with a triangle (sensitivity 100%, 1 − specificity 44%). OD = optical density. (Reprinted from Demma LJ, Winkler AM, Levy JH. A diagnosis of heparin-induced thrombocytopenia with combined clinical and laboratory methods in cardiothoracic surgical intensive care unit patients. Anesth Analg. 2011;113:697-702, with permission from International Anesthesia Research Society.)

immunoassay alone. Furthermore, with an intermediate 4Ts score and positive PF4/heparin antibody test, a confirmatory platelet activation assay such as the SRA is necessary. Physicians treating patients after cardiothoracic surgery should recognize the need for an antibody test and confirmation with a platelet activation assay with even moderate clinical probability of HIT (Fig 2).

▶ The purpose of this study was to assess clinical and laboratory diagnosis of heparin-induced thrombocytopenia (HIT) in a cohort of patients after cardiothoracic surgery. Because alternative anticoagulation therapy with direct thrombin inhibitors is expensive and has increased potential for bleeding complications, a prompt and accurate diagnosis of HIT is important and often challenging in this patient population. Therefore, the authors examined the relationships among the magnitude of anti−platelet factor 4 (PF4)/heparin antibodies, the 4Ts clinical score (The 4Ts in the 4Ts score are: [1] thrombocytopenia with a platelet count decrease greater than 50% and platelet nadir greater than 20 000/microL; [2]

timing of platelet decrease with clear onset between days 5 and 10 or platelet decrease less than 1 day [prior heparin exposure within 30 days]; [3] new thrombosis [confirmed]; and [4] no likely alternative cause for thrombocytopenia), and confirmed HIT cases as defined by a positive serotonin release assay (SRA). They analyzed the sensitivity and specificity of the PF4/heparin optical density (OD) alone and the combined use of 4Ts score and PF4/heparin OD (Fig 2). To improve early detection of HIT in this clinical setting, they also evaluated additional factors that may be associated with HIT, including baseline preoperative platelet count, magnitude of thrombocytopenia, and on- versus off-pump surgery.

M. G. Bissell, MD, PhD, MPH

Report of the first nationally implemented clinical routine screening for fetal *RHD* in D– pregnant women to ascertain the requirement for antenatal RhD prophylaxis

Clausen FB, Christiansen M, Steffensen R, et al (Copenhagen Univ Hosp, Denmark; Aarhus Univ Hosp, Skejby, Denmark; Aalborg Hosp, Denmark; et al)
Transfusion 52:752-758, 2012

Background.—A combination of antenatal and postnatal RhD prophylaxis is more effective in reducing D immunization in pregnancy than postnatal RhD prophylaxis alone. Based on the result from antenatal screening for the fetal *RHD* gene, antenatal RhD prophylaxis in Denmark is given only to those D– women who carry a D+ fetus. We present an evaluation of the first national clinical application of antenatal *RHD* screening.

Study Design and Methods.—In each of the five Danish health care regions, blood samples were drawn from D– women in Gestational Week 25. DNA was extracted from the maternal plasma and analyzed for the presence of the *RHD* gene by real-time polymerase chain reaction targeting two *RHD* exons. Prediction of the fetal RhD type was compared with serologic typing of the newborn in 2312 pregnancies, which represented the first 6 months of routine analysis.

Results.—For the detection of fetal *RHD*, the sensitivity was 99.9%. The accuracy was 96.5%. The recommendation for unnecessary antenatal RhD prophylaxis for women carrying a D– fetus was correctly avoided in 862 cases (37.3%), while 39 women (1.7%) were recommended for antenatal RhD prophylaxis unnecessarily. Two *RHD*+ fetuses (0.087%) were not detected, and antenatal RhIG was not given.

Conclusion.—These data represent the first demonstration of the reliability of routine antenatal fetal *RHD* screening in D–, pregnant women to ascertain the requirement for antenatal RhD prophylaxis. Our findings should encourage the implementation of such screening programs worldwide, to reduce the unnecessary use of RhIG.

▶ Pregnancy-related immunization against the red blood cell D antigen is the major cause of hemolytic disease of the fetus and the newborn (HDFN), a condition marked by fetal anemia, hydrops fetalis, jaundice, kernicterus, and intrauterine death. Since the late 1960s, postnatal prophylactic treatment with Rh immune globulin has prevented maternal immunization with great efficacy and has reduced the incidence of HDFN in D-negative women who are carrying a D-positive fetus. Postnatal RhD prophylaxis has reduced the immunization risk from 16% to 2%. In the late 1970s, the combination of antenatal and postnatal RhD prophylaxis was then reported to reduce the immunization risk even further, and based on these promising results, antenatal prophylaxis was implemented in several countries. A national routine antenatal anti-D prophylaxis program was implemented on January 1, 2010, in Denmark. Antenatal RhD screening is performed by targeting specific exon sequences in the *RHD* gene in DNA extracted from maternal plasma obtained from a blood sample taken in gestational week 25. This screening is conducted in 5 different health care regions in Denmark, and each region employs its own method. The authors present an evaluation of the first 6 months of the antenatal RhD screening program in Denmark. This is the first national clinical application of noninvasive prenatal detection of fetal RhD to ascertain the requirement for antenatal RhD prophylaxis.

M. G. Bissell, MD, PhD, MPH

Is current serologic RhD typing of blood donors sufficient for avoiding immunization of recipients?
Krog GR, Clausen FB, Berkowicz A, et al (Copenhagen Univ Hosp, Denmark)
Transfusion 51:2278-2285, 2011

Background.—Avoiding immunization with clinically important antibodies is a primary objective in transfusion medicine. Therefore, it is central to identify the extent of D antigens that escape routine RhD typing of blood donors and to improve methodology if necessary.

Study Design and Methods.—We screened 5058 D− donors for the presence of the *RHD* gene, targeting Exons 5, 7, and 10 with real-time polymerase chain reaction. Samples that were positive in the screen test were investigated further by adsorption-elution, antibody consumption, flow cytometry, and sequencing of all *RHD* exons with intron-specific primers. Lookback was performed on all recipients of RBCs from *RHD*+ donors.

Results.—We found 13 *RHD*+ samples (0.26%). No variants or chimeras were found. Characterization of DNA revealed a novel *DEL* type (IVS2-2 A>G). In the lookback of the 136 transfusions with subsequent antibody follow-up, of which 13 were from *DEL* donors, one recipient developed anti-D. However, in this case, a competing and more likely cause of immunization was the concurrent transfusion of D+ platelets. Eleven recipients were immunized with 13 antibodies different from anti-D, of which five were anti-K.

Conclusion.—In our laboratory, serologic RhD typing was safe. We detected all D variants and only missed *DEL* types. In assessing the immunization risk we included a *DEL* donor, found previous to this study, that did immunize a recipient with anti-D. We conclude that inadvertent immunization with D antigens in our setting was rare and in the order of 1.4 in 100,000 D− transfusions.

▶ Serologic typing of the RhD blood group can be challenging in donors with weak, minute, or partial D antigens or in chimeric or mosaic donors. To avoid immunization with clinically important antibodies, it is central to identify the extent of D antigens that escape routine RhD typing of blood donors and to improve methodology if necessary. In the last decade, there have been many findings of blood donors with D antigens among the D− blood donor population, detected by molecular analysis: detection of the *RHD* gene in the D− pool, followed by more sensitive serologic methods. Sensitive serologic analysis was performed to discriminate between blood donors with and without D antigens. Molecular analysis was performed to determine and discover new RHD alleles. There have been long-standing discussions of whether RHD genotyping should be implemented in routine RhD typing of blood donors. The aim of this study was to investigate the sufficiency of current serologic determination of the RhD blood group of blood donors in Denmark. The authors analyzed genomic DNA from 4932 D− donors for the presence of the *RHD* gene. Thirteen samples were found RHD + and were further examined by enlarged serologic methods, and extremely weak D antigens were found in 2 samples. They described a novel *DEL* type with a splice site mutation, IVS2-2 A > G. Lookback was done on all donations from the 13 RHD + donors, and from these observations they estimated the risk of immunization.

M. G. Bissell, MD, PhD, MPH

In vitro properties of platelets stored in three different additive solutions
Tynngård N, Trinks M, Berlin G (Linköping Univ, Sweden; County Council of Östergötland, Linköping, Sweden)
Transfusion 52:1003-1009, 2012

Background.—New platelet (PLT) additive solutions (PASs) contain compounds that might improve the storage conditions for PLTs. This study compares the in vitro function, including hemostatic properties (clot formation and elasticity), of PLTs in T-Sol, Composol, or SSP+ during storage for 5 days.

Study Design and Methods.—Fifteen buffy coats were pooled and divided into three parts. PLT concentrates (PCs) with 30% plasma and 70% PAS (T-Sol, Composol, or SSP+) were prepared (n = 10). Swirling, PLT count, blood gases, metabolic variables, PLT activation markers, and coagulation by free oscillation rheometry (FOR) were analyzed on Days 1 and 5.

Results.—Swirling was well preserved and pH acceptable (6.4-7.4) during storage for all PASs. Storage of PLTs in T-Sol led to a decrease in PLT count whereas the number of PLTs was unchanged in Composol or SSP+ PCs. PLTs in T-Sol showed higher glucose metabolism than PLTs in Composol or in SSP+. At the end of storage PLTs in T-Sol had higher spontaneous activation and lower ability to respond to an agonist than PLTs in Composol or SSP+. PLTs in all the PASs had a similar ability to promote clot formation and clot elasticity.

Conclusion.—Storage of PLTs in Composol or in SSP+ improved the quality of PCs in terms of better maintained PLT count, lower glucose metabolism, lower spontaneous activation, and improved response to a PLT agonist compared to PLTs in T-Sol. PLTs stored in the various PASs had similar hemostatic properties. These findings make Composol and SSP+ interesting alternatives as PASs.

▶ Platelets (PLTs) are stored in plasma or in a combination of plasma and a PLT additive solution (PAS). The use of a PAS reduces the risk for transfusion complications caused by substances present in the plasma, leads to more plasma available for other purposes, and could improve the storage conditions. PLTs can generate adenosine triphosphate through the tricarboxylic acid cycle or glycolysis. Glycolysis results in formation of lactate and hydrogen ions that need to be buffered by bicarbonate in plasma. Consumption of bicarbonate results in a pH decrease, which might result in a loss of PLT viability. Thus, a good storage solution should keep glycolysis at a minimal level as well as preserve PLT function. Composol (PAS-D) and SSP+ (PAS-E) are newly developed PASs containing substances that have been suggested to be beneficial for preservation of PLT function, but there is a lack of studies showing the hemostatic properties of PLTs stored in these new PASs. In this study, the authors compare the quality of buffy coat (BC)-derived PLTs stored in T-Sol (PAS-B), Composol, or SSP+. The quality was assessed by in vitro assays, including measurement of the hemostatic function by free oscillation rheometry.

M. G. Bissell, MD, PhD, MPH

Detection of bacterial contamination in prestorage culture-negative apheresis platelets on day of issue with the Pan Genera Detection test
Jacobs MR, the PGD Study Group (Case Western Reserve Univ and Univ Hosps Case Med Ctr, Cleveland, OH; et al)
Transfusion 51:2573-2582, 2011

Background.—Bacterial contamination is currently the most important infectious risk associated with transfusion of platelet (PLT) products. Prestorage culture has reduced but not eliminated this problem.

Study Design and Methods.—Eighteen hospitals studied the Pan Genera Detection (PGD) test, a rapid, lateral-flow immunoassay for the detection of Gram-positive and Gram-negative bacteria. The PGD test was performed on day of issue on apheresis PLTs released by collection centers as culture negative. Confirmatory bacterial culture was performed when PGD tests were repeatedly reactive, with three sites performing culture on all doses studied.

Results.—PGD tests on nine of 27,620 (1:3069, 95% confidence interval [CI] 1:6711 to 1:1617; or 326 per million, 95% CI 149-618 per million) apheresis PLT doses were repeatedly reactive and verified as bacterially contaminated by confirmatory culture. Bacterial species isolated included coagulase-negative staphylococci (n = 6), *Bacillus* sp. (n = 2), and *Enterococcus faecalis* (n = 1). The ages of these contaminated doses were Day 3 (n = 4), Day 4 (n = 2), and Day 5 (n = 3). Two contaminated doses with nonreactive PGD tests were detected among 10,424 doses at hospitals where concurrent culture was performed, and one other was identified via a transfusion reaction investigation. There were 142 PGD false positives (0.51%).

Conclusions.—The PGD test detected bacterial contamination in 1:3069 (9 of 27,620) doses released as negative by prestorage culture in PLTs as young as 3 days old. Three contaminated doses, two clinically insignificant, had nonreactive PGD tests, while 0.51% of tests were false positives. Application of this test on day of issue can interdict contaminated units and prevent transfusion reactions.

▶ The main factor associated with the failure of a culture to detect bacterial contamination near the time of collection is sampling error, which can occur if bacteria are not at a sufficient concentration in platelet (PLT) units to be consistently present in the culture sample. In view of the demonstrated limitations of prestorage culture methods to adequately detect bacterial contamination of PLTs, alternate assays have been pursued. In 2007, the Platelet Pan Genera Detection (PGD) test (Verax Biomedical, Inc, Worcester, MA), a qualitative, rapid, lateral-flow immunoassay for the detection of gram-positive and gram-negative bacteria, received Food and Drug Administration (FDA) clearance as an adjunct test for quality control (QC) testing of single-donor platelets when used in conjunction with another FDA-cleared QC test. The PGD test was subsequently also FDA cleared as a standalone QC test for the detection of bacterial contamination in pools of up to six random-donor PLTs, both leukoreduced and nonleukoreduced. The goal of this study was to determine if the PGD test could detect bacterial contamination in apheresis PLT units, previously released as culture negative by collection centers, at hospitals on the day of transfusion.

M. G. Bissell, MD, PhD, MPH

Normal range of mean platelet volume in healthy subjects: Insight from a large epidemiologic study

Demirin H, Ozhan H, Ucgun T, et al (Duzce Univ, Turkey)
Thromb Res 128:358-360, 2011

Aim.—Mean platelet volume (MPV) in the healthy population has not been studied before. Therefore, the aim of the study was to measure MPV in normal subjects in a large cohort of Turkish adults.

Methods.—A total of 2298 subjects with a mean age of 50 (age range 18 to 92) were interviewed. Subjects who had smoking habit, diabetes, hypertension, coronary artery disease, dyslipidemia, chronic obstructive pulmonary disease, cancer, chronic use of any drugs including antiplatelets, heavy drinkers, metabolic syndrome, ejection fraction < 55%, creatinine > 1.4 in men and > 1.1 in women, abnormal liver function tests and an abnormal TSH were excluded in a in a stepwise manner. Complete blood counts were done on the same day within 6 hours by a CELL-DYN 3700 SL analyzer (Abbott Diagnostics).

Results.—Three hundred twenty-six participants (204 females (63%) and 122 males (37%) with a mean age of 41 ± 16) constituted the final healthy cohort. Mean MPV of the cohort was 8.9 ± 1.4 fL. There was no significant difference among age groups regarding MPV.

Conclusion.—Ninety-five percent of the individuals had a MPV between 7.2 and 11.7 fL. A patient having a MPV beyond this range should be evaluated carefully especially for occlusive arterial diseases.

▶ Platelets play a pivotal role in atherothrombosis, the major cause of most unstable coronary syndromes. Activation of platelets at the site of vascular injury is the main pathogenesis of occlusive arterial disease. Platelets secrete and express a large number of substances that are crucial mediators of coagulation, inflammation, thrombosis, and atherosclerosis. The demonstrated ability of anti-platelet drugs to reduce cardiovascular events has reinforced the major role of platelets in the atherothrombotic process. Circulating platelets vary in both size and functional activity. Larger platelets are probably younger, more reactive, and produce more thrombogenic factors. Mean platelet volume (MPV) is an indicator of platelet activation, and it has been reported to increase in acute myocardial infarction and acute coronary syndromes. Increased MPV is also associated with higher mortality following myocardial infarction. Although measurement of MPV produces clinically useful information, it remains a research tool that is yet to be included in routine clinical decision making. Although analyzed in automated machines, MPV measurement is anticoagulant and time dependent. MPV increases over time as platelets swell in ethylenedia-minetetraacetic acid; therefore, optimal MPV measurement should be within 2 hours of venipuncture. In most of the investigations dealing with platelet reactivity, the mean MPV of patients was compared with that of the subjects who were admitted to the hospital but did not have that specific disease. These control groups were collected from the patients who were admitted to the hospitals and definitely did not contain healthy subjects, causing a bias and uncertainty about the interpretation and clinical utility of the results. The results of epidemiologic studies will supply important support to define the "real normal" range for that specific marker. Therefore, the aim of the current study was to measure reference intervals of MPV in a large cohort of Turkish adults.

M. G. Bissell, MD, PhD, MPH

Blood platelet biochemistry
Broos K, De Meyer SF, Feys HB, et al (IRF Life Sciences, Kortrijk, Belgium)
Thromb Res 129:245-249, 2012

Defects in platelet function or formation increase the risk for bleeding or thrombosis, which indicates the crucial role for platelets in maintaining

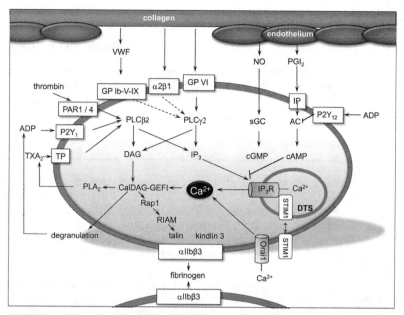

FIGURE 1.—Schematic overview of the main platelet receptors and effectors involved in platelet activation, amplification, aggregation and inhibition. (Reprinted from Broos K, De Meyer SF, Feys HB, et al. Blood platelet biochemistry. *Thromb Res.* 2012;129:245-249, Copyright 2012, with permission from Elsevier.)

haemostasis in normal life. Upon vascular injury, platelets instantly adhere to the exposed extracellular matrix which results in platelet activation and aggregation and the formation a haemostatic plug that stops bleeding. To prevent excessive platelet aggregate formation that eventually would occlude the vessels, this self-amplifying process nevertheless requires a tight control. This review intends to give a comprehensive overview of the currently established main mechanisms in platelet function (Fig 1).

▶ Defects in platelet function or formation increase the risk for bleeding or thrombosis, which indicates the crucial role for platelets in maintaining hemostasis in normal life. Although platelets are involved in different processes, such as triggering inflammation, fighting microbial infection, promoting tumor metastasis, and embryonic blood/lymphatic vessel separation, their principal function still remains stopping hemorrhage following vascular injury (Fig 1). Upon tissue trauma, platelets initially tether and roll over the exposed extracellular matrix, a process that eventually results in firm platelet adhesion and that triggers a signaling cascade mediated by tyrosine kinases and G-protein—coupled receptors, resulting in full platelet activation with concomitant granule release. Released effectors in turn recruit and activate additional platelets, next leading to platelet aggregation and the presentation of a procoagulant surface, promoting formation of a fibrin-rich hemostatic plug. Platelet activation, in addition, also triggers endothelial cells to locally synthesize and secrete molecules that limit thrombus formation.

M. G. Bissell, MD, PhD, MPH

A flow cytometric method for platelet counting in platelet concentrates
van der Meer PF, on behalf of the Biomedical Excellence for Safer Transfusion (BEST) Collaborative (Sanquin Blood Supply, Amsterdam, the Netherlands; et al)
Transfusion 52:173-180, 2012

Background.—The platelets (PLTs) in PLT concentrates are counted with hematology analyzers, but varying results among different hematology analyzers are observed, making comparisons very difficult. Due to the absence of red blood cells in PLT concentrates, the International Council for Standardization in Hematology (ICSH) reference method was modified to be used for PLT concentrates and validated in an international comparative study.

Study Design and Methods.—Five PLT samples were shipped to eight participating centers of the Biomedical Excellence for Safer Transfusion (BEST) Collaborative and counted on the same day. PLTs were stained with fluorescein isothiocyanate—labeled anti-CD41a in tubes (TruCount, BD Biosciences), measured on a flow cytometer, and analyzed with a uniform template. These samples were also counted on 15 hematology analyzers.

Results.—The ICSH method and newly developed BEST method yielded PLT counting results with less than 1% difference (not significant). The intercenter coefficient of variation (CV) of the BEST method was on average 6.3% versus 7.6% on average for hematology analyzers. The CV of individual hematology analyzers was on average 0.9%, which was considerably lower than for the flow cytometers with a mean of 3.7%.

Conclusion.—The BEST flow cytometric method has a smaller intercenter CV and a smaller center-to-center deviation from the group mean compared to hematology analyzers. Conversely, individual hematology analyzers are more precise than the flow cytometric method. Thus, the flow cytometric method provides a calibration tool to allow comparisons between centers, but there is no need to replace routine counting with hematology analyzers.

▶ Hematology analyzers are intended to count (patient) blood samples. Many blood centers use these analyzers to perform quality control on the blood components that they produce. However, the composition of the components differs from that of whole blood: for example, platelet (PLT) concentrates have a 5-fold higher PLT concentration compared with that of whole blood, while red blood cells are (almost) absent. Previous studies of the Biomedical Excellence for Safer Transfusion (BEST) Collaborative have shown that, when counting PLT concentrates, large differences in results are observed. In the previous study, at PLT concentrations relevant for blood centers, the deviation from the group mean could range from an underestimation of 35% to an overestimation of 16% compared with the mean value of all data combined (overall group mean), depending on the type of hematology analyzer. Within a group of analyzers of the same type, the deviation was much smaller, generally in the range of 5% to 10%. Because there was no concordance among the analyzers, a true PLT value could not be established. It was, therefore, necessary to develop a method to count PLTs in PLT concentrates that was independent from that of hematology analyzers. Several laboratories in the BEST Collaborative had separately developed a method to enumerate PLTs in PLT concentrates by flow cytometer. In the first exercise, 4 samples were analyzed by the in-house method of the respective centers as well as counted on hematology analyzers. The different staining and analysis protocols were compared, and critical steps were identified and further evaluated in 1 center. A uniform method was developed that consisted of a standardized dilution, staining, counting, and analysis protocol. The link of this BEST protocol to the official International Council for Standardization in Hematology reference method was established. This uniform method was validated in a second comparative study that included the same 8 laboratories.

M. G. Bissell, MD, PhD, MPH

New allele-specific real-time PCR system for warfarin dose genotyping equipped with an automatic interpretative function that allows rapid, accurate, and user-friendly reporting in clinical laboratories
Kim S, Lee HW, Lee W, et al (Inje Univ College of Medicine, Goyang, South Korea; Univ of Ulsan College of Medicine and Asan Med Ctr, Seoul, South Korea)
Thromb Res 130:104-109, 2012

Introduction.—The optimal dose of the oral anticoagulant warfarin varies with polymorphisms of the vitamin K epoxide reductase complex subunit 1 (*VKORC1*) and cytochrome P450 2C9 (*CYP2C9*) genes. A fast and reliable method of warfarin dose adjustment is required to prevent serious hemorrhagic or thrombotic complications. The aim of this study is to develop and validate a new warfarin dose genotyping system with an automatic interpretation function.

Materials and Methods.—Four *VKORC1* and two *CYP2C9* SNPs were genotyped by real-time PCR using allele-specific primers and probes. Multiple reactions that included internal positive controls were performed in each well, and an automatic interpretative algorithm was developed. This system was validated using 82 clinical specimens previously genotyped by PCR-direct sequencing. The analytical time of the method was calculated.

Results.—No interference was observed when multiple samples were included in each reaction, with all internal positive control reactions being successful. In the genotyping algorithm, Ct differences < 2 and ≥ 2 identified heterozygotes and homozygotes, respectively. All results obtained were concordant with those of the reference method. The overall analytical time for assay of 12 specimens was around 3 hours.

Conclusion.—This rapid, accurate, and user-friendly genotyping system improves the efficacy and safety of anticoagulation therapy in clinical practice.

▶ Warfarin, the most commonly used oral anticoagulant, has a narrow therapeutic range, and hemorrhagic or thromboembolic events may occur even after careful dose titration. The optimal dose of warfarin is dependent on clinical factors; demographic variables; and variations in 2 genes, the cytochrome P450, family 2, subfamily C, polypeptide 9 (CYP2C9), and the vitamin K epoxide reductase complex, sub-unit 1 (VKORC1) genes. The most important genetic variations, VKORC1 haplotype group A and CYP2C9 *2 and *3, have been assessed with regard to warfarin dosing. Carriers of these polymorphic alleles have low-level warfarin metabolism, and consequently lower dose requirements. Genotypes at these loci not only indicate the appropriate initial and maintenance doses of warfarin, but certain genotypes have been associated with adverse events. In 2010, the US Food and Drug Administration updated the labeling recommendations for warfarin to stress that "The patient's CYP2C9 and VKORC1 genotype information, when available, can assist in the selection of the starting dose." To be useful, genotyping test results should be available at the time that warfarin therapy is initiated. Genetic testing before commencement of warfarin therapy is impractical in most centers, however, because results are not available in a timely manner. Only about 60 laboratories participated in the 2009 College of American Pathologists surveys on the pharmacogenetics of CYP2C9 and VKORC1. Although polymerase chain reaction (PCR)-direct sequencing is considered the gold standard method, both the procedure and the interpretation of results are time-consuming and labor-intensive. Moreover, only certain polymorphic sites, such as CYP2C9 *2 and *3 and VKORC1 haplotype group A, are significant in determining warfarin sensitivity or resistance. Therefore, a faster and higher throughput method that covers the essential SNPs may be sufficient to replace the direct sequencing method. Allele-specific real-time PCR may therefore be a good approach. The authors developed and validated a new allele-specific real-time PCR system with an automatic interpretative function to detect VKORCI and CYP2C9 genetic polymorphisms for dose adjustment of warfarin.

M. G. Bissell, MD, PhD, MPH

Development of an ethidium monoazide—enhanced internally controlled universal 16S rDNA real-time polymerase chain reaction assay for detection of bacterial contamination in platelet concentrates
Patel P, Garson JA, Tettmar KI, et al (NHS Blood and Transplant, Colindale, London, UK; Univ College London, UK; Centre for Infections, Colindale, London, UK)
Transfusion 52:1423-1432, 2012

Background.—Bacterial contamination of platelet (PLT) concentrates remains a problem for blood transfusion services. Culture-based bacterial screening techniques are available but offer inadequate speed and sensitivity.

Alternative techniques based on polymerase chain reaction (PCR) amplification have been described but their performance is often compromised by traces of bacterial DNA in reagents.

Study Design and Methods.—Universal 16S rDNA primers were used to develop a real-time PCR assay (TaqMan, Applied Biosystems) and various reagent decontamination strategies were explored. Detection sensitivity was assessed by spiking PLT concentrates with known concentrations of 13 different organisms.

Results.—Restriction enzyme digestion, master mix ultrafiltration, and use of alternative *Taq* polymerases all reduced the level of reagent DNA contamination to some extent but all proved unreliable. In contrast, ethidium monoazide (EMA) treatment of the PCR master mix followed by photoactivation was reliable and effective, permitting a full 40 amplification cycles, and totally eliminated contamination without compromising assay sensitivity. All 13 organisms were efficiently detected and the limit of detection for *Escherichia coli*—spiked PLTs was approximately 1 colony-forming unit/mL. Coamplification of human mitochondrial DNA served to confirm efficient nucleic acid extraction and the absence of PCR inhibition in each sample. One of five automated extraction platforms evaluated was found to be contamination free and capable of high-throughput processing.

Conclusion.—Cross-linking of EMA to DNA via photoactivation solved the previously intractable problem of reagent contamination and permitted the development of a high-sensitivity universal bacterial detection system. Trials are ongoing to assess the suitability of the system for high-throughput screening of PLT concentrates.

▶ The limitations of culture-based screening systems have led to the exploration of alternative strategies for bacterial detection in blood products, primarily nucleic acid amplification by polymerase chain reaction (PCR). The most common target for such assays is the highly conserved 16S ribosomal RNA gene (16S rDNA), which is present as multiple copies in all bacterial genomes. The broad reactivity provided by this target is essential because of the very diverse range of bacterial species that has been associated with sepsis after platelet transfusion. In theory, PCR-based assays should be able to detect a single molecule of 16S rDNA and therefore achieve extraordinarily high sensitivity, but in practice this potential has not been realized because of the intractable problem of contaminating bacterial DNA in consumables and reagents, particularly in Taq polymerases. Many different approaches to PCR reagent decontamination have been described, including DNase I digestion, restriction endonuclease digestion, ultrafiltration, and ultraviolet irradiation in conjunction with 8-methoxypsoralen treatment. Additionally, the use of specially purified or highly diluted Taq polymerases has been advocated by some workers, whereas others have recommended treatment of reagents with ethidium mono azide (EMA). In this study, the authors developed an internally controlled 16S rDNA real-time PCR assay and compared the effectiveness of several of these reagent decontamination methods. The most effective method (EMA treatment) was selected for further optimization and alternative nucleic acid extraction platforms were assessed. After optimization, the performance of the EMA-enhanced PCR assay was evaluated with a panel of bacterial species known to have been involved in transfusion-transmitted infections. Sensitivity and specificity of the novel assay were assessed using spiked platelet concentrates.

M. G. Bissell, MD, PhD, MPH

Artificial microvascular network: a new tool for measuring rheologic properties of stored red blood cells
Burns JM, Yang X, Forouzan O, et al (Tulane Univ, New Orleans, LA)
Transfusion 52:1010-1023, 2012

Background.—The progressive deterioration of red blood cell (RBC) rheologic properties during refrigerated storage may reduce the clinical efficacy of transfusion of older units.

Study Design and Methods.—This article describes the development of a microfluidic device designed to test the rheologic properties of stored RBCs by measuring their ability to perfuse an artificial microvascular network (AMVN) comprised of capillary-size microchannels arranged in a pattern inspired by the real microvasculature. In the AMVN device, the properties of RBCs are evaluated by passing a 40% hematocrit suspension of RBCs through the network and measuring the overall perfusion rate.

Results.—The sensitivity of the AMVN device to the storage-induced change in rheologic properties of RBCs was tested using five prestorage leukoreduced RBC units stored in AS-1 for 41 days. The AMVN perfusion rate for stored RBCs was 26 ± 4% (19%-30%) lower than for fresh RBCs. Washing these stored RBCs in saline improved their performance by 41 ± 6% (the AMVN perfusion rate for washed stored RBCs was still 15 ± 2% lower than for fresh RBCs).

Conclusions.—The measurements performed using the AMVN device confirm a significant decline in the rheologic properties of RBCs in units nearing expiration and demonstrate the sensitivity of the device to these storage-induced changes. The AMVN device may be useful for testing the effect of new storage conditions, additive solutions, and rejuvenation strategies on the rheologic properties of stored RBCs in vitro.

▶ The ability of red blood cells (RBCs) to oxygenate tissues and end organs largely depends on the dynamics of blood flow in capillaries of microvascular networks. RBCs must be able to deform at a variety of physiologic conditions through a wide range of capillaries, arterioles, and venules. Therefore, the ability of the RBC to deform is extremely important for physiologic function. The storage of RBCs may lead to deterioration and loss of this deformity function and, if transfused, may inhibit the effective delivery of oxygen when compared with fresh RBCs. The least deformable stored RBCs are mechanically sensed and retained by the spleen and removed from circulation by the reticuloendothelial system shortly after transfusion. Several tools are used to measure the deformability of RBCs, which are informative for studying the rheologic response under well-defined conditions but have limitations in physiologic conditions. The authors of this study implemented a novel microfluidic device for an integrative assessment of deformability of stored RBCs by measuring their effective ability to perfuse an artificial microvascular network. This device is a microfabricated network of microchannels ranging in size comparable to capillaries, arterioles, and venules and arranged in a pattern inspired by the topologic organization of real microvasculature. The authors subjected the RBCs to a wide range of physiologic relevant deformations under a variety of flow conditions as they transversed this device at physiologic hematocrit concentrations to obtain a single perfusion rate. They were able to demonstrate reproducibility of the measurements using fresh blood test and also test the sensitivity of the device to storage-induced changes in RBC rheologic properties using stored RBC units. A unique property of their device is the ability to compare multiple samples simultaneously so that different storage conditions could be compared at the same time.

H. Signorelli, DO

Molecular blood typing augments serologic testing and allows for enhanced matching of red blood cells for transfusion in patients with sickle cell disease
Wilkinson K, Harris S, Gaur P, et al (Puget Sound Inst of Pathology and the Puget Sound Blood Ctr, Seattle, WA)
Transfusion 52:381-388, 2012

Background.—Sickle cell disease (SCD) patients have dissimilar red blood cell (RBC) phenotypes compared to the primarily Caucasian blood donor base due, in part, to underlying complex Rh and silenced Duffy expression. Gene array—based technology offers high-throughput antigen typing of blood donors and can identify patients with altered genotypes. The purpose of the study was to ascertain if RBC components drawn from predominantly Caucasian donors could provide highly antigen-matched products for molecularly typed SCD patients.

Study Design and Methods.—SCD patients were genotyped by a molecular array (HEA Beadchip, BioArray Solutions). The extended antigen phenotype (C, c, E, e, K, k, Jk^a, Jk^b, Fy^a, Fy^b, S, s) was used to query the inventory using different matching algorithms; the resulting number of products was recorded.

Results.—A mean of 96.2 RBC products was available for each patient at basic-level, 34 at mid-level, and 16.3 at high-level stringency. The number of negative antigens correlated negatively with the number of available products. The Duffy silencing mutation in the promoter region ($67T > C$) (*GATA*) was found in 96.5% of patients. Allowing Fy(b+) products for patients with *GATA* increased the number of available products by up to 180%, although it does not ensure prevention of Duffy antibodies in all patients.

Conclusions.—This feasibility study provides evidence that centers with primarily Caucasian donors may be able to provide highly antigen-matched products. Knowledge of the *GATA* status expands the inventory of antigen-matched products. Further work is needed to determine the most clinically appropriate match level for SCD patients.

▶ Sickle cell disease (SCD) is an autosomal recessive hemoglobinopathy that affects nearly 1 in 500 African Americans. It is characterized by red blood cells (RBCs) that become sickle-shaped when deoxygenated, altering their deformability. Patients with SCD are at an increased risk for anemia and microvascular vasoocclusion throughout the body, which can result in stroke and organ dysfunction. The treatment often includes transfusion to decrease the amount of RBCs with hemoglobin-S as well as restore oxygen-carrying capacity. Patients with SCD often need frequent transfusions and are at a high risk of developing alloantibodies that can result in hemolytic transfusion reactions. This is especially true because African Americans have dissimilar RBC phenotypes when compared with the primarily Caucasian blood donor base. Therefore, extra care must be taken to prevent antibody development. This includes finding a more sophisticated approach to compatibility testing, which can often be more complex and potentially delay the release of blood components for SCD patients. Molecular blood group analysis offers a fast and reproducible means of typing donors and recipients. Most hospitals in North America do not currently determine the RBC antigen phenotype of nonalloimmunized SCD patients beyond ABO and D. Only roughly 40% of hospitals do use additional testing and prophylactic matching, usually C, E, and K. The authors of this study designed an inventory feasibility study to determine if current inventory of antigen-type components could support SCD patients with antigen matching greater than C, c, E, e, and K using molecular genotyping. The study evaluated the number of antigen-matched RBC components that would meet the transfusion needs of the SCD patients based on their molecularly predicted RBC phenotype. Future studies should address which antigens are clinically relevant for prospective matching and if this approach changes clinical outcome. Additional concerns relating to the cost-effectiveness of this method should also be explored.

H. Signorelli, DO

Transfusion of older stored blood and risk of death: a meta analysis
Wang D, Sun J, Solomon SB, et al (Natl Insts of Health, Bethesda, MD; West China Hosp of Sichuan Univ, Cheng Du, China)
Transfusion 52:1184-1195, 2012

Background.—Blood for transfusion is stored for up to 42 days. Older blood develops lesions and accumulates potentially injurious substances. Some studies report increasing toxicity as blood ages. We assessed the safety of transfused older versus newer stored blood.

Study Design and Methods.—PubMed, Scopus, and Embase were searched using terms *new* and *old* and *red blood cell* and *storage* through May 6, 2011, for observational and randomized controlled studies comparing outcomes using transfused blood having longer and shorter storage times. Death was the outcome of interest.

Results.—Twenty-one studies were identified, predominantly in cardiac surgery (n = 6) and trauma (n = 6) patients, including 409,966 patients. A test for heterogeneity of these studies' results was not significant for mortality ($I^2 = 3.7\%$, $p = 0.41$). Older blood was associated with a significantly increased risk of death (odds ratio, 1.16; 95% confidence interval [CI], 1.07-1.24). Using available mortality data, 97 (95% CI, 63-199) patients need to be treated with only new blood to save one life. Subgroup analysis of these trials indicated that the increased risk was not restricted to a particular type of patient, size of trial, or amount of blood transfused.

Conclusion.—Based on available data, use of older stored blood is associated with a significantly increased risk of death.

▶ Transfusion of red blood cells (RBCs) is 1 of the most important therapies in clinical medicine. The World Health Organization reported that 80.7 million units of blood were collected in 167 countries surveyed between 2004 and 2005. Approximately 15 million units of whole blood are collected in the United States each year, all of which are required to be processed, shipped, and stored prior to use. The majority of research and time has been spent over the years trying to extend the life of these units to maximize availability and provide adequate inventories all over the country. Modified storage solutions, containers, and processing procedures have been successful at accomplishing this goal and extending the shelf life of RBCs to 6 weeks. Blood at the end of this time frame meets the Food and Drug Administration (FDA)'s guidelines regarding RBC quality, but over the past few years it has been debated whether this "old" blood is as safe and efficient as blood stored for shorter durations. Refrigeration of RBCs results in "storage lesions" that can lead to a multitude of changes in the RBCs and may also lead to the accumulation of molecules that could cause harm to the recipient.

Recent studies have suggested that patients receiving older blood with storage lesions have an increased mortality risk when compared with patients receiving newer stored units but the data are not conclusive. Current practices dictate that most adult and pediatric patients requiring transfusion receive blood of their specific type with the oldest compatible unit available given first in order to conserve the blood supply. Standard approaches to inventory management would need to be drastically changed if older blood were found to pose clinically significant risks with major operational and fiscal consequences. The authors of this article attempt to summarize previously published transfusion data to analyze the effect of storage on mortality and determine if effects are restricted to any specific patient population. These authors did a formal meta-analysis of more than 20 studies, increasing the overall number of results and credibility of their findings. However, it cannot be overlooked that some of the data used in their analysis were derived largely from observational studies with potential unrecognized biases. Well-designed, multicenter, adequately powered, randomized controlled trials will need to confirm the results presented in this article. This type of study is extremely challenging both from an operational and ethical standpoint, but is necessary to adequately protect patients.

H. Signorelli, DO

In vitro platelet quality in storage containers used for pediatric transfusions

Weiss S, Scammell K, Levin E, et al (Canadian Blood Services Res and Development, Edmonton, Alberta, Canada; Univ of British Columbia Centre for Blood Res, Vancouver, Canada; Univ of British Columbia, Vancouver, Canada; et al)
Transfusion 52:1703-1714, 2012

Background.—The in vitro quality of small-volume platelet (PLT) aliquots for pediatric transfusions was assessed to determine the best practice approach.

Study Design and Methods.—Small volumes (50 mL) of single apheresis PLT components (APCs), collected on either CaridianBCT Trima or Haemonetics MCS+ instruments, were aliquoted on Days 2, 3, 4, and 5 postcollection into Fenwal PL1240 or 4R2014 bags or 60-mL polypropylene syringes. Samples were tested for in vitro quality at their recommended expiry times (4 hr for 4R2014 bags and syringes or Day 5 for PL1240 bags). Assays included pH, CD62P expression, and metabolic measures.

Results.—CD62P expression increased throughout storage in all containers. Among the small-volume containers, pH, pCO_2, lactate, and bicarbonate varied considerably. Regardless of the day of aliquoting, pCO_2 was significantly higher and pO_2 was significantly lower in gas-impermeable syringes than other containers. No bacterial growth was detected in any sample.

Conclusion.—The quality of APCs aliquoted into small-volume containers meets regulatory requirements and is generally equivalent to that of full-volume APCs at expiry.

▶ Transfusions to pediatric patients comprise 1% of blood transfusions and require special guidelines for the small volume of product being transfused. However, there is a wide variation in the preparation and clinical application without a standardized approach for the removal and storage of aliquots for pediatric transfusions. Current practice is to obtain small-volume aliquots from full-volume single donor—derived platelet components (PCs) that can then be removed into transfer bags by sterile docking or aspirated into a syringe. Guidelines have been established in North America, Europe, and elsewhere regarding the maximum storage time of platelets aliquoted for pediatric transfusions. For example, if PCs are transferred using a closed system into gas-permeable platelet bags, storage of PCs for up to the normal expiration time of the source PC (eg, in North America, 5 days after collection) is acceptable. PCs in polypropylene syringes maintain acceptable storage characteristics for up to 6 hours, although transfusion is generally recommended within 4 hours. Currently, the Canadian Blood Services produces single-donor apheresis-derived platelet (APC) products that limit the donor exposure, thereby reducing alloimmunization and infectious disease risk. The authors of this study assessed the quality of PLT aliquots from full-volume APCs, produced by 2 different apheresis machines, and transferred into several different small-volume containers. Although they did conclude that there were observed differences in in vitro quality measures between the different small-volume containers, all still fell within regulated quality control limits and were of comparable quality to full-volume APCs at expiry. Therefore, although the least favorable conditions were found in the syringes, they are currently acceptable based on regulated guidelines for pediatric transfusions.

H. Signorelli, DO

Measuring Direct Thrombin Inhibitors With Routine and Dedicated Coagulation Assays: Which Assay Is Helpful?

Curvers J, van de Kerkhof D, Stroobants AK, et al (Catharina Hosp, Eindhoven, the Netherlands; Academic Med Ctr, Amsterdam, the Netherlands)
Am J Clin Pathol 138:551-558, 2012

The use of direct thrombin inhibitors (DTIs) for prophylactic or therapeutic anticoagulation is increasing because of the predictable bioavailability and short half-life of these DTIs. However, in certain situations, indication of the concentration is warranted. We investigated the effects of 3 DTIs (lepirudin, argatroban, and bivalirudin) in 6 pooled plasma specimens on routine coagulation assays (activated partial thromboplastin time [aPTT], prothrombin time [PT], and thrombin time [TT]) and dedicated DTI assays (Hemoclot, HemosIL, the ecarin clotting time, and a chromogenic ecarin clotting time) on 2 coagulation analyzers. We found routine tests to be nondiscriminative between concentrations of different DTIs in the aPTT. Moreover, for PT and TT, the responses for different DTIs differed. This was similar for ecarin clotting assays. The Hemoclot and HemosIL assays showed identical linear increases for all 3 DTIs. We conclude that dedicated calibrated assays based on a diluted TT (Hemoclot and HemosIL) appear to be the most suitable for monitoring purposes.

▶ Direct thrombin inhibitors (DTIs) are used for anticoagulant therapy in patients with heparin-induced thrombocytopenia (type II), impaired renal function, and antithrombin deficiency. DTIs are also used during coronary artery bypass grafting surgery in patients with atrial fibrillation and in acute venous thrombotic events. Some of the advantages DTIs have over heparins and vitamin K antagonists include a shorter half-life, better bioavailability, and less variation between individuals. Therefore, DTIs shouldn't need regular monitoring. However, these agents do not have an adequate antidote. Although monitoring of anticoagulation therapy may not be required for DTIs, certain patients with an increased risk for bleeding or other complications may still require occasional blood analysis. Additionally, physicians may choose to monitor a patient's coagulation status for compliance or effectiveness. DTIs interfere with the central clotting enzyme thrombin; therefore, almost every coagulation assay will be affected by their presence in the blood. This includes routinely used assays such as the activated partial thromboplastin time (aPTT), prothrombin time (PT), and thrombin time (TT). Different assays are available to specifically measure DTIs such as the diluted thrombin time (dTT), the ecarin clotting time, and the ecarin chromogenic assay. dTT assays include the Hemoclot thrombin inhibitor assay and the HemosIL DTI assay. However, there is no consensus on how DTIs should be monitored and which assay should be used. Here the authors performed a study to look at the in vitro effect of increasing concentration levels of 3 DTIs—lepirudin, bivalirudin, and argatroban—in pooled plasma on different assays. They compared results from routine assays such as aPTT, PT, and TT to dedicated DTA assays such as Hemoclot, HemosIL, ECT, and ECA.

H. Signorelli, DO

Polymerase chain reaction–based tests for pan-species and species-specific detection of human *Plasmodium* parasites

Mahajan B, Zheng H, Pham PT, et al (US Food and Drug Administration, Rockville, MD; Univ of Ghana, Legon, Accra)
Transfusion 52:1949-1956, 2012

Background.—There is still a need to improve the sensitivity of polymerase chain reaction (PCR) tests for malaria to detect submicroscopic asexual stage *Plasmodium* infections during the early phase and chronic, asymptomatic phase of infection when the parasite burden is very low.

Study Design and Methods.—The inhibitory effect of hemoglobin (Hb) on PCR limits the volume of blood that can be used in the PCR-based detection of intraerythrocytic *Plasmodium* parasites. We lysed red blood cells with saponin to reduce the Hb concentration in extracted nucleic acid and, as a result, significantly increased the volume of blood that can be tested by PCR. The analytical sensitivity of the PCR was determined using whole blood spiked with ring-stage *Plasmodium falciparum* parasites, and its clinical sensitivity by testing blood film—positive and blood film—negative samples from individuals living in an endemic area in Ghana.

Results.—We have developed a pan-*Plasmodium* PCR that detects all five human *Plasmodium* species with the highest analytical sensitivity of two *P. falciparum* parasites/mL of whole blood and species-specific PCR tests that distinguished between the five human *Plasmodium* species. Pan-*Plasmodium* PCR detected 78 of 78 (100%) blood film—positive and 19 of 101 (18.81%) blood film—negative samples from asymptomatic individuals living in Ghana. Pan-*Plasmodium* PCR was equally sensitive with samples collected as anticoagulated whole blood and clotted blood and in blood collected by finger stick into capillaries.

Conclusion.—We have developed PCR tests with the highest reported sensitivity to date for pan-*Plasmodium* diagnosis and species-specific diagnosis and detected blood film—negative asymptomatic infections in individuals living in malaria-endemic countries.

▶ When selecting blood donors, it is extremely important to identify those with an infectious disease that can be transmitted by blood. The safety of the blood supply has benefited from the advances in technology that have improved the ability to detect a number of viruses. However, advances in laboratory tests to detect human *Plasmodium* spp. are still limited. The mainstay for detection of parasites such as *Plasmodium* spp. is the inexpensive microscopic examination of blood films. This method remains limited by the need for highly skilled technicians along with a difficulty in diagnosing persons with low-grade infections. Patients that are asymptomatic with low-grade infections are most likely to go undiagnosed and pose a serious risk to blood safety in nonendemic countries. Obstacles for developing a sensitive nucleic acid test (NAT) for malaria include the intra-erythrocytic location of *Plasmodium* parasites and host DNA and hemoglobin interference from lysed red blood cells. The authors from this study developed an assay that attempts to improve the sensitivity of the NAT for *Plasmodium* by adding a saponin lysis step. They hypothesized that this would allow for less contamination by host DNA and allow for processing of larger test volumes. The assay was developed for both anticoagulated and clotted samples of whole venous blood. The clinical sensitivity of the assay was assessed using samples from adults who tested negative or positive for parasites by routine examination of blood films. The assay was capable of detecting and distinguishing between the five known human malarial parasites: *P. falciparum*, *P. vivax*, *P. malariae*, *P. ovale*, and *P. knowlesi*. The clinical sensitivity of the assay was compared with previous NAT tests showing higher sensitivity and the ability to be performed on small and large blood volumes.

H. Signorelli, DO

A Massive Transfusion Protocol Incorporating a Higher FFP/RBC Ratio Is Associated With Decreased Use of Recombinant Activated Factor VII in Trauma Patients

Tan JNM, Burke PA, Agarwal SK, et al (Boston Univ Med Ctr, MA)
Am J Clin Pathol 137:566-571, 2012

We implemented a protocol incorporating a higher fresh frozen plasma (FFP)/RBC ratio for the management of trauma patients requiring massive transfusion in 2007. This study aims to identify issues that affected the effective deployment of the massive transfusion protocol (MTP) and compare outcome variables with a historic cohort. Data from 49 trauma patients who received at least 10 units of packed RBCs within 24 hours were analyzed and compared with a historic massively transfused cohort who had received recombinant activated factor VII (rFVIIa).

Of the patients, 28 received an FFP/RBC ratio of 1:1 to 1:2; 12 received a lower ratio of 1:2 to 1:4; 3 received more than 1:1 and 6 had less than 1:4. Compared with the historic cohort, the 1:1-1:2 group received significantly fewer blood components and did not require rescue rFVIIa. An MTP incorporating a higher FFP/RBC ratio of 1:1 to 1:2 is associated with decreased use of blood components and may obviate the need for rFVII.

▶ Trauma deaths are a leading cause of death in patients younger than age 45 years. Death within the first 6 hours is usually due to hemorrhage from coagulopathy and hyperfibrinolysis. In addition to the use of blood components for hemostasis control, recombinant activated factor VII (rFVIIa) is often used empirically to treat the coagulopathy. However, the use of rFVIIa is not without its complications, including thrombosis and high cost. The institution in this study had recently changed their massive transfusion protocol (MTP) algorithm to implement a higher fresh frozen plasma (FFP)/red blood cell (RBC) ratio that was derived from military experience. Studies have shown that ratios of FFP/RBC are optimal at 1:1 to 1:2, which can lead to an overall decrease in blood component use. This study was designed to assess the blood component use after the implementation of the new MTP and look at the FFP/RBC ratio that patients received. Outcome variables and use of rFVIIa were analyzed for each cohort of patients. The study concluded that at their institution the use of an MTP with higher FFP/RBC ratios resulted in patients receiving fewer blood components and having lower mortality and decreased use of rFVIIa as compared with their previous transfusion protocol.

H. Signorelli, DO

Epidemiologic and laboratory findings from 3 years of testing United States blood donors for _Trypanosoma cruzi_
Custer B, Agapova M, Bruhn R, et al (Blood Systems Res Inst, San Francisco, CA; Univ of Washington, Seattle; Univ of California at San Francisco; et al)
Transfusion 52:1901-1911, 2012

Background.—At most blood centers in the United States routine testing of donations for _Trypanosoma cruzi_ using an enzyme-linked immunosorbent assay (ELISA) is followed by supplemental testing by radioimmunoprecipitation assay (RIPA). The objective of this study was to report the results of routine testing and risk factor data from allogeneic blood donors.

Study Design and Methods.—T. _cruzi_ testing data from January 2007 through December 2009 were analyzed, and risk factor interviews and follow-up studies were conducted on seroreactive donors. Prevalences of confirmed infection and risk factors associated with infection were assessed using logistic and multivariable logistic regression.

Results.—Of 2 940 491 allogeneic donations from 1 183 076 donors, 305 (0.01% per donation tested and 0.026% per blood donor) were repeat reactive (RR) and 89 of those were confirmed positive by RIPA, yielding an overall seroprevalence of 1 per 33 039 donations and 1 per 13 292 donors. Country of birth and US blood center location differences in the seroprevalence of _T. cruzi_ were evident. The odds of confirmed infection were highest if the donor reported having been bitten by the reduviid (kissing) bug (odds ratio [OR], 76.1; 95% confidence interval [CI], 11.1-3173) followed by having lived in a rural area of Latin America (OR, 38.6; 95% CI, 15.1-102.5). In multivariable analyses, having spent 3 months or more in Mexico or Central and/or South America was associated with the highest odds of RIPA-confirmed infection (OR, 8.5; 95% CI, 2.7-26.5). Polymerase chain reaction (PCR) testing of ELISA RR donors exhibited low sensitivity (1/22 [4%] RIPA-confirmed donors was PCR positive).

Conclusion.—Risk factors for confirmed infection in US blood donors are consistent with the known epidemiology of Chagas disease. Blood donors or transfusions do not substantially contribute to the burden of *T. cruzi* infection in the United States.

▶ *Trypanosoma cruzi* is the etiologic agent for Chagas disease, which typically results in a lifelong infection. Persistent infection can lead to cardiomyopathy, which often evolves into congestive heart failure and possibly death. It is estimated that there are 8 to 10 million people infected with *T. cruzi* in the Americas and more than 300 000 individuals infected in the United States. Therefore, the need to characterize the prevalence of *T. cruzi* and the threat to the blood supply is necessary. The *T. cruzi* enzyme-linked immunosorbent assay (ELISA) test is commonly used among blood collectors voluntarily to screen all donations. Donors who test repeat reactive (RR) on a single donation on the ELISA test are deferred and the donation is further tested by supplemental radioimmunoprecipitation assay (RIPA) for confirmation. Here the authors present the results of nearly 3 years of testing and risk factor data from allogeneic donors including the prevalence of *T. cruzi* in US blood donors, characteristics associated with infection in donors and findings from follow-up laboratory studies. During the interval from January 2007 through December 2009, 1120 RIPA-confirmed infections were identified in blood donors in the United States based on the national reporting system maintained by the AABB. Within the first 16 months of this interval, the national seroprevalence of *T. cruzi* was estimated to be 1 in 27 500 donations. This study found the seroprevalence of confirmed *T. cruzi* to be nearly 1 in 13 300 donors screened.

H. Signorelli, DO

Storage time of blood products and transfusion-related acute lung injury
Middelburg RA, Borkent B, Jansen M, et al (Leiden Univ Med Ctr, The Netherlands; UMC Utrecht, The Netherlands; TRIP (Transfusion Reactions in Patients) Dutch National Hemovigilance Office, The Hague, The Netherlands; et al)
Transfusion 52:658-667, 2012

Background.—Besides white blood cell antibodies in plasma-rich products, another cause of transfusion-related acute lung injury (TRALI) could be release of biologically active substances during storage of cellular blood products. We aimed to investigate the association of storage time and risk of TRALI for different product types.

Study Design and Methods.—We compared storage time of blood products transfused within 6 hours before the onset of TRALI to storage time of a representative sample of all blood products transfused in the Netherlands. Generalized linear models were used to correct for confounding variables.

Results.—Platelets (PLTs) in plasma transfused to TRALI patients were stored for 0.7 (95% confidence interval [CI], 0.073 to 1.3) days longer than those transfused to controls. The relative risk of TRALI, after receiving PLTs stored for 4 or 5 days, compared to 3 days or less, was 5.8 (95% CI,

0.99 to 110) and increased to 6.3 (95% CI, 1.1 to 118) after more than 5 days (i.e., 6 or 7 days).

Conclusions.—While longer storage of buffy coat–derived PLTs was associated with an increased risk of TRALI, storage of plasma for up to 2 years and red blood cells for up to 35 days was not associated with the risk of TRALI.

▶ Transfusion-related acute lung injury (TRALI) is defined as an acute lung injury syndrome that occurs within 6 hours of transfusion that cannot be explained by another risk factor. It is a serious adverse event of blood transfusions with a mechanism related to white blood cell (WBC) antibodies. However, exclusion of donors with WBC antibodies from the donor pool has not eliminated all TRALI cases. Some studies have suggested that substances released in the storage of blood products may also contribute to the cause of TRALI. Previous studies have been done looking the storage time on platelets (PLTs) and the associated risk of TRALI. A study analyzing the storage time of fresh frozen plasma (FFP) and red blood cells (RBCs) on the risk of TRALI has not been done clinically. The authors of this study analyzed the risk of TRALI associated with storage time of different types of prestorage leuko-reduced blood components including PLTs, RBCs, and FFP. They prospectively looked at TRALI patients and the blood components that were transfused within 6 hours before the onset of symptoms. They demonstrated that there was no association of TRALI with longer storage times for RBCS and FFP. However, longer storage of PLTs was strongly associated with an increased risk of TRALI.

H. Signorelli, DO

Flow cytometry assessment of apoptotic CD34+ cells by annexin V labeling may improve prediction of cord blood potency for engraftment
Duggleby RC, Querol S, Davy RC, et al (Royal Free Hosp, London, UK; Nottingham Trent Univ, UK; Banc de Sang i Teixits, Barcelona, Spain)
Transfusion 52:549-559, 2012

Background.—Nonviable CD34+ cells are commonly assessed by standard flow cytometry using the nuclear stain 7-aminoactinomycin D (7AAD). 7AAD, however, only detects necrotic and late apoptotic cells, not earlier apoptosis, which engraft poorly in animal models of cord blood (cord) transplantation. The standard method, therefore, may overestimate engraftment potency of cord units under certain conditions.

Study Design and Methods.—To detect apoptotic events, costaining with 7AAD and annexin V (AnnV), in parallel with the quantitative, standard enumeration, was used. Cord units were assessed before and after cryopreservation using both staining methods and colony-forming units (CFU) to determine if graft potency can be predicted using a "functional flow cytometry" approach.

Results.—Significant numbers of CD34+ AnnV+ events were found within the 7AAD-gated population. Nonapoptotic cell dose (CD34+ AnnV−)

correlated well with CFUs in both a small-scale (n = 10) and a large-scale banking study (n = 107). Finally, following samples postthaw with time showed increasing numbers of apoptotic CD34+ cells and consequently the AnnV assessed dose was better at predicting the CFU compared with just the standard enumeration.

Conclusion.—Defining the apoptotic population of CD34+ cells improved the prediction of CFU, making this method a rapid test of potency for assessment of cord units for clinical use.

▶ The time to engraftment after stem cell transplantation and overall outcome largely depends on the stem cell dose in both pediatric and adult patients. The stem cell dose is usually determined using CD34 + cell enumeration. Flow cytometry quantification of CD34 cells remains the most widely used tool but is inferior to colony-forming unit (CFU) assays at predicting time to engraftment and graft survival in umbilical cord blood (cord) transplantation. However, CFU assays are impractical in a routine clinical setting because they have long readout times and are difficult to standardize. Different techniques have been developed to try and improve flow cytometry quantification of CD34 cells. One includes adding forward-scatter low, 7-aminoactinomycin D (7AAD) + CD34 + events for cord units which results in an inverse correlation with CFUs. However, this method fails to discount a population of apoptotic cells that are no longer capable of engraftment. It is postulated that this method continues to measure cells with early changes of irreversible apoptosis. Annexin V (AnnV) is a stain that can also be used to indicate loss of cellular functionality on apoptotic cells and may be better at discriminating between engrafting and nonengrafting cells than the 7AAD method. This study proposed that AnnV + cells are committed to apoptosis and unlikely to engraft and therefore do not have the ability to generate colonies in a CFU assay. The authors from this study used data from standard CD34 + enumeration assays along with data from AnnV assays to correct the CD34 + enumeration for apoptotic cells. This assessment was correlated with CFUs as a measure of graft potency. One challenge in the study that was overcome included AnnV not properly working with the lysis buffer used in the standard enumeration assay. An additional concern included the possibility of apoptotic cells being induced after thawing and causing false positives, but this variable was thought to be minimal if samples were run quickly and in parallel with each other. The use of AnnV as a potential apoptotic marker to improve CD34 enumeration would be a useful test and further studies could identify the predictive capabilities in a clinical setting.

H. Signorelli, DO

Treatment of whole blood with riboflavin plus ultraviolet light, an alternative to gamma irradiation in the prevention of transfusion-associated graft-versus-host disease?

Fast LD, Nevola M, Tavares J, et al (Rhode Island Hosp/Brown Univ, Providence; TerumoBCT Biotechnologies, Lakewood, CO)
Transfusion 2012 [Epub ahead of print]

Background.—Exposure of blood products to gamma irradiation is currently the standard of care in the prevention of transfusion-associated graft-versus-host disease (TA-GVHD). Regulatory, technical, and clinical challenges associated with the use of gamma irradiators are driving efforts to develop alternatives. Pathogen reduction methods were initially developed to reduce the risk of microbial transmission by blood components. Through modifications of nucleic acids, these technologies interfere with the replication of both pathogens and white blood cells (WBCs). To date, systems for pathogen and WBC inactivation of products containing red blood cells are less well established than those for platelets and plasma.

Study Design and Methods.—In this study, the in vitro and in vivo function of WBCs present in whole blood after exposure to riboflavin plus ultraviolet light (Rb-UV) was examined and compared to responses of WBCs obtained from untreated or gamma-irradiated blood by measuring proliferation, cytokine production, activation, and antigen presentation and xenogeneic (X-)GVHD responses in an in vivo mouse model.

Results.—In vitro studies demonstrated that treatment of whole blood with Rb-UV was as effective as gamma irradiation in preventing WBC proliferation, but was more effective in preventing antigen presentation, cytokine production, and T-cell activation. Consistent with in vitro findings, treatment with Rb-UV was as effective as gamma irradiation in preventing X-GVHD, a mouse model for TA-GVHD.

Conclusion.—The ability to effectively inactivate WBCs in fresh whole blood using Rb-UV, prior to separation into components, provides the transfusion medicine community with a potential alternative to gamma irradiation.

▶ Transfusion-associated graft-versus-host disease (TA-GVHD) is a serious and often fatal complication of transfusing blood components with viable white blood cells (WBCs). This occurs in patients who are unable to mount an immune response to the allogeneic donor cells because of immunosuppression or to human leukocyte antigen (HLA) compatibility. Additional adverse events caused by transfused donor WBCs include alloimmunization, platelet refractoriness, and transfusion-related immune modulation (TRIM). TRIM is a transient suppression of the immune system related to circulating donor WBCs within the recipient. For the past 40 years, gamma irradiation has been the standard of care used to treat blood components for patients susceptible to TA-GVHD. However, growing concerns over the use of cesium source irradiators and the risk of terrorist activity have led the US Nuclear Regulatory Commission to call for efforts to develop alternate forms of treatment. Riboflavin plus ultraviolet light (Rb-UV) originally developed to inactivate pathogens in the blood supply has been shown to also inhibit immunologic response mediated by WBCs. Riboflavin is added to the blood component and activated by UV light, which causes irreparable modifications in nucleic acids. This method has been difficult to implement with red blood cell (RBC) components or whole blood because of the absorption of UV light by hemoglobin. This study looked at the in vitro and in vivo WBC functionality after treatment of whole blood with Rb-UV in comparison to gamma irradiation. The authors also assessed lower UV energy doses and the ability to cause WBC inactivation. The study demonstrated that although gamma-irradiation was able to prevent proliferation of lymphocytes, it was much less effective than treatment with Rb-UV in preventing lymphocyte activation, cytokine production, and the ability of the cells to act as antigen-presenting cells. The study also showed that the mice that were injected with both gamma-irradiated and Rb-UV treated mononuclear cells did not show signs of GVHD. This study showed that Rb-UV treatment could be a potential alternative to gamma irradiation and could eliminate the use of highly regulated irradiators. Studies to test the quality of the RBCs and the function in human subjects need to be explored before this method can be accepted. Additional areas that also should be explored include the ability of the Rb-UV treatment to prevent alloimmunization, platelet refractoriness, and TRIM.

H. Signorelli, DO

The clinical relevance of persistent recombinant immunoblot assay—indeterminate reactions: insights into the natural history of hepatitis C virus infection and implications for donor counseling

Makuria AT, Raghuraman S, Burbelo PD, et al (Natl Inst for Diabetes and Digestive and Kidney Diseases, Bethesda, MD; Natl Insts of Health, Bethesda, MD; The Greater Chesapeake and Potomac Region American Red Cross, Baltimore, MD)
Transfusion 52:1940-1948, 2012

Background.—Recombinant immunoblot assay (RIBA) is used to determine the specificity of antibody to hepatitis C virus (anti-HCV). The RIBA result is recorded as positive, negative, or indeterminate. The interpretation and significance of RIBA-indeterminate reactions are unclear. We addressed the clinical relevance of these reactions in the context of the natural history of HCV infection in a prospectively followed cohort of anti-HCV—positive blood donors.

Study Design and Methods.—Donor demographics, exposure history, and humoral and cell-mediated immunity (CMI) were compared in 15 RIBA-indeterminate subjects, nine chronic HCV carriers, and eight spontaneously recovered subjects. Serum samples were tested for anti-HCV by a quantitative, liquid luciferase immunoprecipitation system (LIPS). CMI was assessed by interferon-γ enzyme-linked immunosorbent spot assay.

Results.—In the LIPS assay, the sum of antibody responses to six HCV antigens showed significant ($p < 0.001$) stepwise diminution progressing from chronic carriers to spontaneously recovered to RIBA-indeterminate subjects. CMI responses in RIBA-indeterminate subjects were similar to spontaneously recovered subjects and greater than chronic carriers and controls ($p < 0.008$). A parenteral risk factor was identified in only 13% of RIBA-indeterminate subjects compared to 89% of chronic carriers and 87% of spontaneously recovered subjects. RIBA-indeterminate donors were older than the other groups.

Conclusion.—The CMI and LIPS results suggest that persistent RIBA-indeterminate reactions represent waning anti-HCV responses in persons who have recovered from a remote HCV infection. In such cases, detectable antibody may ultimately disappear leaving no residual serologic evidence of prior HCV infection, as reported in a minority of long-term HCV-recovered subjects.

▶ Although screening for hepatitis C (HCV) has reduced the incidence of HCV infection associated with blood transfusions from 3.84% to 0.57% per recipient, rare cases of transfusion-transmitted HCV infection still occur. The Centers for Disease Control and Prevention estimates 17 000 new HCV infections in 2007. Most patients infected with HCV remain asymptomatic and therefore may present as healthy blood donors and present a risk to the blood supply. Currently, the testing for HCV includes a highly sensitive enzyme immunoassay (EIA) for anti-HCV along with a molecular amplification assay for HCV RNA. Even though the immunoassay is very sensitive, it can still miss individuals with an early infection or those with remote past infections because of low antibody levels. Additionally, the EIA test is prone to false positives. A recombinant immunoblot assay (RIBA) is used to confirm a repeat reactive EIA result in blood donors, especially in those who are HCV RNA negative. However, indeterminate RIBA results create a controversy for blood utilization and donor counseling. In this study, the authors examined the relevance and clinical interpretation of reproducible RIBA-indeterminate results. Cell-mediated immune responses to HCV antigens were assessed along with anti-HCV levels by an immunoprecipitation method. They concluded that persistent RIBA-indeterminate reactions could indicate a false positive but more likely indicate recovery from a remote HCV infection.

H. Signorelli, MD

Report of the first nationally implemented clinical routine screening for fetal *RHD* in D− pregnant women to ascertain the requirement for antenatal RhD prophylaxis
Clausen FB, Christiansen M, Steffensen R, et al (Copenhagen Univ Hosp, Denmark; Aarhus Univ Hosp, Skejby, Denmark; Aalborg Hospital, Denmark; et al)
Transfusion 52:752-758, 2012

Background.—A combination of antenatal and postnatal RhD prophylaxis is more effective in reducing D immunization in pregnancy than postnatal RhD prophylaxis alone. Based on the result from antenatal screening for the fetal *RHD* gene, antenatal RhD prophylaxis in Denmark is given only to those D− women who carry a D+ fetus. We present an evaluation of the first national clinical application of antenatal *RHD* screening.

Study Design and Methods.—In each of the five Danish health care regions, blood samples were drawn from D− women in gestational Week 25. DNA was extracted from the maternal plasma and analyzed for the presence of the *RHD* gene by real-time polymerase chain reaction targeting two *RHD* exons. Prediction of the fetal RhD type was compared with serologic typing of the newborn in 2312 pregnancies, which represented the first 6 months of routine analysis.

Results.—For the detection of fetal *RHD*, the sensitivity was 99.9%. The accuracy was 96.5%. The recommendation for unnecessary antenatal RhD prophylaxis for women carrying a D− fetus was correctly avoided in 862 cases (37.3%), while 39 women (1.7%) were recommended for antenatal RhD prophylaxis unnecessarily. Two *RHD*+ fetuses (0.087%) were not detected, and antenatal RhIG was not given.

Conclusion.—These data represent the first demonstration of the reliability of routine antenatal fetal *RHD* screening in D−, pregnant women to ascertain the requirement for antenatal RhD prophylaxis. Our findings should encourage the implementation of such screening programs worldwide, to reduce the unnecessary use of RhIG.

▶ Hemolytic disease of the fetus and newborn (HDFN) is characterized by fetal anemia, hydrops fetalis, jaundice, kernicterus, and intrauterine death. A major cause is pregnancy-related immunization against the red blood cell D antigens. Current prophylactic treatment with Rh immune globulin (RhIG) prevents maternal immunization and has reduced the incidence of HDFN in D− women who are carrying a D+ fetus.

According to current practice of routine antenatal anti-D prophylaxis (RAADP) in Denmark, RhIG is given to all D− pregnant women, which is unnecessary for D− women who are carrying a D− fetus. This occurs in approximately 40% of pregnancies in Europe. The discovery of cell-free fetal DNA circulating in maternal plasma provides a tool for noninvasive prenatal prediction of the fetal RhD type. Consequently, it is possible to identify D− women who are carrying a D+ fetus and to include only those women in the RAADP program to receive RhIG and avoid unnecessary, costly treatment. Detection of the fetal RHD gene is done by real-time polymerase chain reaction (PCR) and has been shown to be exceedingly reliable, especially with improvements in DNA extraction and assay development.

The authors of this study present data from the evaluation of the first 6 months of an antenatal RHD screen program in Denmark. This is the first national clinical application of noninvasive routine antenatal screening for fetal RHD in D− women using cell-free fetal DNA extracted from maternal plasma. Their results of an extremely sensitive assay demonstrate the reliability of method and program. One hurdle that continues to be an issue is low quantities of fetal DNA in maternal plasma, which leads to false-negative results and leaves women with undetected D+ fetuses at risk of immunization. However, the method used in this study was developed to avoid false-negative results by using an automated DNA extraction method on samples at gestation week 25 when the concentration of cell-free fetal DNA in the maternal plasma is significantly higher than earlier in pregnancy. This compromised the specificity of the method leading to the unnecessary administration of anti-D in a small number of cases. Unfortunately, there remained a large group of patients with inconclusive results that were mostly likely related to variant D types, weak PCR amplification, and failed PCR procedures. Therefore, the study decided to include women with inconclusive results in the antenatal RhD prophylaxis program because variant D women, although rare, may be immunized by a D + fetus. Their calculations show that the expenses for routine antenatal screening are covered by the reduction in anti-D usage. However, the study will need to be followed for many years to assess the clinical effect of the program and if participants are being compliant with the study algorithm.

H. Signorelli, DO

Comparative in vitro evaluation of apheresis platelets stored with 100% plasma or 65% platelet additive solution III/35% plasma and including periods without agitation under simulated shipping conditions
Moroff G, Kurtz J, Seetharaman S, et al (American Red Cross Biomedical Services and Holland Laboratory, Rockville, MD)
Transfusion 52:834-843, 2012

Background.—A comparative study evaluated the retention of apheresis platelet (A-PLT) in vitro properties prepared with PLT additive solution (PAS)-III or 100% plasma and stored with continuous agitation (CA) and without continuous agitation (WCA).

Study Design and Methods.—PLTs collected with the Amicus cell separator (Fenwal, Inc.) were utilized to prepare two matched components, each with approximately 4×10^{11} PLTs. In the primary study, one component contained 65% PAS-III/35% plasma and the other 100% plasma. Four storage scenarios were used, one with CA and three with periods without agitation under simulated shipping conditions. In vitro assays were used early and after 5 days of storage.

Results.—pH levels after 5 days with CA were less with PAS-III components than 100% plasma components, with levels always above 6.6 in any component. With CA, a number of other variables were reduced even early during storage with PAS-III including morphology, extent of shape change, hypotonic stress response, adhesion, and aggregation. Storage WCA resulted in only a limited increase in the magnitude of the assay differences between PAS-III and 100% plasma components. Periods WCA did not reduce the pH below 6.6. The thromboelastograph variable associated with the strengthening of clots by PLTs was essentially comparable with PAS-III and plasma components throughout storage with CA or WCA.

Conclusion.—The data indicate that a 100% plasma medium provides for better retention of specific in vitro PLT properties, with CA and WCA, although the clinical significance of these in vitro decrements due to PAS-III is unknown.

▶ Apheresis platelets (A-PLTs) in the United States are traditionally collected and stored in 100% plasma. In countries in Europe and in Australia, platelets (PLTs) are prepared in a platelet additive solution (PAS). PASs contain salts and metabolic nutrients and have replaced a major part of the plasma volume in PLTs. The use of PASs has many potential benefits. First, the use of PAS allows for more plasma to be recovered and used for clinical use. Reducing the volume of plasma in a unit of PLTs has the potential to reduce adverse events. Some of the adverse events that have been implicated by the plasma component include allergic transfusion reactions and transfusion-related acute lung injury (TRALI). PAS-III is a PAS that was recently approved in the United States for A-PLTs collected using the Amicus cell separator. This solution contains sodium chloride, sodium citrate, sodium phosphate, and sodium acetate. Glucose is not present in the solution because acetate serves as the substance that is metabolized. Recent studies have evaluated the PAS-III in both in vitro and in vivo assays and concluded that recovery and survival met current standards. The PLT units in those previous studies were stored with continuous agitation (CA). The authors of this study compared the in vitro properties of Amicus A-PLTs as single-unit equivalents in 100% plasma or 65% PAS-III/35% plasma after preparation from double-apheresis collections. They also wanted to address the question of whether CA was necessary because PLTs are often required to be shipped without equipment to provide CA. Prior studies have shown that in vitro changes after 5 days of storage were acceptable with 24 hours without agitation. Therefore, they used 4 scenarios for their study so they could understand the combined influence of storage medium and interruption of agitation. Their results are represented in Fig 1 in the original article looking at 2 of the scenarios. Scenario 1 involved CA of the units and scenario 2 involved interruption of agitation for a continuous period of 24 hours. Their study concluded that PLT storage in 65% PAS-III is associated with a lesser quality profile compared with storage in 100% plasma and that periods without agitation did not greatly alter the results. However, other studies have shown that PAS can be an effective substitute for plasma and even increase storage time of the platelets. More studies that directly compare the recovery and survival of PLTs stored in 100% plasma and PASs will be necessary to demonstrate the effect on clinical outcomes.

H. Signorelli, DO

21 Cytogenetics and Molecular Pathology

Digital PCR Analysis of Maternal Plasma for Noninvasive Detection of Sickle Cell Anemia

Barrett AN, McDonnell TCR, Chan KCA, et al (Great Ormond Street Hosp for Children, London, UK; Chinese Univ of Hong Kong, Shatin, SAR, China; et al)
Clin Chem 58:1026-1032, 2012

Background.—Cell-free fetal DNA (cffDNA) constitutes approximately 10% of the cell-free DNA in maternal plasma and is a suitable source of fetal genetic material for noninvasive prenatal diagnosis (NIPD). The objective of this study was to determine the feasibility of using digital PCR for NIPD in pregnancies at risk of sickle cell anemia.

Methods.—Minor-groove binder (MGB) TaqMan probes were designed to discriminate between wild-type hemoglobin A and mutant (hemoglobin S) alleles encoded by the *HBB* (hemoglobin, beta) gene in cffDNA isolated from maternal plasma samples obtained from pregnancies at risk of sickle cell anemia. The fractional fetal DNA concentration was assessed in male-bearing pregnancies with a digital PCR assay for the Y chromosome—specific marker DYS14. In pregnancies with a female fetus, a panel of biallelic insertion/deletion polymorphism (indel) markers was developed for the quantification of the fetal DNA fraction. We used digital real-time PCR to analyze the dosage of the variant encoding hemoglobin S relative to that encoding wild-type hemoglobin A.

Results.—The sickle cell genotype was correctly determined in 82% (37 of 45) of male fetuses and 75% (15 of 20) of female fetuses. Mutation status was determined correctly in 100% of the cases (25 samples) with fractional fetal DNA concentrations > 7%. The panel of indels was informative in 65% of the female-bearing pregnancies.

Conclusions.—Digital PCR can be used to determine the genotype of fetuses at risk for sickle cell anemia. Optimization of the fractional fetal DNA concentration is essential. More-informative indel markers are needed for this assay's comprehensive use in cases of a female fetus.

▶ Digital polymerase chain reaction has been used successfully to detect trisomy 21 via analysis of relative chromosome dosage, which looks for overrepresentation of chromosome 21 sequences in maternal plasma compared with reference DNA sequences. This technique has been refined for use in diagnosing single-gene

413

disorders and has been referred to as "relative mutation dosage." Digital PCR and relative mutation dosage are used to determine allelic balance in 10 pregnancies at risk of beta-thalassemia in which both parents carried the same mutation in the beta-globin gene. The same group has also described the successful application of this technique for hemophilia in 7 pregnancies at risk because the mothers were carriers of this X-linked condition. Noninvasive prenatal diagnosis based on detection of allelic imbalance requires accurate measurement of the fractional fetal DNA concentration, which can be estimated only by using a DNA sequence not present in the mother. The studies reported in the literature to date have been limited to male-bearing pregnancies and have used Y chromosome sequences for fractional cell-free fetal DNA assessment. The development of an assay for assessing the fractional cell-free fetal DNA content of female-bearing pregnancies is essential for allowing testing of all pregnancies at risk for sickle cell anemia. The authors describe the use of digital polymerase chain reaction and relative mutation dosage for prenatal detection of sickle cell anemia in both male- and female-bearing pregnancies.

M. G. Bissell, MD, PhD, MPH

Newborn Screening for Spinal Muscular Atrophy by Calibrated Short-Amplicon Melt Profiling

Dobrowolski SF, Pham HT, Downes FP, et al (Children's Hosp of Pittsburgh, PA; ARUP Laboratories, Salt Lake City, UT; Michigan Dept of Community Health, Lansing; et al)
Clin Chem 58:1033-1039, 2012

Background.—The management options for the autosomal recessive neurodegenerative disorder spinal muscular atrophy (SMA) are evolving; however, their efficacy may require presymptom diagnosis and continuous treatment. To identify presymptomatic SMA patients, we created a DNA-based newborn screening assay to identify the homozygous deletions of the *SMN1* (survival of motor neuron 1, telomeric) gene observed in 95%–98% of affected patients.

Methods.—We developed primers that amplify a 52-bp PCR product from homologous regions in the *SMN1* and *SMN2* (survival of motor neuron 2, centromeric) genes that flank a divergent site at site c.840. Post-PCR high-resolution melt profiling assessed the amplification product, and we used a unique means of melt calibration to normalize profiles. Samples that we had previously characterized for the numbers of *SMN1* and *SMN2* copies established genotypes associated with particular profiles. The system was evaluated with approximately 1000 purified DNA samples, 100 self-created dried blood spots, and >1200 dried blood spots from newborn screening tests.

Results.—Homozygous deletion of *SMN1* exon 7 produced a distinctive melt profile that identified SMA patients. Samples with different numbers of *SMN1* and *SMN2* copies were resolved by their profiles. All samples with homozygous deletions were unambiguously recognized, and no normal sample was misidentified as a positive.

Conclusions.—This assay has characteristics suitable for population-based screening. A reliable screening test will facilitate the identification of an SMA-affected cohort to receive early intervention to maximize the benefit from treatment. A prospective screening trial will allow the efficacy of treatment options to be assessed, which may justify the inclusion of SMA as a target for population screening.

▶ Several therapeutic regimens for treating spinal muscular atrophy (SMA) are being evaluated. The common thread among the potential therapies is that early and continuous intervention is required. In type I SMA (severe infantile variant and the most common form of the disease), the window of opportunity for treatment intervention is small, because substantial denervation occurs by 3 months of age. For patients to derive the maximal benefit from promising new treatments, intervention is almost certainly required before disease manifestation. The optimal scenario is to genetically identify the infants at the highest risk of disease progression shortly after birth and to enter them in a treatment regimen during the first few weeks of life. To facilitate the identification of a presymptomatic cohort of SMA-affected patients, the authors have developed an assay suitable for prospective newborn screening. The assay is DNA-based and leverages site c.840, where the SMN1 and SMN2 genes are divergent. Post—polymerase chain reaction high-resolution melt profiling produces unique melting profiles resulting from the differences in SMN1 and SMN2 copy numbers, and patients with homozygous SMN1 deletion are readily identified.

M. G. Bissell, MD, PhD, MPH

Development of Plasmid Calibrators for Absolute Quantification of miRNAs by Using Real-Time qPCR

Formisano-Tréziny C, de san Feliciano M, Gabert J (Univ of the Mediterranean (Aix-Marseille II), France; et al)
J Mol Diagn 14:314-321, 2012

MicroRNAs (miRNAs) are small noncoding RNAs of approximately 18 to 25 nucleotides in length that negatively regulate gene expression via either the degradation or translational inhibition of their target mRNAs. Because miRNAs are essential for the regulation of critical physiological processes as well as a variety of pathological events, they have emerged as a novel class of molecular diagnostic biomarkers and therapeutic agents or targets. Accordingly, the need for novel methods for the quantification of miRNA has increased due to interest in their clinical implications. Currently, real-time quantitative polymerase chain reaction (qPCR) is considered the most robust technology for nucleic acid quantification. Different tools for miRNA quantification by using qPCR are now commercially available, but only relative quantification strategies have been reported. This situation may be partly due to the difficulty in obtaining an appropriate molecule with which to establish an miRNA calibration range. Here, we describe a rapid and convenient strategy for the development of a calibrator, which enables the absolute quantification of miRNAs by using qPCR and allows the cloning of a synthetic sequence of interest instead of a PCR product into a plasmid.

▶ MicroRNAs (miRNAs) are highly conserved families of small (18 to 25 nucleotides [nt] in length) noncoding RNAs. They down-regulate gene expression by translational repression or mRNA degradation. miRNAs are transcribed as large RNA precursor molecules with hairpin structures, and they undergo a stepwise maturation process through the nucleus and cytoplasm. The seed region, located between nts 2 to 8 of the mature miRNA, then binds to its complementary regions in the 3′ untranslated region of target mRNA. miRNA pairing with its mRNA target in the cytoplasm conditions its effect on posttranscriptional regulation. To date, more than 1000 human miRNAs have been identified, regulating more than 50% of human genes. miRNAs are involved in the regulation of critical physiological processes, such as embryonic development, cell survival and cycle, cell differentiation, apoptosis, and immunity. Growing evidence indicates that miRNAs are also involved in a variety of human diseases, and abnormal patterns of miRNA expression level have been described in viral infection, cancer development and aggressiveness, and immune and cardiovascular diseases. Their potential role as diagnostic biomarkers, therapeutic agents, or targets is emerging and has led to several patents concerning technology for miRNA investigation and miRNAs used as biomarkers, therapeutic targets, or agents. In this context, precise quantification of miRNAs is essential for research and clinical applications. Different studies argue in favor of the use of plasmid standard curves for absolute quantitative polymerase chain reaction (qPCR) quantification. However, plasmid standard curves for absolute miRNA qPCR constitute a challenging goal. In fact, because of their short length and the high sequence homology between miRNAs of the same family, specific miRNA amplification and cloning require extensive effort. The authors present an alternative method for miRNA cloning in which an in vitro synthesized molecule is cloned instead of a PCR product. miRNA hsa-let-7b is used as the model to demonstrate the proof of principle and confirmed by using a second miRNA (hsa-mir-141).

M. G. Bissell, MD, PhD, MPH

Performance and Clinical Evaluation of the 92-Gene Real-Time PCR Assay for Tumor Classification
Erlander MG, Ma X-J, Kesty NC, et al (BioTheranostics, Inc, San Diego, CA)
J Mol Diagn 13:493-503, 2011

Accurate determination of cancer origin is necessary to guide optimal treatment but remains a diagnostic challenge. Gene expression profiling technologies have aided the classification of tumors and, therefore, could be applied in conjunction with clinicopathologic correlates to improve accuracy. We report an expanded version of the previously described 92-gene assay to classify 30 main tumor types and 54 histological subtypes, with coverage of ≥95% of all solid tumors based on incidence. Increased tissue coverage was achieved through expansion of a reference tumor database containing 2206 specimens, with a median of 62 samples per main tumor type. The 92-gene classification algorithm demonstrated sensitivities of 87% and 85% for 30 main types and 54 histological subtypes, respectively, in leave-one-out cross validation, and 83% in a test set of 187 tumors representing 28 of the 30 main cancer types. These findings provide further support that broad and diverse tumor classification can be performed using a relatively compact gene set. An additional 300 consecutive cases submitted for clinical testing were profiled to characterize clinical utility in a real-world setting: the 92-gene assay confirmed 78% of samples having a single suspected primary tumor and provided a single molecular prediction in 74% of cases with two or more differential diagnoses. Further development of the 92-gene RT-PCR assay has resulted in a significant expansion in reportable tumor types and histological features with strong performance characteristics and supports the use of molecular classification as an objective standardized adjunct to current methods.

▶ Current paradigms of evidence-based patient management require more accurate diagnosis and better classification of tumors. In addition to broad site-directed treatments, newer strategies include agents that selectively target molecular pathways within a specific cellular context or tissue. As such, precise determination of the site of tumor origin is an important step toward improving diagnosis and optimizing treatment selection. In the context of metastatic disease, pathologic diagnosis is challenging when the morphologic features or clinical presentation of the tumor is overlapping or atypical. Here the authors report the use of their previously described 92-gene assay for the generation of a reference tumor database, with a significant increase in tumor coverage and depth. In addition, a novel 2-step classification algorithm was developed to enable the classification of 30 main cancer types and 54 histologic subtypes. The performance and preliminary clinical utility of this second-generation version of the 92-gene reverse transcription polymerase chain reaction assay are also presented.

M. G. Bissell, MD, PhD, MPH

Influence of RNA Labeling on Expression Profiling of MicroRNAs

Kaddis JS, Wai DH, Bowers J, et al (Univ of Southern California, Los Angeles, CA; Genisphere LLC, Hatfield, PA; et al)
J Mol Diagn 14:12-21, 2012

Although a number of technical parameters are now being examined to optimize microRNA profiling experiments, it is unknown whether reagent or component changes to the labeling step affect starting RNA requirements or microarray performance. Human brain/lung samples were each labeled in duplicate, at 1.0, 0.5, 0.2, and 0.1 μg of total RNA, by means of two kits that use the same labeling procedure but differ in the reagent composition used to label microRNAs. Statistical measures of reliability and validity were used to evaluate microarray data. Cross-platform confirmation was accomplished using TaqMan microRNA assays. Synthetic microRNA spike-in experiments were also performed to establish the microarray signal dynamic range using the ligation-modified kit. Technical replicate correlations of signal intensity values were high using both kits, but improved with the ligation-modified assay. The drop in detection call sensitivity and miRNA gene list correlations, when using reduced amounts of standard-labeled RNA, was considerably improved with the ligation-modified kit. Microarray signal dynamic range was found to be linear across three orders of magnitude from 4.88 to 5000 attomoles. Thus, optimization of the microRNA labeling reagent can result in at least a 10-fold decrease in microarray total RNA requirements with little compromise to data quality. Clinical investigations bottlenecked by the amount of starting material may use a ligation mix modification strategy to reduce total RNA requirements.

▶ MicroRNA (miRNA) expression profiling platforms have burgeoned in the past decade and promise to aid in the diagnosis, prognosis, and therapeutic treatment of human diseases such as cancer, cardiovascular disease, and diabetes. In response, intra-, inter-, and cross-platform comparisons have recently emerged that examine the use of microarray technology alone or in contrast to other profiling methods. Such studies have reported on the reliability and validity of widely used miRNA discovery tools and to highlight the advantages and limitations of these platforms. However, there also remains a need to evaluate pre-experimental factors, such as sample handling, processing, storage, and nucleic acid quality, which may influence miRNA expression profiling experiments. The authors therefore conducted a study to directly compare the Genisphere FlashTag biotin-HSR (biotin-HSR) labeling kit with the previously recommended FlashTag biotin-only (biotin-only) assay (Genisphere, Hatfield, PA) for the Affymetrix GeneChip miRNA Arrays. The biotin-HSR kit is a modified version of the biotin-only assay. More specifically, a smaller, more efficient labeling molecule having a higher number of biotins per unit mass of DNA has been used in the biotin-HSR kit compared with the DNA dendrimer of the original FlashTag biotin kit. Thirty-two chips were used for this evaluation, followed by cross-platform validation using TaqMan miRNA assays. In addition, the linear dynamic range of the GeneChip was assessed using synthetic miRNA spiked in at different amounts, labeled with the biotin-HSR kit, on 12 chips. A total of 44 microarray chips were used in this study.

M. G. Bissell, MD, PhD, MPH

Mutant Enrichment with 3′-Modified Oligonucleotides: A Practical PCR Method for Detecting Trace Mutant DNAs
Lee S-T, Kim J-Y, Kown M-J, et al (Sungkyunkwan Univ School of Medicine, Seoul, Korea)
J Mol Diagn 13:657-668, 2011

Many clinical situations necessitate highly sensitive and reliable molecular assays; however, the achievement of such assays remains a challenge due to the inherent limitations of molecular testing methods. Here, we describe a simple and inexpensive enrichment technique that we call mutant enrichment with 3′-modified oligonucleotides (MEMO). The method is based on the use of a 3′-modified oligonucleotide primer that blocks extension of the normal allele but enables extension of the mutated allele. The performance of the technique was evaluated with respect to its ability to detect common cancer mutations in the *EGFR, KRAS, BRAF, TP53, JAK2,* and *NPM1* genes. We achieved sensitivities of 10^{-2} to 10^{-6} using downstream Sanger sequencing, depending on the concentrations and thermodynamics of the primers. MEMO may be applicable to the quantitative real-time PCR platform and other downstream assays. This technique may be practically applicable to various medical situations.

▶ Molecular characterization of disease-associated alleles has become an essential part of medicine and serves as a powerful tool for early or confirmatory diagnoses, therapeutic decisions, disease monitoring, and prognostic stratification, as exemplified in the case of epidermal growth factor mutations in lung cancers. The strength of this methodology lies in the sensitive and confident detection of trace mutant alleles among an excess of normal alleles. Many clinical situations necessitate high levels of selectivity in diagnostic assays; however, this remains challenging because of the dilemma of balancing high sensitivity with reliability and practicality of use. Sanger sequencing, the robust standard method, can only detect approximately 20% of mutant alleles in a background of normal alleles, whereas other, more sensitive, polymerase chain reaction (PCR)—based assays, such as restriction fragment length polymorphism, amplification refractory mutation system PCR, denaturing high-performance liquid chromatography, and real-time PCR, are more limited, with accuracies below a certain level of allele minority. Amplification refractory mutation system PCR, the most widely used method, is an amplification strategy in which a PCR primer is designed to discriminate among templates that differ by a single nucleotide residue. This method is simple and time efficient but sometimes produces serious false-positive results because the mutant specific primer may induce false sequences. There have been efforts to develop new molecular technologies aimed at overcoming the inherent drawbacks of prior methods. There has been particular interest in the innovation of PCR stages that enable nondestructive selection and enrichment of mutant alleles, as this can improve sensitivity and credibility of downstream assays, such as standard sequencing analysis. These recent enrichment PCR techniques include thermostable restriction endonuclease-mediated selective PCR, PCR clamping mediated by peptide nucleic acid or locked nucleic acid, and coamplification at lower denaturation temperature PCR. Each technique has its own strengths and limitations in regard to the cost, availability, or enrichment efficiency. In this study, the authors describe a simple and practical enrichment technique, mutant enrichment with 3′-modified oligonucleotides, and they evaluate its use for detection of cancer mutations in medical specimens.

M. G. Bissell, MD, PhD, MPH

Novel, Improved Sample Preparation for Rapid, Direct Identification from Positive Blood Cultures Using Matrix-Assisted Laser Desorption/Ionization Time-of-Flight (MALDI-TOF) Mass Spectrometry

Schubert S, Weinert K, Wagner C, et al (Ludwig-Maximilians-Univ, Munich, Germany; et al)
J Mol Diagn 13:701-706, 2011

Matrix-assisted laser desorption ionization time-of-flight mass spectrometry (MALDI-TOF MS) is widely used for rapid and reliable identification of bacteria and yeast grown on agar plates. Moreover, MALDI-TOF MS also holds promise for bacterial identification from blood culture (BC) broths in hospital laboratories. The most important technical step for the identification of bacteria from positive BCs by MALDI-TOF MS is sample preparation to remove blood cells and host proteins. We present a method for novel, rapid sample preparation using differential lysis of blood cells. We demonstrate the efficacy and ease of use of this sample preparation and subsequent MALDI-TOF MS identification, applying it to a total of 500 aerobic and anaerobic BCs reported to be positive by a Bactec 9240 system. In 86.5% of all BCs, the microorganism species were correctly identified. Moreover, in 18/27 mixed cultures at least one isolate was correctly identified. A novel method that adjusts the score value for MALDI-TOF MS results is proposed, further improving the proportion of correctly identified samples. The results of the present study show that the MALDI-TOF MS-based method allows rapid (< 20 minutes) bacterial identification directly from positive BCs and with high accuracy.

▶ A few years ago, matrix-assisted laser-desorption ionization time-of-flight mass spectrometry (MALDI-TOF MS) was introduced as a rapid and reliable method for bacterial identification from plate cultures, based on protein profiles characteristic for each organism. This approach has been used to identify a broad spectrum of organisms, including gram-positive and gram-negative bacteria, mycobacteria, yeasts, and molds. The rapid and reproducible MALDI-TOF MS technology occasions only minimal consumable costs and has already replaced biochemical differentiation in several microbiologic routine laboratories. More recently, MALDI-TOF MS has been successfully used as a rapid method for the direct identification of bacteria and yeasts from positive blood culture (BC) bottles. The host proteins and blood cells have to be substantially removed to reveal species-specific protein spectra of bacteria and yeasts. Thus, the sample preparation of BCs for MALDI-TOF MS proves to be a key step for the successful identification. In previous studies, sample preparation protocols relying on differential centrifugation were applied. Under these protocols, collection tubes with separator gels are used to separate bacteria and yeasts from blood cells. Others have applied centrifugation or lysis of blood cells by adding sterile water, trifluoroacetic acid, or formic acid. In this study, the authors established and applied an easy-to-perform sample preparation protocol in combination with a commercially available mass spectrometry typing system for the rapid and reliable identification of bacteria from positive

BC bottles. Using the new protocol, the time for sample preparation could be reduced from up to 30 minutes to less than 10 minutes. They evaluated this novel sample preparation method in a prospective survey of 500 positive BC bottles over a 3-month period.

M. G. Bissell, MD, PhD, MPH

Design and Analytical Validation of Clinical DNA Sequencing Assays
Pont-Kingdon G, for the Biochemical and Molecular Genetic Resource Committee of the College of American Pathologists (ARUP Laboratories, Salt Lake City, UT; et al)
Arch Pathol Lab Med 136:41-46, 2012

Context.—DNA sequencing is the method of choice for mutation detection in many genes.

Objectives.—To demonstrate the analytical accuracy and reliability of DNA sequencing assays developed in clinical laboratories. Only general guidelines exist for the validation of these tests. We provide examples of assay validation strategies for DNA sequencing tests.

Design.—We discuss important design and validation considerations.

Results.—The validation examples include an accuracy study to evaluate concordance between results obtained by the newly designed assay and analyzed by another method or laboratory. Precision (reproducibility) studies are performed to determine the robustness of the assay. To assess the quality of sequencing assays, several sequence quality measures are available. In addition, assessing the ability of primers to specifically and robustly amplify target regions before sequencing is important.

Conclusion.—Protocols for validation of laboratory-developed sequencing assays may vary between laboratories. An example summary of a validation is provided.

▶ As more genes are implicated in disease, the desire and need to analyze genetic information from patient samples have increased dramatically in recent years. Some genes, especially for common diseases, have been extensively studied, whereas others are relatively newly discovered and need further study. Sanger dideoxy terminator DNA sequencing is a widely used technique to interrogate genes for small mutations and is considered a gold standard for detecting these sequence changes. Other technologies are required for detection of large rearrangements or copy-number variations, such as large deletions or duplications. Sequencing is especially useful when mutations are scattered across the entire gene or when genes have not been sufficiently studied to determine mutational hot spots. With the increased development of clinical sequencing assays, the question arises how to validate such assays. There are general guidelines published by the American College of Medical Genetics, the College of American Pathologists, the Clinical and Laboratory Standards Institute, the Association for Molecular Pathology, and others regarding what is required for analytical test validations. With those established general guidelines in mind the authors describe an approach for analytical validation of clinical sequencing assays. Sequencing assay design, validation criteria, and quality measures are addressed, using examples of assays that were developed for the MECP2 and the SMAD4 genes to demonstrate specific challenges associated with the validation of DNA sequencing assays. In addition, they include a summary for the complete sequence-based assay validation for PTEN, which is used to aid in diagnosing PTEN hamartoma tumor syndrome.

M. G. Bissell, MD, PhD, MPH

A Locked Nucleic Acid Clamp-Mediated PCR Assay for Detection of a p53 Codon 249 Hotspot Mutation in Urine
Lin SY, Dhillon V, Jain S, et al (Drexel Univ College of Medicine, Doylestown, PA; et al)
J Mol Diagn 13:474-484, 2011

Hepatocellular carcinoma (HCC) has a 5-year survival rate of <10% because it is difficult to diagnose early. Mutations in the *TP53* gene are associated with approximately 50% of human cancers. A hotspot mutation, a G:C to T:A transversion at codon 249 (249T), may be a potential DNA marker for HCC screening because of its exclusive presence in HCC and its detection in the circulation of some patients with HCC. A locked nucleic acid clamp-mediated PCR assay, followed by melting curve analysis (using the SimpleProbe), was developed to detect the *TP53* 249T mutation. In this assay, the locked nucleic acid clamp suppressed 10^7 copies of wild-type templates and permitted detection of 249-T mutated template, with a sensitivity of 0.1% (1:1000) of the mutant/wild-type ratio, assessed by a reconstituted standard within 2 hours. With an amplicon size of 41 bp, it detects target DNA sequences in short fragmented DNA templates. The detected mutations were validated by DNA sequencing analysis. We then tested DNA isolated from urine samples of patients with HCC for p53 mutations and identified positive *TP53* mutations in 9 of 17 samples. The possibility of using this novel *TP53* 249T assay to develop a urine or blood test for HCC screening is discussed (Fig 1).

▶ Hepatocellular carcinoma (HCC) is the fourth leading cause of cancer and the third leading cause of cancer deaths worldwide. The 5-year survival rate is 26% among patients in whom cancer is found at an early stage compared with only 2% when it is found after spreading to distant organs. A better method for detecting HCC at an early curable stage is needed to improve the prognosis of this disease. Mutations in the *TP53* gene are associated with approximately 50% of human cancers. Although the mutations have been found in many sites of the *TP53* gene in cancers, a specific missense mutation, resulting from a guanine to thymine (G > T) transversion at the third position of codon 249 (249T) of the exon 7 of the gene, is the particular hotspot mutation found almost exclusively in patients with HCC. Approximately 50% of patients with HCC have this p53 hotspot mutation; in some patients with HCC, this p53

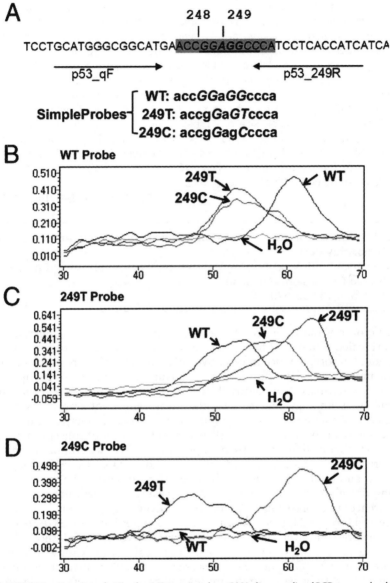

FIGURE 1.—Detection of p53 codon 249 mutations by an LNA clamp-mediated PCR assay and melting curve analysis with SimpleProbes. A: Locations and sequences of primers (**arrows**), clamp (underlined), and probes (shaded) used in the assay. Codons 248 and 249 are indicated by vertical lines. LNAs are italicized. SimpleProbe sequences shown with LNA are italicized and capitalized. PCR products derived from plasmids p53 WT, p53_249T, p53_249C, or H_2O (**arrows**) were determined by melting curve analysis with the SimpleProbes 249WT (B), 249T (C), and 249C (D). (Reprinted from Lin SY, Dhillon V, Jain S, et al. A locked nucleic acid clamp-mediated PCR assay for detection of a p53 codon 249 hotspot mutation in urine. *J Mol Diagn*. 2011;13:474-484, Copyright 2011, with permission from American Society for Investigative Pathology and the Association for Molecular Pathology.)

hotspot mutation is also found in the circulation. Thus, the *TP53* 249T hotspot mutation could possibly be a DNA marker for HCC screening. The authors applied 3 strategies for the development of an assay for detecting the circulation-derived *TP53* 249T mutation in the urine of patients with HCC (Fig 1): 1) a locked nucleic acid (LNA) clamp to suppress the amplification of the wild type (WT) template to allow the detection of a small fraction of mutated sequences, 2) a SimpleProbe to characterize the polymerase chain reaction (PCR) product by melting curve analysis at the completion of the PCR, and 3) an amplicon size of 41 base pair to enhance the sensitivity of the assay for detecting circulating DNA markers. They demonstrate that this LNA-clamp mediated PCR assay successfully detected the *TP53* codon 249 mutation in the urine of patients with HCC, suggesting that a urine test for HCC screening could be possible.

M. G. Bissell, MD, PhD, MPH

Proof of Concept Study to Assess Fetal Gene Expression in Amniotic Fluid by NanoArray PCR
Massingham LJ, Johnson KL, Bianchi DW, et al (Floating Hosp for Children at Tufts Med Ctr, Boston, MA; et al)
J Mol Diagn 13:565-570, 2011

Microarray analysis of cell-free RNA in amniotic fluid (AF) supernatant has revealed differential fetal gene expression as a function of gestational age and karyotype. Once informative genes are identified, research moves to a more focused platform such as quantitative reverse transcriptase-PCR. Standardized NanoArray PCR (SNAP) is a recently developed gene profiling technology that enables the measurement of transcripts from samples containing reduced quantities or degraded nucleic acids. We used a previously developed SNAP gene panel as proof of concept to determine whether fetal functional gene expression could be ascertained from AF supernatant. RNA was extracted and converted to cDNA from 19 AF supernatant samples of euploid fetuses between 15 to 20 weeks of gestation, and transcript abundance of 21 genes was measured. Statistically significant differences in expression, as a function of advancing gestational age, were observed for 5 of 21 genes. *ANXA5*, *GUSB*, and *PPIA* showed decreasing gene expression over time, whereas *CASC3* and *ZNF264* showed increasing gene expression over time. Statistically significantly increased expression of *MTOR* and *STAT2* was seen in female compared with male fetuses. This study demonstrates the feasibility of focused fetal gene expression analysis using SNAP technology. In the future, this technique could be optimized to examine specific genes instrumental in fetal organ system function, which could be a useful addition to prenatal care (Fig 2).

▶ Cell-free nucleic acids in second-trimester amniotic fluid (AF) supernatant derive almost exclusively from the fetus. Transcriptomic analyses of gene expression from AF supernatant may be useful in assessing fetal organ system

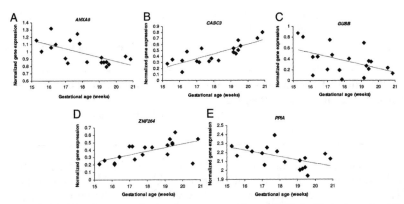

FIGURE 2.—Regression curves showing the genes among the panel with significant expression differences by gestational age. **A:** *ANXA5* ($P = 0.005$). **B:** *CASC3* ($P < 0.0001$). **C:** *GUSB* ($P = 0.03$). **D:** *ZNF264* ($P = 0.005$). **E:** *PPIA* ($P = 0.018$). *ANXA5*, *GUSB*, and PPIA show decreasing expression with increasing gestational age, and *CASC3* and *ZNF264* show increasing gene expression with increasing gestational age. (Reprinted from Massingham LJ, Johnson KL, Bianchi DW, et al. Proof of concept study to assess fetal gene expression in amniotic fluid by NanoArray PCR. *J Mol Diagn.* 2011;13:565-570, with permission from American Society for Investigative Pathology and the Association for Molecular Pathology.)

function. Standardized NanoArray PCR (SNAP) is a new technology that may provide the necessary attributes for the assessment of fetal organ system function. SNAP uses internal standard (IS) sequences to reproducibly measure the abundance of gene transcript. This technology uses a unique assay design for the simultaneous analysis of up to 3072 genes (or 384 samples at 8 genes per sample). SNAP uses the sensitivity and specificity of quantitative real-time polymerase chain reaction (qRT-PCR) and the design of array technology for the assessment of a sufficient number of genes to evaluate fetal organ system function. The SNAP approach has several technical advantages. First, the IS sequences provide a control for analytical false-negative results, and the melting curve provides an additional source of specificity to reduce analytical false-positive results. Second, IS sequences are supplied by a single manufacturer, ensuring a high degree of interlaboratory concordance. Third, IS sequences control for PCR inhibitors that are common in clinical samples. Fourth, SNAP requires very little sample volume but is capable of delivering 10s to 100s of transcript measurements. The SNAP approach has been previously validated by comparison with standard qRT-PCR techniques. These qualities are highly desirable and necessary when developing and implementing molecular diagnostics. The authors applied a previously developed gene panel with five additional genes (CASC3, GUSB, PPIA, TBP, and UBE2O2) to the SNAP array to examine the effectiveness of this technology in the prenatal setting (Fig 2). The previously developed panel correlates with survival among patients with non-small-cell lung cancer. Genes associated with carcinogenesis also are associated with fetal development. After the measurement of RNA isolated from amniocytes to assess the performance (eg, dynamic range, accuracy) of SNAP technology, the objective of the current study was to use this lung gene panel with SNAP as proof of concept to evaluate the effectiveness of this technique with cell-free AF supernatant.

M. G. Bissell, MD, PhD, MPH

Identification of Recombinant Alleles Using Quantitative Real-Time PCR: Implications for Gaucher Disease

Velayati A, Knight MA, Stubblefield BK, et al (Natl Insts of Health, Bethesda, MD)
J Mol Diagn 13:401-405, 2011

Pseudogenes, resulting from duplications of functional genes, contribute to the functional complexity of their parental genes. The glucocerebrosidase gene (*GBA*), located in a gene-rich region on chromosome 1q 21, is mutated in Gaucher disease. The presence of contiguous, highly homologous pseudogenes for both *GBA* and *metaxin 1* at this locus increases the likelihood of DNA rearrangement. We describe a facile method to identify and analyze recombinant alleles in patients with Gaucher disease. Genomic DNA from 20 patients with recombinant *GBA* alleles and five controls was evaluated to identify DNA rearrangements or copy number variation using six probes specific for either the *GBA* gene or pseudogene. Quantitative real-time PCR was performed on genomic DNA, and Southern blot analyses using HincII together with sequencing confirmed the real-time results. Both *GBA* fusions and duplications could be detected. Different sites of crossover were identified, and alleles resulting from gene conversion could be distinguished from reciprocal recombinant alleles. Quantitative real-time PCR is a sensitive and rapid method to detect fusions and duplications in patients with recombinant *GBA* alleles. This technique is more sensitive, faster, and cheaper than Southern blot analysis, and can be used in diagnostic laboratories, and to detect other recombinant alleles within the genome (Fig 1).

▶ DNA rearrangement, occurring by chromosomal pairing, breakage, and crossover between 2 non-sister chromatids during meiosis, is a cellular process essential for genetic diversity. Recombination between homologous sequences may also introduce harmful mutations. DNA rearrangement is influenced by the degree of sequence homology between corresponding segments and can be prompted by the presence of a pseudogene. Gaucher disease (GD), the most common lipidosis and the most frequently inherited disorder among Ashkenazi Jewish individuals, presents with hepatosplenomegaly, anemia, thrombocytopenia, bone involvement, and neurological symptoms (types 2 and 3). This disorder is caused by a deficiency of the lysosomal enzyme glucocerebrosidase, which degrades glucocerebroside, a membrane glycolipid, to ceramide and glucose. The gene for glucocerebrosidase (GBA) is located on 1 q21, a gene-rich region encompassing 7 genes and 2 pseudogenes within 85 kb; 1-3 GBA, spanning 7,6 kb, has 11 exons and 10 introns. A highly homologous 5.7-kb pseudogene (GBAP) is located 16 kb downstream, with the same organization of exons and introns. Another gene, metaxin (MTX), encoding for a mitochondrial membrane protein,

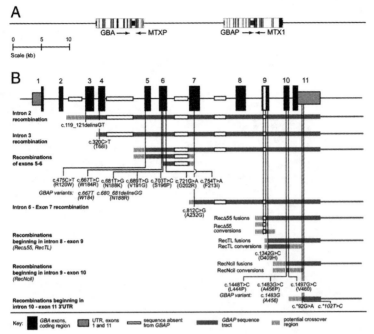

FIGURE 1.—A: The location of glucocerebrosidase gene (*GBA*) and its pseudogene, *metaxin* and *metaxin* pseudogene on chromosome 1. **B:** Exonic and intronic structure of *GBA*, pseudogenederived mismatches, and amino acid changes associated with the allele are indicated. Typical nonreciprocal (gene conversion) and reciprocal (gene fusion or duplication) recombinants are shown. The sequences absent in pseudogene are also shown. (Reproduced from Hruska et al, 2008.[9]) *Editor's Note*: Please refer to original journal article for full references. (Reprinted from Velayati A, Knight MA, Stubblefield BK, et al. Identification of recombinant alleles using quantitative real-time PCR: implications for gaucher disease. *J Mol Diagn.* 2011;13:401-405, Copyright 2011, with permission from Elsevier.)

is convergently transcribed and located immediately downstream of GBAP, with a pseudogene (pMTX) located between GBA and GBAP (Fig 1). To accurately describe a recombinant allele, a combination of direct sequencing and Southern blot analyses often performed using several restriction enzymes has been required. Because both of these techniques are time-consuming and expensive, they are not commonly used in diagnostic laboratories, and the detection of recombinant alleles in diagnostic settings has been challenging. The authors report the optimization of a facile method to identify and analyze recombinant alleles in patients with GD using quantitative real-time polymerase chain reaction.

M. G. Bissell, MD, PhD, MPH

Article Index

Chapter 1: Outcomes Analysis

Chapter 2: Breast

Chapter 3: Gastrointestinal System

Chapter 4: Hepatobiliary System and Pancreas

Chapter 5: Dermatopathology

Chapter 6: Lung and Mediastinum

Chapter 7: Cardiovascular

Chapter 8: Soft Tissue and Bone

Chapter 9: Female Genital Tract

Chapter 10: Urinary Bladder and Male Genital Tract

Chapter 11: Kidney

Chapter 14: Cytopathology

Chapter 15: Techniques/Molecular

Chapter 16: Laboratory Management and Outcomes

Chapter 17: Clinical Chemistry

Chapter 18: Clinical Microbiology

Chapter 19: Hematology and Immunology

Chapter 20: Transfusion Medicine and Coagulation

Chapter 21: Cytogenetics and Molecular Pathology

Author Index

A

Adsay V, 45
Agaimy A, 73
Agapova M, 402
Agarwal SK, 401
Aghemo A, 89
Ahnen DJ, 48
Akay OM, 379
Alexander EK, 10, 271
Ali RH, 167
Allison KH, 160
Alston EA, 280
Alves V, 87
Amin A, 179, 200
Amundsen EK, 351
Anagnostou VK, 114
André F, 20
Andreoni K, 86
Angelini A, 129
Anguita J, 363
Antic T, 80
Arcidiacono PG, 77
Arnold CA, 71
Ashrafian H, 115
Assaad A, 232
Atkinson AB, 325
Austin RM, 276

B

Bailey LC, 356
Bains A, 375
Baker SN, 323
Baloch ZW, 10, 271
Baron JA, 48
Barrau V, 91
Barrett AN, 413
Basu A, 219
Baxter R, 341
Becker K, 73
Behrens C, 109
Ben-Artzi A, 349
Ben-Baruch S, 354
Bénet C, 102
Benirschke K, 173
Benn DE, 68
Bennett MR, 215
Bercovitch L, 315
Beriwal S, 38
Berkowicz A, 384
Berlin G, 385
Bernacki KD, 313
Bianchi DW, 424
Bioulac-Sage P, 82

Blankenstein MA, 329
Boland JM, 124, 147
Bolliger S, 136
Borkent B, 403
Botsis T, 114
Boulos FI, 22
Bowers J, 417
Bradford CR, 277
Brase C, 247
Braunstein R, 354
Bray RA, 358
Brevnov MG, 345
Broos K, 388
Brown DFM, 340
Brown JM, 122
Bruhn R, 402
Brunner HI, 215
Bunyan RF, 264
Burbelo PD, 407
Burd EM, 346
Burk RD, 278
Burke PA, 401
Burns JM, 394
Büttner R, 118

C

Calvo KR, 374
Campbell WS, 15
Canaani J, 354
Cannizzo E, 376
Cao D, 177
Cao Q, 50
Capp R, 340
Caragea M, 149
Carr RA, 5
Carrara S, 77
Carulli G, 376
Celi AC, 175
Chan JKC, 59
Chan KCA, 413
Chan MK, 321
Chang A, 179
Chang Y, 340
Chapman S, 289
Chaux A, 186, 200
Chen P, 344
Chen SS, 369
Cheville JC, 226
Chiosea SI, 232
Chitale DA, 182
Cho GS, 241
Christiansen M, 383, 408
Chromecki TF, 225
Chu H, 19

Chung DC, 47
Clarke W, 333
Clarkson A, 68
Clausen FB, 383, 384, 408
Coe BP, 285
Cohen D, 276
Cohen P, 6
Colantonio DA, 321
Colby TV, 124, 147
Collet B, 265
Conces MR, 192
Cornejo K, 169
Cornell LD, 213
Cortes JE, 355
Cosio FG, 210
Couthouis J, 266
Crowder CD, 63
Cubel G, 82
Cunha LL, 253
Curvers J, 399
Custer B, 402
Cuzick J, 204

D

Dabbs DJ, 38
Daimon M, 140
D'Ambrosio R, 89
Daniels TE, 229
Darcy T, 309
Darragh TM, 55, 153
Davy RC, 404
De Brot M, 16, 31
de Feraudy S, 97
de Graaff AA, 158
De Meyer SF, 388
de Noronha SV, 134
de san Feliciano M, 415
Deetz CO, 328
Del Vecchio L, 376
Delvoux B, 158
Demehin AA, 3
Demirin H, 387
Demma LJ, 381
Deshpande V, 59, 293
Dhillon V, 422
Dickason TJ, 370
Dimou AT, 114
Dinis-Ribeiro M, 44
Dintzis SM, 23
Dobrowolski SF, 414
Doern GV, 339
Doherty D, 171
Douville NJ, 277
Downes FP, 414

443